COLOR ATLAS
& SYNOPSIS
OF
PEDIATRIC
DERMATOLOGY

Kay Shou-Mei Kane, M.D.

Clinical Instructor in Dermatology
Harvard Medical School

Associate Physician (Dermatology)
Division of Dermatology, Children's Hospital

Associate Physician (Dermatology)
Mt. Auburn Hospital
Boston, Massachusetts

Jen Bissonette Ryder, M.D.

Intern in Medicine
Strong Memorial Hospital
Rochester, New York

Richard Allen Johnson, M.D.

Clinical Instructor in Dermatology
Harvard Medical School

Clinical Associate in Dermatology
Division of Dermatology
Massachusetts General Hospital
Boston, Massachusetts

Howard P. Baden, M.D.

Professor in Dermatology
Harvard Medical School

Clinical Associate in Dermatology
Massachusetts General Hospital
Boston, Massachusetts

Alexander Stratigos, M.D.

Instructor in Dermatology-Venereology
University of Athens School of Medicine
Andreas Syngros Hospital for Skin and Venereal Diseases
Athens, Greece

COLOR ATLAS & SYNOPSIS OF PEDIATRIC DERMATOLOGY

Kay Shou-Mei Kane, M.D.

Jen Bissonette Ryder, M.D.

Richard Allen Johnson, M.D.

Howard P. Baden, M.D.

Alexander Stratigos, M.D.

McGraw-Hill

MEDICAL PUBLISHING DIVISION

New York   Chicago   San Francisco   Lisbon   London
Madrid   Mexico City   Milan   New Delhi   San Juan
Seoul   Singapore   Sydney   Toronto

McGraw-Hill

*A Division of The **McGraw·Hill** Companies*

COLOR ATLAS & SYNOPSIS OF PEDIATRIC DERMATOLOGY

567890 IMP IMP 0987654

ISBN 0-07-006294-3

This book was set in Times Roman by York Graphic Services, Inc.
The editors were Darlene Cooke, Nicky Panton, and Susan Noujaim.
The production supervisor was Richard Ruzycka.
The cover designer was Marsha Cohen.
The index was prepared by Jerry Ralya.

Imago was printer and binder.

This book is printed on acid-free paper.

Library of Congress Cataloging-in-Publication Data are on file for this title at the Library of Congress.

INTERNATIONAL EDITION ISBN 112452-7

To David, Michaela, and Cassandra,
the ones who ultimately contributed the most.

C O N T E N T S

The First Edition of the *Color Atlas & Synopsis of Pediatric Dermatology* fills a much-needed void in the current medical bookshelf. It encompasses a myriad of sources pooled together to provide detailed, large, color photographs of skin diseases in children alongside up-to-date pediatric management and treatment recommendations. Of particular interest is the new addition of topical immunomodulators to our armamentarium of skin therapies. Topical FK506 (tacrolimus or Protopic) has been approved for use in moderate to severe atopic dermatitis, and topical imiquimod, risiquimod, and ascomycin are new immunomodulators being used for HPV infections. Up-to-date therapies and pediatric doses have been included in this edition such as the new Accutane dosing and systemic antifungal therapies.

Modeled after the successful *Fitzpatrick Color Atlas & Synopsis of Clinical Dermatology*, the *Pediatric Atlas* strives to give primary-care specialists, residents, and medical students a helpful, easy-to-read, picture book to aid in the in-office recognition and diagnosis of pediatric skin disorders. Dr. T. B. Fitzpatrick defined the format with his first book over 40 years ago. Dr. Klaus Wolff added to the *Atlas* with his wonderful clinical images. Despite the overlap between the two books in topics, the *Pediatric Atlas* demonstrates the differences in presentation of skin diseases in children, the cutaneous disorders unique to children, and most importantly, the therapies approved for pediatric usage. The authors have made every attempt to provide accurate information regarding the disease entities and recommended pediatric dosages for therapy at the time of publication. However, in this world of ever-changing medicine, it is recommended that the reader confirm information contained herein with other sources.

Every blade of grass has its angel that bends over it and whispers "Grow, grow."

The Talmud

I am fortunate to have two such angels. The first is Stephen E. Gellis, MD, who inspired the writing of the book and contributed many of the wonderful photographs. Much of the book encompasses his thoughts, his recommendations, and teachings. All mistakes, blunders, and typographical errors are mine. The second major influence on this book is Thomas B. Fitzpatrick, MD. Dr. Fitzpatrick is an inspiration to many and I, like others, learned a lot about dermatology from him, and much, much more about life. As far as this book is concerned, TBF asked me to write several "précis" during my residency, convinced me that teaching was the key to learning, and from there, this book was born.

I'd also like to thank my colleagues at Boston Children's Hospital, Belmont Medical Associates and the SkinCare Physicians of Chestnut Hill: Marilyn Liang, MD; Jeffrey Dover, MD; Kenneth Arndt, MD; Jeanine Maglione, RN; Diane Lysak; Donna Cresta; Patricia Leahy, RN; Michelle Andrade; Roberta O'Connor; and many others. Drs. Lisa Cohen and Karen Wiss are to be credited for help with obtaining certain clinical photographs.

Finally, a special thanks to the editors and publishing staff at McGraw-Hill. My life wouldn't be complete without a daily e-mail or Fed-ex from Martin Wonsiewicz, Publisher; Nicky Panton, Editing Supervisor; Susan Noujaim, Development Editor; or Krishma Tuli, Editorial Assistant. And if it weren't for Darlene Cooke, Executive Editor, sitting me down one day and saying "finish the book", this book would not be finished.

Kay S. Kane

COLOR ATLAS
& SYNOPSIS
OF
PEDIATRIC
DERMATOLOGY

CUTANEOUS FINDINGS IN THE NEWBORN

PHYSIOLOGIC SKIN FINDINGS IN THE NEWBORN

VERNIX CASEOSA

The skin of a newborn is covered with a whitish-gray vernix that is thought to be a protective covering comprised of degenerated fetal epidermis and sebaceous secretions.

EPIDEMIOLOGY

Age Newborns.

Gender M = F.

Prevalence Seen in all infants.

PATHOPHYSIOLOGY

The vernix caseosa is thought to be a protective covering for the newborn skin and should be left to fall off by itself over the first few weeks of life.

PHYSICAL EXAMINATION

Skin Findings

Type of Lesion Adherent greasy membrane-like material which dries and desquamates (Fig. 1-1) after birth.

Color Gray-to-white.

Distribution Generalized.

DIFFERENTIAL DIAGNOSIS

Clinically, the vernix caseosa must be differentiated from other membranous coverings. The collodion baby and the harlequin fetus both have much thicker, rigid skin at birth.

COURSE AND PROGNOSIS

In an otherwise healthy newborn, the vernix caseosa will fall off in 1 to 2 weeks with simple handling and diaper changes.

TREATMENT

No treatment is necessary. The vernix caseosa is usually wiped from the face at birth and with the first few feedings. The rest of the vernix is shed over the first few weeks of life.

Current newborn skin care recommendations are as follows.

1. Full immersion baths are not recommended until the umbilical stump is fully healed and detached.
2. At birth, blood and meconium can be gently removed with warm water and cotton balls.
3. Umbilical cord care and/or circumcision varies from hospital to hospital. Several methods include a local application of alcohol (alcohol wipes), topical antibiotic (bacitracin, polysporin, or neosporin), or silver sulfadiazine cream (Silvadene) to the area(s) with each diaper change. The umbilical cord typically falls off in 7 to 14 d.
4. Until the umbilical and/or circumcision sites are healed, spot cleaning the baby with

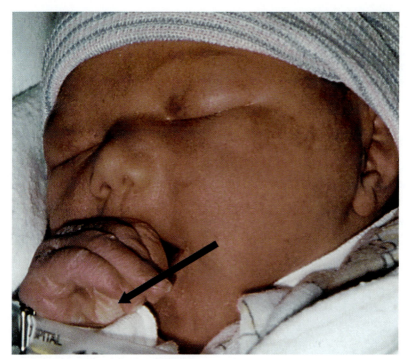

Figure 1-1   Vernix caseosa   *White, peeling vernix caseosa on the hand of a 1-day old baby.*

cotton balls and warm water is recommended. After the open sites have healed, the baby can be gently immersed in lukewarm water and rinsed from head to toe.

5. Avoiding perfumed soaps and bubble baths is best. Dove fragrance-free soap or soap-free cleansers (Aquanil, Cetaphil, and Aveeno) are the least irritating. Soaps should be used only on dirty areas and rinsed off immediately.

6. After bathing, newborn skin should be patted dry (not rubbed). Again, the vernix caseosa may still be present and adherent for several weeks. Hence topical moisturizers are usually not recommended.

CUTIS MARMORATA

A normal red-blue reticulated mottling of the skin of newborn infants. Seen as an immature physiologic response to cold with resultant dilatation of capillaries and small venules. Skin findings usually disappear with rewarming. Skin findings resolve as the child gets older.

EPIDEMIOLOGY

Age   Onset during first 2 to 4 weeks of life; associated with cold exposure.

Gender   M = F.

Prevalence   More prevalent in premature infants.

PATHOPHYSIOLOGY

Thought to be due to the immaturity of the autonomic nervous system of newborns. Physiologically normal and resolves as child gets older.

HISTORY

Reticulating mottling of the skin resolves with warming.

PHYSICAL EXAMINATION

Skin Findings

Type   Reticulated mottling (Fig. 1-2).

Color   Reddish-blue.

Distribution   Diffuse, symmetric involvement of the trunk and extremities.

DIFFERENTIAL DIAGNOSIS

Cutis marmorata is benign and self-limited. It can be confused with cutis marmorata telangiectasia congenita (CMTC), a more severe condition that can also present as reticulated vascular changes at birth. CMTC is a rare, chronic, relapsing, severe form of vascular disease that can lead to permanent scarring skin changes.

COURSE AND PROGNOSIS

Recurrence unusual after 1 month of age. Persistence beyond neonatal period is possible marker for trisomy 18, Down's syndrome, Cornelia de Lange syndrome, hypothyroidism, or CMTC.

TREATMENT AND PREVENTION

Disorder usually self-resolves, which renders treatment unnecessary.

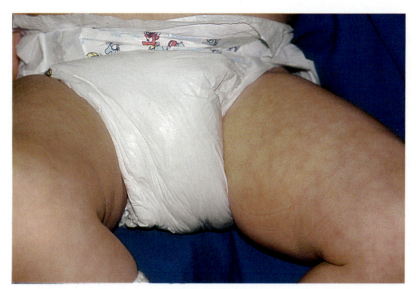

Figure 1-2   Cutis marmorata   *Reticulated vascular mottling on the legs of a healthy newborn which improves with age.*

NEONATAL HAIR LOSS

Neonatal hair at birth is actively growing in the anagen phase, but within the first few days of life convert to telogen (dying and shedding) hairs. Consequently, there is normally a large amount of hair shed during the first 3 to 4 months of life.

Synonym   Telogen effluvium of the newborn.

EPIDEMIOLOGY

Age   Newborns, can be seen at 3 to 4 months of age.

Gender   M = F.

Prevalence   Affects all infants to some degree.

PATHOPHYSIOLOGY

The hair has three stages of its life cycle.

1. Anagen (the active growing phase that typically lasts 2 to 6 years).
2. Catagen (a short partial degeneration phase that lasts 10 to 14 d).
3. Telogen (resting and shedding phase that lasts 3 to 4 months).

At any given time in a normal scalp, 89% of the hairs are in anagen phase, 1% are in catagen phase and 10% are in telogen phase. Neonatal hair loss occurs because all the anagen hair at birth simultaneously converts to catagen then telogen phases in the first few days of life. This results in whole-scalp shedding of the birth hair in 3 to 4 months. The shedding is gradually counteracted by regrowing new hairs.

HISTORY

During the first 3 to 6 months of life, there will be physiologic shedding of all the newborn hair. In some individuals, the new hair growing in will mask the shedding hair and the process will be barely noticeable. In most infants, some degree of loss, even total baldness, will be seen.

PHYSICAL EXAMINATION

Skin Findings

Type of Lesion   Non-scarring alopecia (Fig. 1-3).

Distribution   Diffuse involving the entire scalp.

DIFFERENTIAL DIAGNOSIS

Neonatal hair loss is a normal physiologic process that is diagnosed clinically by history and physical examination. Another benign form of hair loss that may be seen in the newborn period is rubbing or traumatic alopecia, typically seen on the posterior of the scalp of babies who sleep on their backs.

COURSE AND PROGNOSIS

In an otherwise healthy newborn, the hair loss self-resolves by age 6 to 12 months.

TREATMENT

No treatment is necessary. The parents should be reassured that neonatal hair loss is a normal physiologic process and that the hair will grow back by age 6 to 12 months without treatment.

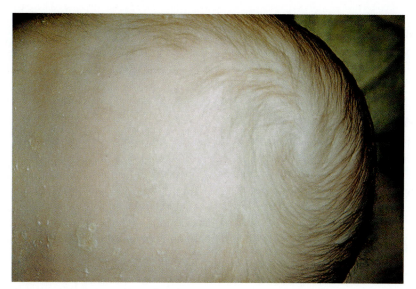

Figure 1-3   Neonatal hair loss   *Frontal and vertex scalp hair loss of the newborn hair in a healthy 4-month old baby. Slight scale is mild seborrheic dermatitis.*

MISCELLANEOUS CUTANEOUS DISORDERS OF THE NEWBORN

MILIARIA, NEWBORN

Miliaria is a common neonatal dermatosis resulting from sweat retention caused by incomplete differentiation of the epidermis and its appendages. Obstruction and rupture of epidermal sweat ducts is manifested by a vesicular eruption.

Synonyms Prickly heat, heat rash.

EPIDEMIOLOGY

Age Newborn.

Gender M = F.

Incidence Greatest in the first few weeks of life.

Prevalence Virtually all infants develop miliaria in appropriate settings.

Etiology Immature appendages and keratin plugging of eccrine duct leads to vesicular eruption.

PATHOPHYSIOLOGY

Incomplete differentiation of the epidermis and its appendages at birth leads to keratinous plugging of eccrine ducts and subsequent leakage of eccrine sweat into the surrounding tissue.

PHYSICAL EXAMINATION

Skin Findings

Miliaria Crystallina (Sudamina)

Type Superficial pinpoint clear vesicles (Fig. 1-4).

Color Skin, pink.

Distribution Generalized in crops.

Sites of Predilection Intertriginous areas, commonly neck and axillae, or clothing covered truncal areas.

Miliaria Rubra (Prickly Heat)

Type Pinpoint papules/vesicles.

Color Erythematous.

Sites of Predilection Covered parts of the skin, forehead, upper trunk, volar aspects of the arms and body folds.

DIFFERENTIAL DIAGNOSIS

The diagnosis of miliaria is made based on observation of characteristic lesions. Vesicles may be ruptured with a fine needle, yielding clear, entrapped sweat. Miliaria rubra requires close inspection to ascertain its extrafollicular nature. Miliaria can be confused with folliculitis, candidiasis, and acne.

LABORATORY EXAMINATIONS

In miliaria crystallina, vesicles are often found superficially in the stratum corneum and serial sectioning demonstrates direct communication with ruptured sweat ducts. Miliaria rubra histologically demonstrates degrees of spongiosis and vesicle formation within the epidermal sweat duct.

MANAGEMENT

Prevention Avoid excessive heat and humidity. Lightweight clothing, cool baths and air conditioning help prevent build-up of sweat and retention in closed pores.

Treatment Lesions will resolve with these measures.

Figure 1-4 Miliaria *Superficial clear pinpoint vesicles of miliaria crystallina on the back of an infant.*

MILIA

Multiple 1- to 2-mm white/yellow superficial tiny cysts seen over the forehead, cheeks, and nose of infants. They may be present in the oral cavity as well where they are called Epstein's pearls.

EPIDEMIOLOGY

Age All ages, especially newborns.

Gender M = F.

Prevalence Up to 40% of infants have milia on the skin, up to 85% of infants have the intraoral counterpart (Epstein's pearls) on the palate.

Etiology May be related to trauma to the skin surface during delivery.

PATHOPHYSIOLOGY

Milia and Epstein's pearls are caused by the cystic retention of keratin in the superficial epidermis.

PHYSICAL EXAMINATION

Skin Findings

Type Few to numerous pinpoint white papules (Fig. 1-5).

Size 1 to 2 mm.

Color Yellow to pearly white.

Distribution Forehead, nose, cheeks, gingiva, midline palate (Epstein's pearls), rarely on the penis, and at sites of trauma.

DIFFERENTIAL DIAGNOSIS

Milia must be differentiated from molluscum contagiosum and sebaceous hyperplasia. Molluscum contagiosum does not typically appear in the immediate neonatal period and is characterized by dome-shaped papules with central umbilication. Sebaceous hyperplasia is more yellowish rather than whitish in color. Epstein's pearls can be differentiated from intraoral mucinous cysts by their typical midline palate location and spontaneous resolution.

LABORATORY EXAMINATIONS

Dermatopathology Superficial tiny epithelial cysts containing keratin and developing in connection with the pilosebaceous follicle.

COURSE AND PROGNOSIS

Milia and Epstein's pearls should spontaneously exfoliate during the first few weeks of life. Unusually, persistent milia or widespread milia can be seen in conjunction with more severe developmental problems, namely, oral-facial-digital syndrome and hereditary trichodysplasia.

TREATMENT AND PREVENTION

No treatment is necessary. Cosmetically, lesions may be incised and expressed.

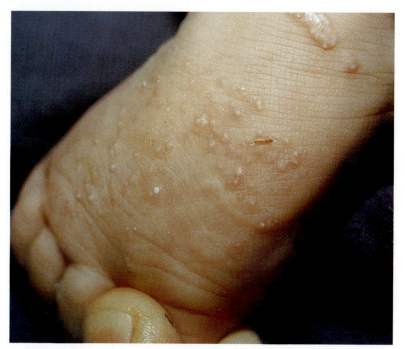

Figure 1-5 Milia *Numerous pinpoint white papules on the foot of a premature infant.*

ACNE NEONATORUM

Acne neonatorum is a benign, self-limited, acneform eruption that develops within the first 30 days of life.

EPIDEMIOLOGY

Age Rare at birth, peaks between ages 2 to 4 weeks of life.

Gender M = F.

Prevalence Up to 50% of infants.

PATHOPHYSIOLOGY

Neonatal sebaceous glands are hyperplastic, and hydroxysteroid dehydrogenase activity in these structures is high in the 2 months just before and at birth. It is also thought that transient increases in circulatory androgens may contribute to neonatal acne.

HISTORY

Multiple discrete papules develop between ages 2 to 4 weeks of life, evolve into pustules and spontaneously resolve.

PHYSICAL EXAMINATION

Skin Findings

Type Comedones, inflammatory papules and pustules (Fig. 1-6).

Color Red.

Distribution Face, chest, back, and groin.

DIFFERENTIAL DIAGNOSIS

Clinically, comedones and inflammatory papules are characteristic for this condition.

LABORATORY EXAMINATIONS

Dermatopathology Increased number of sebaceous glands and keratin-plugged pilosebaceous orifices lead to rupturing and neutrophilic or granulomatous inflammation.

COURSE AND PROGNOSIS

Neonatal acne may persist up to 8 months of age. There is some suggestion that infants with extensive neonatal acne may experience severe acne as adults.

TREATMENT AND PREVENTION

Neonatal acne typically resolves spontaneously. For severe involvement, 2.5% benzoyl peroxide gel may be used.

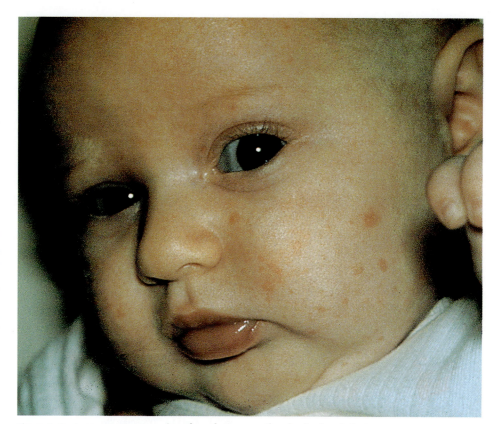

Figure 1-6 **Acne neonatorum** *Acneform lesions on the cheek of an infant.*

ERYTHEMA TOXICUM NEONATORUM

Benign transient, blotchy erythema with central vesiculation seen in newborns.

EPIDEMIOLOGY

Age Newborns.

Gender M = F.

Prevalence Unclear, reports range from 4.5 to 70% of term infants. Less common in premature infants.

PATHOPHYSIOLOGY

The cause of erythema toxicum is unknown. The eosinophil response is suggestive of a hypersensitivity reaction, but specific allergens have not been identified.

HISTORY

Macular erythema with central vesicles and pustules appear between 24 to 48 h of age.

PHYSICAL EXAMINATION

Skin Findings

Type Blotchy erythematous macules 2 to 3 cm in diameter with a central 1- to 4-mm central papule, vesicle or pustule (Fig. 1-7).

Color Hyperpigmented macules may develop at the site of resolving vesicles and pustules.

Distribution Chest, back, face and proximal extremities, sparing the palms and soles.

DIAGNOSIS AND DIFFERENTIAL DIAGNOSIS

Diagnosis Wright's stain of a vesicle will reveal a predominance of eosinophils. Gram's stain will be negative.

Differential Diagnosis Erythema toxicum must be differentiated from miliaria rubra and transient neonatal pustular melanosis. Erythema toxicum has a larger 2- to 3-cm area of erythema as compared to the 2- to 3-mm erythema of miliaria rubra lesions. Transient neonatal pustular melanosis has a predominance of neutrophils rather than eosinophils in the vesicles and typically heals with residual pigmentation. Bacterial and fungal culture of erythema toxicum lesions will be negative differentiating it from neonatal bacterial infections and congenital candidiasis.

LABORATORY EXAMINATIONS

Wright's Stain A smear of a vesicle and Wright's stain reveals numerous eosinophils.

Gram's Stain Negative.

Dermatopathology Intraepidermal vesicle filled with eosinophils.

Hematologic Examination Peripheral eosinophilia of up to 20% may be seen in 7 to 15% of cases.

COURSE AND PROGNOSIS

Lesions may occur from birth to the tenth day of life and individual lesions clear in 5 d. By 2 weeks of age, all lesions are resolved.

TREATMENT

No treatment is necessary.

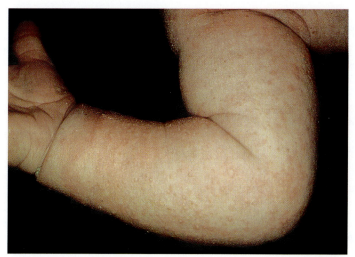

Figure 1-7 **Erythema toxicum neonatorum** *Erythematous macules with central vesicles scattered diffusely over the entire body of a newborn. A smear of the vesicle contents would show a predominance of eosinophils.*

TRANSIENT NEONATAL PUSTULAR MELANOSIS

A benign and self-limited condition characterized by blotchy erythema and superficial pustules of the newborn that heal with residual pigmentation.

EPIDEMIOLOGY

Age   Newborns.

Gender   M = F.

Race   More common in black infants.

Prevalence   0.2 to 4% of the newborns.

PATHOPHYSIOLOGY

Transient neonatal pustulosis is thought to be associated with obstruction of the pilosebaceous orifice.

HISTORY

Idiopathic, superficial, sterile vesicles and pustules that are present at birth, rupture in 24 to 48 h, and heal with pigmented macules that slowly fade over several months.

PHYSICAL EXAMINATION

Skin Findings

Type   Tiny vesicles, pustules (Fig. 1-8) or ruptured lesions with a collarette of scale.

Color   Hyperpigmented macules may develop at the site of resolving vesicles and pustules.

Distribution   Clusters on face, trunk, and proximal extremities, rarely palms and soles may be involved.

DIAGNOSIS AND DIFFERENTIAL DIAGNOSIS

Diagnosis   Wright's stain of a vesicle will reveal a predominance of neutrophils. Gram's stain will be negative.

Differential Diagnosis   Transient neonatal pustulosis must be differentiated from acne neonatorum and staphylococcal and herpetic infections.

LABORATORY EXAMINATIONS

Wright's Stain   A smear of a vesicle and Wright's stain reveals numerous neutrophils and an occasional eosinophil.

Gram's Stain   Negative.

Dermatopathology   Vesicular lesions show intraepidermal vesicles filled with neutrophils. Macular hyperpigmented lesions show mild hyperkeratosis and basilar hyperpigmentation.

COURSE AND PROGNOSIS

The vesicles and pustules usually disappear by 5 d of age and the pigmented macules fade over 3 months time.

TREATMENT

No treatment is necessary.

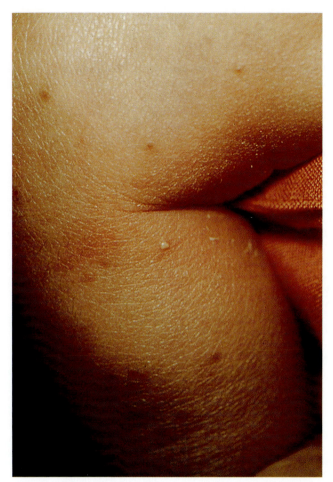

Figure 1-8   Transient neonatal pustulosis   *Vesicles and pustules scattered diffusely on the leg of an infant. Note the hyperpigmented areas at sites of resolved lesions. A smear of the vesicle contents would reveal a predominance of neutrophils.*

NEONATAL LUPUS ERYTHEMATOSUS

Neonatal lupus erythematosus (NLE) is an uncommon autoimmune disease caused by the transplacental antibodies of an affected mother being passed onto an unaffected fetus. The infant manifests skin lesions of nonscarring subacute cutaneous lupus erythematosus (SCLE) or congenital heart block, or both.

EPIDEMIOLOGY

Age Skin lesions appear at birth or, more commonly, within a few weeks of birth. Lesions typically last a few weeks to months. Disease activity typically resolves by 6 months of age. Heart block appears typically during gestation (as early as 16 weeks of gestational age, but may occur later) and is irreversible.

Gender M = F.

Incidence Unknown. One estimate, based on the incidence of congenital heart block with NLE being the most frequent etiology, approximates the incidence of NLE to be near 1:20,000 births.

Etiology and Transmission Maternal autoantibodies cross the placenta during pregnancy and are thought to produce both the cutaneous and systemic findings of NLE.

PATHOPHYSIOLOGY

Mothers of babies with NLE possess autoantibodies (95% of cases possess anti-Ro/SSA, others may have anti-La/SSb or anti-U$_1$RNP antibodies). These IgG autoantibodies pass through the placenta from mother to fetus and can be found in the neonate's sera. It is felt that these autoantibodies are implicated in the development of cutaneous and systemic findings of NLE. The skin lesions are temporary and begin to resolve at or before the time that maternal autoantibodies are cleared from the child's system (typically at 6 months of age). Heart block is caused by antibody-induced fibrosis of the atrioventricular node (or in some cases the sinoatrial node) and is irreversible.

PHYSICAL EXAMINATION

About half of the NLE cases report exhibited skin disease and about half exhibit congenital heart block. Approximately 10% have both skin disease and heart block.

Skin Findings

Type Scaly, erythematous plaques, epidermal atrophy. No scarring or follicular plugging.

Color Pink, red. May be hypopigmented.

Shape Round or elliptical.

Distribution Frequently on face and scalp. Lesions may be concentrated in the periorbital and malar areas (Fig. 1-9). Widespread involvement may occur.

General Findings

Heart block is present in about half of cases. Typically, disease presents with complete heart block that begins during gestation (as early as 16 weeks of gestational age, but may occur later). Uncommonly, babies can have lesser degrees of heart block. Fibrosis of the AV node (in rare instances, the SA node) leads to a slowed heart rate. NLE typically presents with isolated heart block and no associated cardiac anomaly although there are reports of NLE and a concurrent patent ductus arteriosus. Other findings include liver disease, thrombocytopenia, and leukopenia.

DIFFERENTIAL DIAGNOSIS

The skin findings of the newborn may be confused with other scaly, erythematous plaques such as seborrhea, eczema, psoriasis, or tinea. Heart block may be detected during routine obstetrical examination because the fetal heart rate will be slow. This can be confirmed by fetal ultrasound. Finally, the diagnosis can be confirmed by serological studies.

LABORATORY EXAMINATIONS

Histopathology Biopsy of lesional skin reveals findings similar to that of SCLE lesions. There is basal cell damage in the epidermis and a sparse mononuclear cell infiltrate in the superficial dermis. Immunofluorescence studies

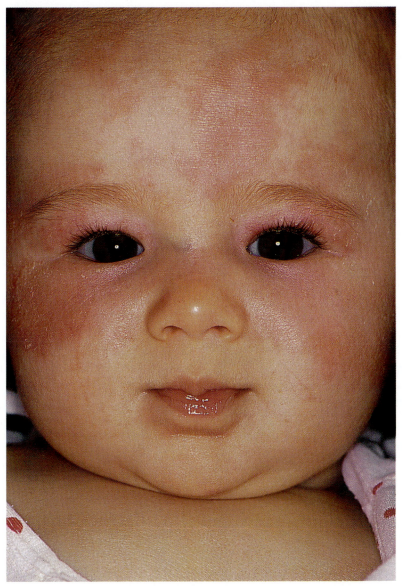

Figure 1-9 Neonatal lupus erythematous *Erythematous, annular plaques on the face of a healthy 6-week-old baby. Skin lesions self-resolved after 6 months.*

demonstrate a particulate deposit of IgG in the epidermis.

Serology Sera of mother and baby should be tested for autoantibodies. Ninety-five percent of cases are due to anti-Ro/SSA antibodies. Anti-La/SSB antibodies may also be present but almost never without the presence of anti-Ro/SSA antibodies. Anti-U_1RNP autoantibodies account for the NLE cases that do not have anti-Ro/SSA antibodies present. The positive serology of any of these autoantibodies with any appropriate clinical finding is strong evidence to favor the diagnosis of NLE.

Other Obstetrical detection of slowed fetal heart rate or ultrasound documentation of heart block may be found as early as 16 weeks of gestational age.

COURSE AND PROGNOSIS

Babies with NLE who survive the neonatal period have a good prognosis and rarely go on to develop autoimmune disease. The estimated mortality rate is 10%, with deaths being secondary to intractable heart failure during the neonatal period.

Mothers with babies who develop NLE do not have an increased rate of spontaneous abortion but often develop autoimmune disease, on average, 5 years after delivery.

Skin Findings

The cutaneous lesions of NLE in the neonate are benign and transient, usually lasting weeks to months and regress by age 6 months, occasionally with residual postinflammatory hypopigmentation or atrophy that gradually improves.

General Findings

Despite complete heart block and a subsequent slowed heart rate, babies with cardiac involvement of NLE tend to be well compensated. Half do not require any treatment, the other half need pacemakers. About 10% do not respond despite pacemaker placement likely due to coexistent myocardial disease, and die of intractable heart failure.

MANAGEMENT

During Gestation

Testing for autoantibodies during pregnancy is appropriate for women with anti-Ro/SSA autoantibody symptomatology: Sjögren's syndrome, SCLE, SLE, arthralgias, dry eyes, dry mouth, or photosensitivity. Women with previous births with heart block or other signs/symptoms suggestive of NLE should also be tested. It is important to keep in mind that 50% of women with babies with NLE are asymptomatic at delivery and conversely, most women with anti-Ro/SSA antibodies will have normal babies. It is estimated that only 1 to 2% of women with anti-Ro/SSA autoantibodies will have a baby with NLE. Risk factors that increase these percentages include a previous baby with NLE and mothers with the diagnosis of SLE. Screening tests should include fluorescent antibody tests for anti-Ro/SSA, anti-La/SSB, and anti-U_1RNP autoantibodies.

Obstetrical screening for a slowed fetal heart rate is also important and if heart block is confirmed, the fetus should be monitored carefully for the development of hydrops fetalis. The delivery room should be equipped to manage a newborn with possible heart failure. The use of systemic steroids or plasmapheresis during gestation has been utilized in life-threatening circumstances.

Neonatal Period

Skin Findings   Skin disease is benign and self-limited. Supportive care includes protection from sun exposure and topical steroids for more severe cutaneous involvement. Systemic treatment is not indicated.

General Findings   Treatment of heart disease is not always indicated. For those children with heart failure due to a slowed heart rate, pacemaker implantation is the treatment of choice. Rarely, will the children go on to develop autoimmune disease.

APLASIA CUTIS CONGENITA

Aplasia cutis congenita is a congenital defect of the scalp characterized by localized loss of the epidermis, dermis, and sometimes, subcutaneous tissue.

EPIDEMIOLOGY

Age   Present at birth.

Gender   M = F.

Incidence   Rare.

Etiology   Unknown.

Genetics   Most cases are sporadic, some familial cases are reported.

PATHOPHYSIOLOGY

The exact mechanism of this disorder is not known. It is hypothesized that aplasia cutis congenita results from incomplete neural tube closure or an embryonic arrest of skin development.

HISTORY

Aplasia cutis congenita presents as an asymptomatic ulceration of the scalp at birth that heals with scarring.

PHYSICAL EXAMINATION

Skin Findings

Type of Lesion   Denuded ulceration that is replaced with scarred tissue. In the scar, no hair or appendages are present (Fig. 1-10).

Size   1 to 3 cm.

Shape   Round, oval, or stellate.

Number   Solitary lesion (70% of cases), two lesions (20% of cases), three or more lesions (10% of cases).

Color   Pink to red healing to white-gray.

Distribution   Scalp vertex, midline (50% of cases) or adjacent areas (30%). Can also rarely be seen on the face, trunk, or extremities.

General Findings

Typically, aplasia cutis congenita is an isolated skin finding. In rare instances it may be seen with other developmental abnormalities such as skeletal, cardiac, neurologic, or vascular malformations.

DIFFERENTIAL DIAGNOSIS

The diagnosis of aplasia cutis congenita is made by history and physical examination. It should be differentiated from scalp electrode monitors, forceps, or other iatrogenic birthing injuries.

LABORATORY EXAMINATIONS

Dermatopathology   Skin biopsy would reveal an absence of the epidermis and appendageal structures. There is a decrease in dermal elastic tissue, and, in some deep cases, a loss of all skin layers and subcutaneous tissues.

COURSE AND PROGNOSIS

The prognosis of cutis aplasia congenita as an isolated finding is good. The ulceration typically heals with scarring in a few weeks. The scarred area will persist as an asymptomatic lesion for life.

TREATMENT

Localized care of the ulcerated area at birth includes:

1. Gentle cleansing of the area with warm water and cotton balls.
2. A thin layer of topical antibiotic (bactroban, bacitracin, polysporin, or neosporin) to prevent secondary infection.
3. Protective coverings to prevent further trauma to the area. The area will heal with

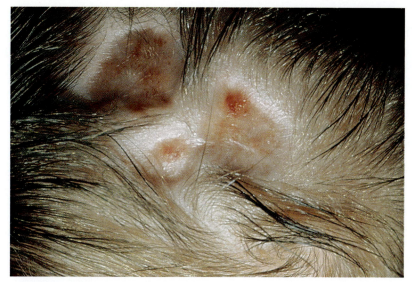

Figure 1-10 Cutis aplasia congenita *Three localized areas of scarring alopecia on the vertex of the scalp. These areas began as ulcerated lesions at birth and are otherwise asymptomatic.*

scarring and as the child grows, the scar usually becomes inconspicuous and covered with surrounding hair.

Management options include:

1. No treatment. The scarred area should be examined annually for any changes since scarred areas do have a higher risk of neoplastic transformation.

2. Surgical correction of the area by excision or hair transplant.

PRE-AURICULAR SKIN TAG

Pre-auricular skin tags result when a brachial arch or cleft fails to fuse or close properly. Defects occur unilaterally or bilaterally and may have accompanying facial anomalies.

Synonym   Peri-auricular tag.

EPIDEMIOLOGY

Age   Newborn.

Gender   M = F.

Prevalence   Uncommon.

Etiology   Developmental defect of first two branchial arches or clefts.

PATHOPHYSIOLOGY

Caused by first or second branchial arch fusion abnormality during embryonic development.

HISTORY

Noted at birth or presents when secondarily infected and persists asymptomatically for life. Usually pre-auricular skin tags are an isolated congenital defect. Rarely, there may be other associated branchial arch abnormalities.

PHYSICAL EXAMINATION

Skin Findings

Type   Small, pedunculated papilloma or papule (Fig. 1-11).

Color   Skin color, tan to brown.

Size   1 to 7 mm.

Shape   Pedunculated, round to oval lesions.

Sites of Predilection   Pre-auricular area.

DIFFERENTIAL DIAGNOSIS

Differential diagnosis includes an accessory tragus (soft cartilaginous pedunculated pre-auricular lesions).

LABORATORY EXAMINATIONS

Dermatopathology   Skin biopsy or removal would show a loose fibrous stroma with overlying thinned epidermis.

COURSE AND PROGNOSIS

Skin tags are typically asymptomatic but persist for life, occasionally getting inflamed. The presence of pre-auricular skin tags should alert the clinician to check for a more serious associated first arch developmental anomaly.

MANAGEMENT

Solitary, uncomplicated lesions may be tied off shortly after birth but otherwise can be excised during childhood for cosmetic purposes.

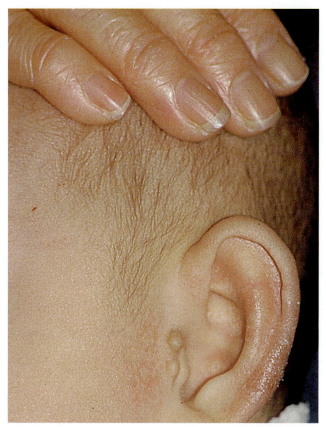

Figure 1-11 Pre-auricular skin tag *Asymptomatic flesh-colored papule in the pre-auricular region of an otherwise healthy infant.*

BRANCHIAL CLEFT CYST

An epithelial cyst on the lateral neck caused by an incomplete obliteration of the branchial clefts in embryologic development.

Synonyms   Branchial cyst, branchial sinus.

EPIDEMIOLOGY

Age   Newborn.

Gender   M = F.

Prevalence   Uncommon.

Etiology   Arises from incomplete closure of the second or third branchial clefts. Remains of the cleft membrane form cysts or sinuses.

Genetics   Most are sporadic but case reports of autosomal dominant inheritance patterns exist.

PATHOPHYSIOLOGY

Branchial cleft cysts are nonregressed remnants of the embryonic second and third branchial clefts. Similar lesions, thyroglossal ducts, and/or sinuses, can be seen more near the midline of the neck.

HISTORY

Onset   Lesions are evident at birth or appear in early childhood as cystic swellings in the neck, deep to the sternomastoid muscle. Occasionally, they can become infected and painful.

PHYSICAL EXAMINATION

Skin Findings

Type   Fluctuant papule or nodule.

Color   Flesh-colored.

Size   2 to 10 mm.

Distribution   Unilateral or bilateral swellings in the neck, deep to the sternomastoid muscle (Fig. 1-12).

DIFFERENTIAL DIAGNOSIS

Branchial cleft cysts can be confused with other nodular lesions on the neck such as lymph nodes or epidermal or pilar cysts. The location and presence at birth can help distinguish them from other neck lesions.

LABORATORY EXAMINATIONS

Dermatopathology   On skin biopsy, the cyst will have a stratified squamous epithelial lining.

COURSE AND PROGNOSIS

Cysts often form sinuses or fistulae, draining mucus internally to the pharynx and/or externally through the skin of the neck along the anterior edge of the sternomastoid muscle. Cysts and associated sinuses may also become infected.

MANAGEMENT

These lesions are benign, however, can be symptomatic with recurrent infections and swelling. Symptomatic lesions can be surgically corrected.

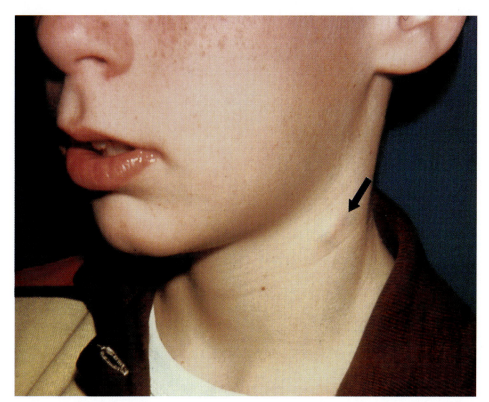

Figure 1-12 Branchial cleft cyst *An asymptomatic, unilateral cystic swelling on the neck present since birth.*

ACCESSORY NIPPLE

An additional nipple appearing anywhere along an imaginary line drawn from the mid-axilla to the inguinal area. Nipples may appear unilaterally or bilaterally and with or without areolae.

Synonyms Supernumerary nipple, polythelia.

EPIDEMIOLOGY

Age Newborn.

Gender M = F.

Prevalence Common.

Etiology Developmental defect with persistence of the embryonic milkline.

PATHOPHYSIOLOGY

Accessory nipples represent persistent fetal embryonic milkline lesions.

HISTORY

Lesions are present at birth, asymptomatic, and persist for life.

PHYSICAL EXAMINATION

Skin Findings

Type Papule with or without surrounding areola.

Color Pinkish-brown.

Size Usually smaller than normal anatomically placed nipples.

Shape Often round to oval in shape.

Distribution Chest, abdomen, face, neck, shoulder, back, vulva, thigh.

Sites of Predilection Along a line from the mid-axillae to the inguinal area (Fig. 1-13).

DIFFERENTIAL DIAGNOSIS

When occurring without an areola, the nipple may be misdiagnosed as a congenital nevus.

LABORATORY EXAMINATIONS

Dermatopathology Skin biopsy would reveal lactation ducts and glands, histologic findings of a normal nipple.

DIAGNOSIS

The diagnosis of an accessory nipple can be made clinically, especially if it is present along the anterior milkline. Other ectopically placed lesions may need a biopsy confirmation.

COURSE AND PROGNOSIS

Accessory nipples are present at birth and persist asymptomatically for life. Malignant degeneration is rare.

MANAGEMENT

Accessory nipples do not need treatment but should be monitored since those with associated breast tissue can have the same malignant potentials as normal breast tissue. Surgical removal can be performed for diagnostic, cosmetic, or therapeutic purposes.

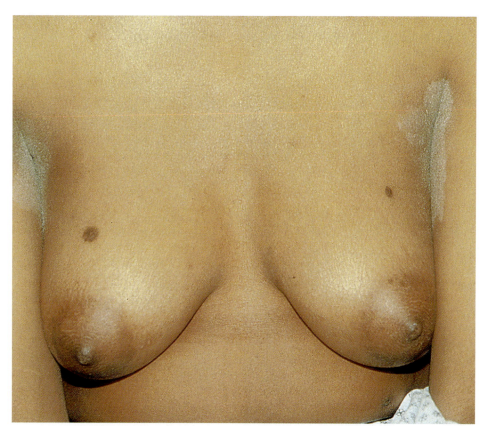

Figure 1-13   Accessory nipple   *Asymptomatic, symmetric brown papules present since birth along the milk-line above the breasts.*

CONGENITAL INFECTIONS OF THE NEWBORN

NEONATAL HERPES SIMPLEX VIRUS INFECTION

Neonatal herpes simplex infection is a frequently fatal disease of infants born vaginally to mothers who have a genital herpetic infection. Neonatal herpes has a broad clinical spectrum and may be categorized into three patterns: localized infection confined to the skin, eyes, or mouth; central nervous system disease; and disseminated disease.

EPIDEMIOLOGY

Age Localized infection typically presents between 10 to 11 days of life. CNS infection typically presents between 16 to 17 days of life. Disseminated infection typically presents between day 9 to 11 days of life.

Gender M = F.

Prevalence Approximately 1 per 2000 live births.

Etiology 80% result from herpes simplex virus-2 (HSV-2) infection, 20% result from herpes simplex virus-1 (HSV-1) infection.

Transmission Herpes virus is inoculated onto the baby's mucous membranes during its passage through the birth canal.

PATHOPHYSIOLOGY

Herpes viral inoculation occurs as the baby passes through the birth canal during vaginal delivery and systemic infection can ensue with disease limited to the brain or diffuse hematogenous dissemination.

HISTORY

Pregnant women with recurrent genital herpes are at risk of transmitting HSV to their babies during vaginal delivery.

The current recommendations for the management of infants exposed to herpes simplex virus at delivery are:

1. If the infant has been exposed to a first episode of maternal genital herpes, the following steps are recommended:

   a. Obtain specimens of urine, stool, and cerebrospinal fluid as well as specimen from the eyes and throat for culture.
   b. Instruct the parents to report signs of lethargy, poor feeding, fever, or lesions.
   c. If the results of a culture are positive or if findings on examination of cerebrospinal fluid are abnormal, initiate therapy with intravenous acyclovir.

2. If the infant has been exposed to recurrent maternal genital herpes, the following steps are recommended:

   a. Instruct the parents to report signs of lethargy, poor feeding, fever, or lesions.
   b. Perform weekly surveillance cultures of specimens from the eyes, nose, mouth, and skin for 4 to 6 weeks after delivery.

PHYSICAL EXAMINATION

It is important to realize that as many as 70% of infants with CNS and disseminated neonatal herpes present with severe symptoms in the *absence* of cutaneous lesions.

Skin Findings

Type of Lesion Skin lesions begin as 2- to 8-mm macules or papules that progress to single or grouped vesicles that break leaving an open sore, which crusts over and heals.

Color Pink to red.

Shape Round to oval.

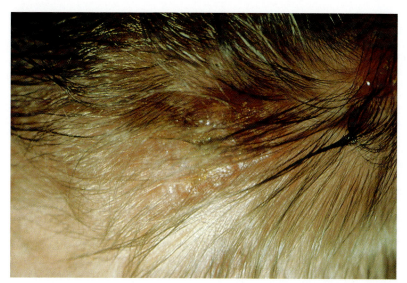

Figure 1-14   Congenital herpes simplex virus, localized   *Grouped vesicles on an erythematous base on the scalp of a newborn.*

Distribution Oral lesions are most frequently located on the tongue, palate, gingiva, lips, and buccal mucosa. Ocular lesions appear as erosions on the conjuctiva and cornea. Skin lesions occur at sites of inoculation and infant monitoring scalp electrodes may produce enough skin trauma to allow invasion by the herpes virus (Fig. 1-14). At birth in vertex deliveries, the scalp is a common site for the development of initial herpetic lesions and conversely, in breech deliveries, the buttocks and perianal area typically manifest the first lesions. The vesicular rash may become generalized in the disseminated pattern of the disease.

General Findings

Early in the infection, infants typically present with nonspecific symptoms such as lethargy, poor feeding, and fever. CNS involvement is manifested by isolated encephalitis with frequent seizures that are nonfocal in nature. Eye involvement is seen in 10 to 20% of these patients and is noted characteristically between age 2 days and age 2 weeks of life. Disseminated infection presents with irritability, respiratory distress, jaundice, and seizures from viral infection of the brain, lungs, liver, and adrenal glands.

DIFFERENTIAL DIAGNOSIS

The diagnosis of neonatal herpes is made by history and clinical presentation and confirmed by detection of the herpes virus. The differential diagnosis includes other blistering diseases of the newborn such as congenital varicella, bullous impetigo, pemphigus vulgaris, and other causes of neonatal sepsis.

LABORATORY EXAMINATIONS

Tzanck Preparation Cells scraped from the base of vesicular lesions are positive for multinucleated giant cells in 60% of culture proven HSV.

Histopathology Intraepidermal vesicle produced by ballooning degeneration, typical of virally induced vesicles. Inclusion bodies (eosinophilic structures with a surrounding clear halo) are frequently seen in the center of enlarged, round nuclei of balloon cells.

Direct Immunofluorescence Cells scraped from the base of vesicular lesions can be tested for the presence of herpes virus infection using HSV-2 or HSV-1 specific monoclonal antibodies. Sensitivity and specificity correlates 88% with tissue culture results.

Serology Antibody measurement in the baby is of little value because the seropositive rate for HSV among all women of child-bearing age exceeds 10%.

Culture HSV may be cultured within 2 to 5 days from infected samples of skin, throat, conjuctiva, cerebrospinal fluid, blood, urine, and stool. Cultures are positive about 85 to 90% of the time.

Polymerase Chain Reaction Herpes simplex DNA can be detected in the CSF using the polymerase chain reaction, an extremely sensitive technique that enzymatically replicates small amounts of nucleic acid to allow its detection and analysis.

COURSE AND PROGNOSIS

Mortality of neonatal herpes is strongly associated with disease classification.

Localized Infection Treated infants with cutaneous infection have virtually a 100% survival rate, although a very high proportion of them will suffer a cutaneous relapse in the first year of life. Approximately 10% will manifest herpetic lesions in the oropharynx. Up to 40% will have persistent ocular pathology, although this is seen most frequently in children suffering from severe neurologic residua (see below.)

CNS Infection Untreated cases have a mortality rate of 50% and treated cases have a mortality rate of 15%. HSV-2 causes significantly worse encephalitis as compared to HSV-1. These cases sustain permanent neurologic impairment. Only 23% of the infants treated with HSV-2 encephalitis are normal at follow-up as compared to all those treated with HSV-1 encephalitis. Many infants after CNS herpetic infection will have ocular pathology, with up to 20% suffering from visual compromise secondary to eye-movement disorders.

Disseminated Infection Babies frequently progress to cardiovascular compromise, coagulopathy, and, in the absence of therapy, 80% of cases result in death. With antiviral therapy, the mortality rate is reduced to 50%.

MANAGEMENT

In light of the varied clinical manifestations of neonatal herpetic infections and the severe consequences of untreated disease, immediate institution of antiviral chemotherapy has been recommended for any infant presenting with signs of severe, unidentified infection in the first month of life, even in the absence of a vesicular rash. Antiviral therapy consists of either:

1. IV acyclovir 30 mg/kg divided into 3 equal doses and administered every 8 h for 10 to 14 d.
2. IV vidarabine 30 mg/kg administered over 12 h once a d for 10 to 14 d.

For acyclovir-resistant HSV:

1. IV foscarnet 40 mg/kg twice a d for 10 to 14 d.

Infants with CNS or disseminated disease that have been treated successfully may require long-term suppressive antiviral therapy to prevent subclinical CNS recurrences although this has not yet been evaluated in a controlled manner.

CONGENITAL VARICELLA ZOSTER VIRUS

The majority of infants exposed to varicella zoster virus (VZV) infection during pregnancy are asymptomatic and normal. There are two exceptions: congenital varicella zoster syndrome and neonatal varicella.

Congenital VZV syndrome occurs if a mother is infected in the first 20 weeks of pregnancy and transplacental infection of fetus occurs before maternal immunity can protect the infant. This acquired infection leads to severe fetal sequelae.

Neonatal varicella occurs if the mother gets VZV 4 days before or 2 days after delivery. Since the infant is born before maternal antibodies have been generated, the infant has no immunity and will have a severe infection between day 5 to 10 days of life with pneumonitis, hepatitis, meningoencephalitis, and 30% mortality.

EPIDEMIOLOGY

Age   Newborn.

Gender   M = F.

Incidence   Only 5 to 16% of women of childbearing age are not VZV immune. Both congenital VZV and neonatal VZV are rare with <40 case reports.

Etiology   Varicella zoster virus.

PHYSICAL EXAMINATION

Congenital VZV Syndrome
Skin Findings

Type   Cicatricial scars, limb contractures.

General Findings   Low birth weight, eye defects, encephalomyelitis, hypoplastic limbs, micrognathia, pneumonitis.

Neonatal Varicella

Type   Monomorphic progression from macule, papules, vesicles, to crust (Fig. 1-15).

Color   Erythematous.

Distribution   Generalized.

General Findings   Pneumonitis, hepatitis, and meningoencephalitis.

DIFFERENTIAL DIAGNOSIS

Congenital HSV, other TORCH (Toxoplasmosis, Other (syphilis), Rubella, CMV, HSV) infections, sepsis.

LABORATORY EXAMINATIONS

DFA (direct immunofluorescence) or skin biopsy of cutaneous lesions can show VZV. Cultures of tissue, CSF, can grow VZV, but very low yield and slow to culture. IgG and IgM antibodies to VZV can be demonstrated in the mother's sera to determine either previous immunity or active infection.

DIAGNOSIS

Based on history or maternal infection, clinical appearance of the newborn, and laboratory findings.

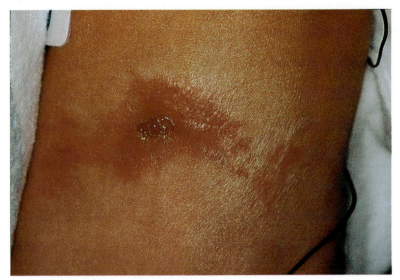

Figure 1-15 Congenital varicella zoster virus infection *T5 dermatomal erythematous plaque on the right side of a newborn's body.* (Slide courtesy of Karen Wiss).

COURSE AND PROGNOSIS

Infants in utero of mothers with VZV are protected by the transplacental acquired antibodies generated during maternal VZV infection. Thus, most infants are unaffected and born normal. These infants may develop unusual manifestations of attenuated immunity later in life such as herpes zoster at an early age. Such children are immunocompetent but had in utero primary VZV infection (chicken pox) and an attenuated immune response since maternal antibodies were present to help fight the infection.

Congenital VZV syndrome and neonatal varicella are more severe and rare outcomes from VZV infection during the first 20 weeks of pregnancy or near delivery, respectively. The course and prognosis is much worse, with 30% mortality.

MANAGEMENT

Any susceptible pregnant woman exposed to varicella should be given VZIG (varicella zoster immune globulin) and/or systemic acyclovir within 96 h to reduce chance of transmission to the fetus and attenuate the course of infection in the mother.

Neonates, once born, can also be treated with VZIG and acyclovir systemically within 48 h of delivery.

BLUEBERRY MUFFIN BABY

The "blueberry muffin baby" is so-called because of the baby's clinical presentation, with disseminated red-blue papules and nodules all over the body representing islands of extramedullary hematopoiesis. The blueberry muffin baby can be seen with in utero infections with toxoplasmosis, varicella, cytomegalovirus (CMV), human immunodeficiency virus (HIV), and rubella.

EPIDEMIOLOGY

Age   Newborn.

Gender   M = F.

Incidence   Rare.

Etiology   Maternal infection during pregnancy and transplacental infection with toxoplasmosis, varicella, CMV, HIV, or rubella.

PHYSICAL EXAMINATION

Skin Findings

Type   Petechiae, scattered purpuric macules and papules (Fig. 1-16).

Color   Bluish-red to purple.

Size   2 to 8 mm in diameter.

Shape   Circular to oval.

Palpation   Infiltrated, larger lesions are palpable 1 to 2 mm above the skin's surface.

Distribution   Head, neck, trunk, extremities.

General Findings

Toxoplasmosis   Lymphadenopathy, hepatosplenomegaly, hydrocephaly, microcephaly, cataracts, pneumonitis, chorioretinitis, convulsions.

Varicella   See "Congenital and Neonatal Varicella."

CMV   Jaundice, hepatosplenomegaly, anemia, thrombocytopenia, respiratory distress, convulsions, and chorioretinitis.

HIV   Hepatosplenomegaly, other opportunistic infections.

Rubella   Cataracts, deafness, growth retardation, hepatosplenomegaly, cardiac defects, and meningoencephalitis.

DIFFERENTIAL DIAGNOSIS

The differential diagnosis of a blueberry muffin baby is typically the infectious causes of extramedullary dermal hematopoiesis: toxoplasmosis, varicella, CMV, HIV, and rubella. The diagnosis is typically made by maternal history and detection of one of the above-named infectious agents.

LABORATORY EXAMINATIONS

Dermatopathology   Blueberry muffin lesions show aggregates of large nucleated and non-nucleated erythrocytes.

Toxoplasmosis

Serology   Infant antitoxoplasma IgM higher than maternal IgM is diagnostic of congenital infection.

Wright's or Giemsa Stain   CSF or lymph node, spleen or liver demonstrating toxoplasmosis organism.

Skull Films   Diffuse punctate comma-shaped intracranial calcifications.

CMV

Culture   Urine, liver, CSF, gastric washing, and pharynx will show characteristic large cells with intranuclear and cytoplasmic inclusions.

Rubella

Serology   Elevated antirubella IgM in infant or persistent antirubella IgG in infants ≥6 months of age or older. Fourfold or greater increase in acute and convalescent sera is also diagnostic.

Culture   Virus can be isolated from nasopharynx, urine, CSF, skin, stool, or eyes.

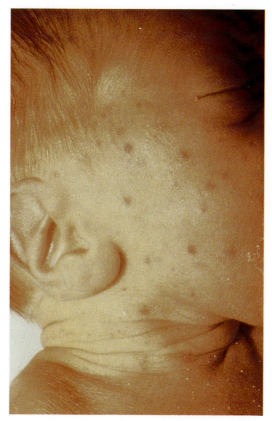

Figure 1-16 Blueberry muffin baby *Scattered red-blue papules and nodules on the face of a newborn. The lesions represent sites of extramedullary hematopoiesis.*

COURSE AND PROGNOSIS

Toxoplasmosis Infected infants may be stillborn, premature, or full term. At birth, they present with malaise, fever, rash, lymphadenopathy, hepatosplenomegaly, convulsions, and chorioretinitis. Overall prognosis is poor, especially with infants that have liver and bone marrow involvement.

CMV Sixty-five percent of affected infants will have sensorineural hearing loss, mental retardation, learning disabilities, and seizures. Poor prognosis, especially with intracranial calcifications or hydrocephalus.

Rubella Rubella acquired during the first trimester may lead to low-birth weight, microcephaly, mental retardation, cataracts, deafness, and heart abnormalities. Rubella acquired during second or third trimester can lead to he-patosplenomegaly, pneumonitis, myocarditis, encephalitis, osteomyelitis, or retinopathy.

MANAGEMENT

Toxoplasmosis 30+ days of sulfadiazine (150 to 200 mg/kg per day divided qid) plus pyrimethamine (1 to 2 mg/kg per day divided bid). Infants with chorioretinitis or high CSF protein levels may need systemic steroids.

CMV Ganciclovir can be used to treat retinitis and organ involvement. Cytarabine and vidarabine have been used experimentally.

Rubella Immune globulin administered to exposed pregnant mother within 22 h of onset can prevent/reduce fetal infection. Neonatal rubella needs ophthalmologic and supportive care. It is important to keep in mind that infected infants can shed the virus for up to a year.

CONGENITAL SYPHILIS

A prenatal spirochetal infection with characteristic early and late signs and symptoms. Clinical manifestations of early congenital syphilis (< age 2) include anemia, fever, wasting, hepatosplenomegaly, lymphadenopathy, rhinitis (snuffles), mucocutaneous eruptions (rhagades), and pseudoparalysis. Symptoms of late congenital syphilis, that persist beyond 2 years of age, include interstitial keratitis, Hutchinson's incisors, mulberry or Moon's molars, and eighth nerve deafness.

Synonym   Prenatal syphilis.

EPIDEMIOLOGY

Age   Within first month of life.

Gender   M = F.

Incidence   Since detection, and treatment, incidence had dropped to insignificant levels in 1959, but since then, a resurgence has occurred.

Etiology   Spirochete *Treponema pallidum* crosses the placenta to infect the fetus.

HISTORY

Neonates with syphilis are often born without signs of disease at time of birth. Clinical manifestation in first month of life common, prematurity more common. Skin findings include maculopapular, papulosquamous, and vesicobullous lesions. Desquamation of entire body possible (Fig. 1-17). Mucocutaneous involvement of mouth and lips. Systemically, there is lymphadenopathy, hepatosplenomegaly, and pseudoparalysis.

PHYSICAL EXAMINATION

Early Congenital Syphilis   Signs and symptoms appearing before 2 years of age.

Skin Findings

Noted in one-third to one-half of affected infants. Skin lesions are infectious.

Type   Maculopapular or papulosquamous lesions on body. Patches on mucous membranes, raised verrucous plaques on anogenital or oral membranes.

Color   Bright pink to red; fades to coppery-brown.

Size and Shape   Large, round or oval.

Distribution   Any part of body.

Sites of Predilection   Face, dorsal surface of trunk and legs, diaper area, palms, and soles.

General Findings

Hepatomegaly, lymphadenopathy (especially epitrochlear), splenomegaly, jaundice, anemia, thrombocytopenia, osteochondritis, and meningitis. "Barber-pole umbilical cord" spiral red, white, and black discoloration of necrotizing umbilical cord.

Late Congenital Syphilis   Signs and symptoms appearing after 2 years of age.

Skin Findings

Hypersensitivity type reaction or scars/deformities related to infection. Skin lesions no longer infectious.

General Findings

Hutchinson's triad: (1) interstitial keratitis, (2) Hutchinson incisors, (3) eighth nerve deafness; dental changes (Moon or mulberry molars or bony gums that progress to necrotic ulcers), Higoumenakia sign (unilateral, thickened inner one-third of clavicle), arthritis, paroxysmal cold hemoglobinuria, and eye changes (chorioditis, retinitis, and optic atrophy).

DIFFERENTIAL DIAGNOSIS

The diagnosis of congenital syphilis can be made based on clinical suspicion and confirmed by positive dark-field microscopy of the umbilical vein or skin lesions, by radiologic bony changes, and positive serology for syphilis. A serologic titer in the newborn higher than the mother is diagnostic of congenital syphilis.

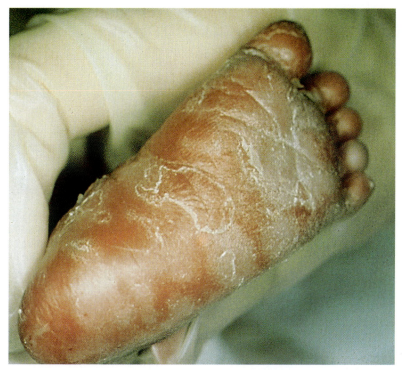

Figure 1-17   Neonatal syphilis   *Copper-colored macules and diffuse desquamation on the plantar surface of a newborn with secondary syphilis.*

LABORATORY EXAMINATIONS

Dark-field microscopy of the umbilical vein, skin lesions, or mucous membranes for *Treponema*.

Radiologic studies for bone abnormalities: widening of the epiphyseal line with increased density of the shafts.

Placental changes include focal villositis, endovascular and perivascular proliferation in villous vessels, and relative immaturity of villi.

COURSE AND PROGNOSIS

Relative to time during pregnancy of maternal spirochetemia and subsequent fetal inoculation. At 4 months of gestation, fetus often dies in utero resulting in spontaneous abortion. Infection after 4 months of gestation results in stillborn or fatally ill neonate. Prognosis with contracted disease is dependent on early and proper diagnosis and adequate treatment.

MANAGEMENT

Treatment without CNS involvement:

1. Aqueous crystalline penicillin G: (100,000 to 150,000 units/kg) IM or (50,000 units/kg IV q 8 to 12 h) × 14 d.
2. Procaine penicillin G: (50,000 units/kg IM q 24 h × 10 to 14 d).
3. Benzathine penicillin G: (50,000 units/kg IM × 1 dose).

Treatment with CNS involvement:

1. Crystalline penicillin G: (30,000 to 50,000 units/kg) divided bid–tid × 3 weeks.
2. Procaine penicillin G: (50,000 units/kg) qd × 3 weeks.

CONGENITAL CUTANEOUS CANDIDIASIS

An intrauterine contracted infection that presents at time of birth as erythematous or generalized eczematous, scaly skin.

Synonym Moniliasis.

EPIDEMIOLOGY

Age Birth.

Gender M = F.

Etiology Candida organisms, most commonly *Candida albicans,* exist in microflora of mouth, GI, and vaginal tracts of mother and infants harbor *C. albicans* in mouth or GI tract and recurrently on skin.

Other Features Endocrine disorders, genetic disorders (Down syndrome, acrodermatitis, enteropathica, chronic mucocutaneous candidiasis, chronic granulomatosus disease) and immune disorder or systemic antibiotics can predispose an individual to candidiasis.

HISTORY

Onset Present at birth or shortly thereafter.

Review of Symptoms Usually no constitutional symptoms.

PHYSICAL EXAMINATION

Skin Findings

Type Erythema and pustules, papules, pustules to exfoliative lesions (Fig. 1-18).

Color Red or white.

Size 1 to 2 mm.

Distribution Head, face, neck, trunk, and extremities. Occasional nail, palm, and sole involvement. Spares diaper area.

Sites of Predilection Intertriginous areas, posterior aspect of trunk and extensor surfaces of extremities.

DIFFERENTIAL DIAGNOSIS

The diagnosis of cutaneous candidiasis is based on clinical signs and demonstration of *Candida* organisms. Clinical period similar to erythema toxicum, transient neonatal pustular melanosis, bacterial folliculitis, bullous impetigo, congenital herpes, varicella, syphilis, or acne neonatorum. Course of congenital candidiasis, however, is progressive but relatively benign and without constitutional symptoms.

LABORATORY EXAMINATIONS

Direct microscopic examination of pustules and culture from the cutaneous lesions yield yeast forms.

COURSE AND PROGNOSIS

Congenital candidiasis clears spontaneously after several weeks.

MANAGEMENT

Systemic (50,000 to 100,000 units qid) and topical nystatin hasten resolution of lesions in 3 to 10 d. In more severe cases, fluconazole (3 to 6 mg/kg PO QD may be needed.

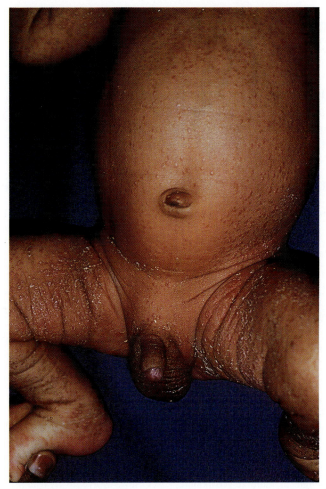

Figure 1-18 Congenital candidiasis *Diffuse erythematous papules, pustules and exfoliation on a newborn with congenital candidiasis.*

ABNORMALITIES OF SUBCUTANEOUS TISSUE

SUBCUTANEOUS FAT NECROSIS

A benign self-limited condition in which a cold-induced rupturing of fat cells results in a subcutaneous nodule in an otherwise healthy newborn.

EPIDEMIOLOGY

Age   Newborns.

Gender   M = F.

Prevalence   Rare.

Etiology   Cold injury, trauma at delivery, asphyxia, and rarely, hypercalcemia.

PATHOPHYSIOLOGY

The fat of neonates contain more saturated fatty acids, which have a higher melting point than adult fatty acids. Once the temperature of the skin drops below the melting point of the fat, crystallization occurs within the fat of the dermal fat cells and a granulomatous reaction ensues.

HISTORY

Asymptomatic single or multiple red nodules that begin within the first 2 weeks of life and resolve spontaneously over several weeks.

PHYSICAL EXAMINATION

Skin Findings

Type of Lesion   Small, sharply demarcated nodules coalescing into larger plaques (Fig. 1-19).

Color   Reddish to purple.

Palpation   Firm to palpation.

Distribution   Cheeks, buttocks, back, arms, or thighs.

General Findings

Infrequently, hypercalcemia can occur with associated irritability, vomiting, weight loss, and failure to thrive.

DIFFERENTIAL DIAGNOSIS

Subcutanous fat necrosis must be differentiated from bacterial cellulitis or septicemic lesions. Babies with subcutaneous fat necrosis have several separate lesions sites and they appear healthy and nurse vigorously, all of which would be unusual in a systemic infection.

LABORATORY EXAMINATIONS

Dermatopathology   Ruptured fat cells surrounded by granulomatous inflammation and necrosis. Needle-shaped clefts within the fat cells with necrosis and crystallization of the saturated fat may be detected.

Laboratory Examination of Blood   Rarely, hypercalcemia may be found.

COURSE AND PROGNOSIS

Lesions evolve slowly over several months from red nodules, to bruise-like discoloration, to a hard subcutaneous mass that resolves in 2 to 4 weeks, usually without atrophy or scarring.

MANAGEMENT

Since the lesion is self-limited, no treatment is necessary. Fluctuant lesions can be aspirated to avoid subsequent scarring. The calcium level should be monitored in these infants as the skin lesions resolve since transient hypercalcemia can occur and should be treated.

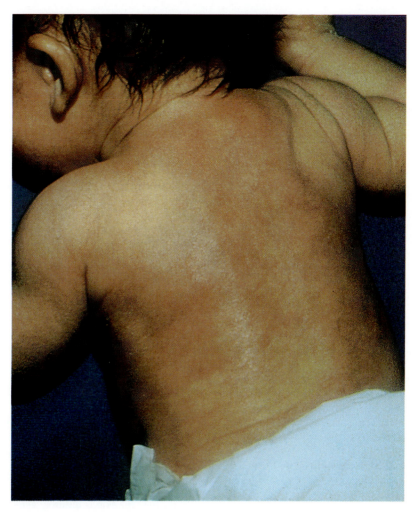

Figure 1-19 Subcutaneous fat necrosis *Confluent erythematous well-demarcated subcutaneous nodules of fat on the back of a newborn.*

SCLEREMA NEONATORUM

Diffuse skin hardening seen in septic, hypothermic, and severely ill newborns.

EPIDEMIOLOGY

Age Newborns, premature infants are more susceptible.

Gender M = F.

Incidence Rare.

Etiology Sclerema can result from a number of physiologic insults and is a nonspecific sign of poor prognostic outcome rather than a primary disease. In 25% of affected infants, the mother is severely ill at the time of delivery.

PATHOPHYSIOLOGY

Cold exposure with vascular collapse and an increase in saturated fat relative to unsaturated fat leads to a diffuse solidification of the tissues.

HISTORY

Onset typically after 24 h of age in severely ill infants with sepsis, hypoglycemia, hypothermia, or severe metabolic abnormalities.

PHYSICAL EXAMINATION

Skin Findings

Type of Lesion Diffuse wood-like hardening and thickening of the skin (Fig. 1-20).

Color Yellow-white mottled appearance.

Palpation Stony, hard, and cold.

Distribution Symmetrical, beginning on the legs and progressing upward to involve the buttocks and trunk.

General Findings

Infant is severely ill with an underlying medical condition such as sepsis, cardiac or respiratory problems, hypothermia, or metabolic abnormality. Infants are weak, lethargic, and feed poorly.

DIFFERENTIAL DIAGNOSIS

Clinically, the diffuse skin thickening and hardening are characteristic of sclerema. It can be confused with scleroderma but the newborn's age and severe illness is characteristic of sclerema neonatorum. Sclerema neonatorum may be confused with subcutaneous fat necrosis of the newborn. Several distinguishing features include: (1) appearance of the infant: in sclerema neonatorum, the infant appears extremely ill; in subcutaneous fat necrosis, the infant appears remarkably well; (2) general appearance of the lesion: in sclerema neonatorum, the sclerosis is diffuse and in subcutaneous fat necrosis, the lesions are localized.

LABORATORY EXAMINATIONS

Dermatopathology Edema of fibrous septa surrounding fat lobules.

COURSE AND PROGNOSIS

The prognosis of sclerema neonatorum is poor. By the time the skin is diffusely hardened, the infant is usually very ill with high morbidity and mortality.

TREATMENT AND PREVENTION

Careful neonatal monitoring of premature infants with precise temperature control, appropriate antibiotic therapy, and correction of metabolic abnormalities, possibly with repeated exchange transfusions or systemic corticosteroids may arrest and reverse the process.

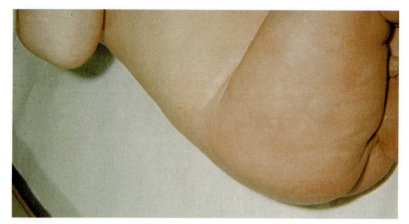

Figure 1-20 Sclerema neonatorum *Diffuse wood-like hardening of the thigh in a sick newborn infant.*

ECZEMATOUS DERMATITIS

ATOPIC DERMATITIS

Atopic dermatitis is an acute, subacute, but usually chronic, pruritic inflammation of the epidermis and dermis, often occurring in association with a personal or family history of hay fever, asthma, allergic rhinitis, or atopic dermatitis. It can be divided into three phases based on the age of the individual: infantile, childhood, and adolescent.

EPIDEMIOLOGY

Age Onset usually in first 2 months of life, by age 1 in 60% of patients, and by age 5 in another 30% of patients. 75% of patients improve by age 10 to 14 years.

Gender M = F.

Incidence Common.

Hereditary Predisposition Over two-thirds have personal or family history of allergic rhinitis, hay fever, or asthma. Thirty to 50% of children with atopic dermatitis develop asthma and/or hay fever later in life.

Prevalence 10 to 15% of the childhood population.

PATHOPHYSIOLOGY

The cause of atopic dermatitis is unknown. In some atopics, a type I (IgE-mediated) hypersensitivity reaction occurs as a result of the release of vasoactive substances from both mast cells and basophils that have been sensitized by the interaction of the antigen with IgE (reaginic or skin-sensitizing antibody); however, the role of IgE in atopic dermatitis is still not clarified. In others, an ingested allergen (particularly milk, eggs, nuts, soy, wheat, or fish) precipitates the itching and leads to the eczematous skin eruptions.

HISTORY

Dry skin and itching are found in all patients. Scratching the skin leads to rash/lichenification and a vicious cycle of itch-scratch-itching. Itching is aggravated by cold weather, frequent bathing, wool, detergent, soap, and stress.

PHYSICAL EXAMINATION

Skin Findings

Type Papules and plaques with scale, crust, and lichenification. Lesions usually confluent and ill defined.

Color Erythematous.

Special Clinical Features

Atopic children may demonstrate increased palmar markings, periorbital atopic pleats (Dennie–Morgan lines), keratosis pilaris, or white dermatographism. They also can develop widespread herpetic, wart, molluscum, or tinea infections because of their impaired skin integrity.

DIFFERENTIAL DIAGNOSIS

Atopic dermatitis can be confused with seborrheic dermatitis, contact dermatitis, psoriasis, or scabies. Certain rare metabolic disorders are associated with atopic dermatitis and these should be considered: acrodermatitis enteropathica, histidinemia, biotin deficiency, phenylketonuria; also some immunologic disorders including Wiskott–Aldrich syndrome, sex-linked agammaglobulinemia, hyper-IgE syndrome, and Letterer–Siwe disease.

DERMATOPATHOLOGY

Acute lesions have varying degrees of acanthosis with rare intraepidermal intercellular edema (spongiosis). The dermal infiltrate is comprised of lymphocytes, monocytes, and mast cells with few or no eosinophils. Chronic lesions show hyperkeratosis, parakeratosis, and papillomatosus.

LABORATORY EXAMINATION

May have an increased IgE or eosinophilia in the serum. RAST testing for systemic allergies is sometimes useful in severe cases.

COURSE AND PROGNOSIS

Two-thirds of children with atopic dermatitis improve by preschool age. However, in some cases, atopic dermatitis may last a long time, requiring life-long management. Thirty to 50% of children may develop asthma or hayfever later in life.

MANAGEMENT

Aggravating Factors

Because atopic dermatitis cannot be cured (although it does go away spontaneously in most cases), the goal is to keep the condition under control. Because each child is different, skin care treatment is individualized. Patients and parents need to be educated about factors that may **aggravate** atopic dermatitis. These include:

1. Excessive bathing or prolonged contact with water; repeated wetting and drying of skin.
2. Extremes in humidity or sudden temperature changes; tends to flare in winter.
3. Wool, acrylic, or fur material in clothing, carpeting, and furniture.
4. Exposure to pillows, comforters, or mattresses filled with feathers or down.
5. Exposure to cats, dogs, rabbits, airborne dust, or pollen.

6. Ingestion (rarely) of certain foods: cow's milk, eggs, wheat, peanuts, fish, or soy.
7. Skin contact with tomatoes or citrus fruits.
8. Skin contact with perfumed or alcohol-containing creams and soaps.
9. Perspiration from physical activity or overheating.
10. Exposure to sandboxes or chlorinated swimming pools.
11. Fatigue, illness, or emotional frustration.
12. Some eczema patients are sensitive to certain environmental substances, such as dust, pollen, and pets. The most common reaction is nose and eye itching, but not a prolonged reaction of the skin. Efforts to avoid these can be attempted.
13. Certain foods may seem to worsen eczema, especially in infants and young children, but elimination of foods rarely brings about a lasting improvement. If a certain food is suspected of causing flare-ups and itching, it can be avoided for a few weeks on a trial basis to see if improvement *occurs*. Prolonged elimination of any food could contribute to malnutrition, and testing for allergies may not always be reliable.

General Principles

The goals of treatment are to reduce the inflammation and itching of the skin and to retain the skin's moisture. Guidelines are as follows:

1. *Baths*. Baths are helpful in soothing itching and removing crusting. They should be lukewarm and limited to 10 min duration. For some, it may be helpful to add an oil containing tar to the water (Balnetar bath oil or Polytar). Immediately after bathing is the most useful time to apply prescription ointments and moisturizers.
2. *Soaps*. Avoiding soap and bubble bath is best. Dove fragrance-free soap is acceptable. Alternative skin cleansers that may be less irritating include Aquanil lotion, Cetaphil cleanser, and Aveeno. Soaps should be used only on dirty areas and rinsed off immediately, as most soaps are irritating and drying to sensitive areas.
3. *Moisturizers*. Moisturizers work to reduce dryness in the skin by trapping moisture. They should be applied to normal and abnormal (affected) skin after prescription ointments have been applied. The most useful time to apply these is immediately

after bathing or showering. Some moisturizers contain perfumes, alcohol, and preservatives—these should be avoided if possible. Generally, for dry skin, the more greasy creams and lotions are best. Some moisturizers are hydrated petrolatum (you must ask the pharmacist to get it), Vaseline, mineral oil, Aquaphor, Lubriderm, Moisturel, and Eucerin creams.

4. *Tar preparations.* Tar ointments, creams, and bath emulsions may be suggested to reduce mild inflammation of the skin. The ointments and creams should be applied just to affected areas once or twice daily. Prolonged use should be avoided.

Topical Corticosteroids **Topical steroids** are effective if used in appropriate strengths:

a. Low-potency steroids (Desowen, 1% hydrocortisone, 2.5% hydrocortisone) should be used on face or groin area, no more than bid × 2 weeks.

b. Medium-potency steroids (Elocon, Dermatop, Cutivate) should be used on the body or extremities no more than bid × 2 weeks.

c. Strong steroids (Ultravate, Psorcon, Diprolene) are reserved for older children/adults on severely affected areas bid for no more than 2 weeks.

Patients need to be cautioned about steroid side effects. Continued use of very strong topical steroids can cause thinning of the skin, stretch marks, accentuation of blood vessels in the skin, and absorption of cortisone into the body. Infants are at greater risk for increased absorption because of their increased body surface-area-to-weight ratio. Prolonged steroid use can also lead to tachyphylaxis (the steroid becomes less and less effective for the skin condition treated), requiring another class of steroids for efficacy. Finally, steroid creams on the eyelid area may lead to cataracts and glaucoma.

Topical Immunomodulators Recently, topical immunomodulators have been developed for the treatment of atopic dermatitis. In November 2000, the FDA approved Protopic (topical FK506 or tacrolimus) for use in patients with moderate to severe atopic dermatitis.

a. Protopic 0.03% ointment bid to affected areas is currently approved for use in children 2 to 15 years of age.

b. Protopic 0.1% ointment bid to affected areas is approved for use in adolescents or adults (>15 years of age).

Side effects reported include burning (~26%) and itching (~23%) in some patients, which decreases as the skin improves. The benefits of topical immunomodulators include safe long-term use and steroid-sparing effects.

Antihistamines. These oral medications may be somewhat helpful in controlling itching. They are particularly useful at bedtime, when itching is usually the worst. They often have the side effect of producing drowsiness and, in rare instances, hyperactivity. The most commonly prescribed antihistamines are Atarax (hydroxyzine, 2 to 4 mg/kg/d divided tid or qid) and Benadryl (diphenhydramine, 5 mg/kg 4 mg/kg/d divided tid or qid, not to exceed 300 mg/d). With continued use, antihistamines may lose their effectiveness, and higher doses may be required. Therefore, use of these should be limited to times of greatest discomfort.

Antibiotics. Topical or oral antibiotics may be needed if the skin becomes infected. Signs of infection include open and moist areas, which may weep or become crusted; extensive redness; or small bumps filled with clear fluid or pus. Topical antibiotics include mupirocin (Bactroban), bacitracin, or polysporin and can be used bid–tid on impetiginized areas. Oral antibiotics are taken for 7 to 10 d. In patients with recurrent infections or severe eczema, a longer maintenance course of antibiotics may be prescribed. The most commonly prescribed antibiotics include Keflex (25 to 50 mg/kg per day divided qid, not to exceed 4 g/d); dicloxacillin (25 to 50 mg/kg/d divided qid, not to exceed 2 g/d); Duricef (30 mg/kg/d divided bid); and erythromycin (30 to 50 mg/kg/d divided qid, not to exceed 2 g/d).

INFANTILE ATOPIC DERMATITIS

Infantile atopic dermatitis is one of the most troublesome skin eruptions in children. There is an "atopic" background without a clearly defined immunologic pattern. Skin lesions seem to be a reaction to itching and rubbing.

EPIDEMIOLOGY

Age   Symptoms appear between 2 to 6 months and 50% clear by age 2 to 3 years.

PHYSICAL EXAMINATION

Skin Lesions

Type   Tiny vesicles on "puffy" surface, scaling, exudation with wet crusts, and cracks (fissures).

Color   Erythematous pink to red.

Distribution   Begins on face (cheeks, forehead, scalp) and then spreads to body, usually sparing diaper area (Fig. 2-1).

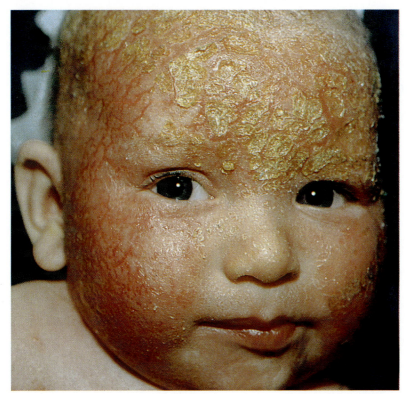

Figure 2-1 Infantile atopic dermatitis *Erythematous crusted scaling exudative rash predominantly on the face of a newborn.*

CHILDHOOD-TYPE ATOPIC DERMATITIS

EPIDEMIOLOGY

Age Typically follows infantile atopic dermatitis and is seen from age 4 to 10 years.

PHYSICAL EXAMINATION

Skin Lesions

Type Papules coalescing into lichenified plaques with erosions and crusts (Fig. 2-2).

Distribution Wrists, ankles, antecubital and popliteal fossae.

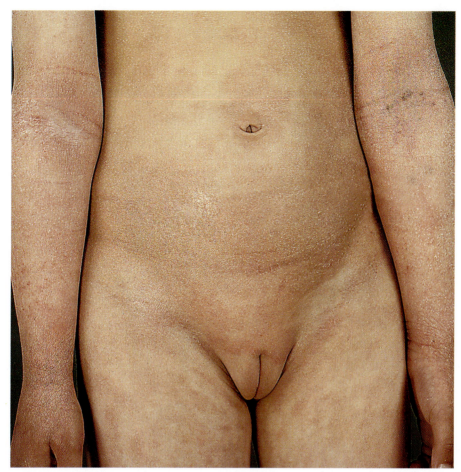

Figure 2-2   Atopic dermatitis, childhood-type   *Ill-defined erythema, papules, excoriations, lichenification (thickening of the skin with accentuation of the skin lines) in the antecubital fossae, with less severe changes on the trunk and thighs.* (Reproduced with permission from TB Fitzpatrick et al., Color Atlas and Synopsis of Clinical Dermatology, 4th edition. New York: McGraw-Hill, 2001).

ADOLESCENT-TYPE ATOPIC DERMATITIS

EPIDEMIOLOGY

Age   Begins at age 12 and continues into the 20s. Cases that begin in the 20s are more refractory to cure.

PHYSICAL EXAMINATION

Skin Lesions

Type   Papules coalescing into lichenified plaques.

Distribution   Flexor folds, face, neck, upper back, hands, and feet (Fig. 2-3).

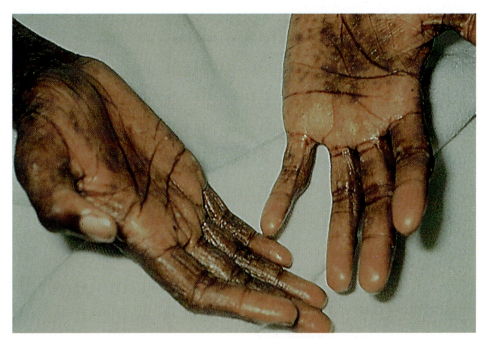

Figure 2-3 Atopic dermatitis, adolescent-type *Papules and vesicles on the palms of an adolescent with atopic dermatitis.* (Reproduced with permission from IM Freedberg et al., Dermatology in General Medicine, 5th edition. New York: McGraw-Hill, 1999).

LICHEN SIMPLEX CHRONICUS

Lichen simplex chronicus (LSC) is a localized, well-circumscribed area of lichenification (thickened skin) resulting from repeated rubbing, itching, and scratching of the skin. It can occur on normal skin of individuals with atopic, seborrheic, contact dermatitis, or psoriasis.

EPIDEMIOLOGY

Age   Rarely seen in young children. Occurs in adolescents and adults.

Gender   F > M.

Incidence   Common.

PATHOPHYSIOLOGY

A special predilection of the skin to respond to physical trauma by epidermal hyperplasia; skin becomes highly sensitive to touch, which is probably related to proliferation of nerves in the epidermis. This leads to a vicious itch-scratch-itch cycle that is difficult to stop.

HISTORY

Duration of Lesion(s)   Weeks to months.

PHYSICAL EXAMINATION

Skin Lesions

Type   Well-delineated plaque of lichenification (Fig. 2-4); at times with scales or excoriations.

Size   5 to 15 cm.

Color   Brown or black hyper- or hypopigmentation.

Shape   Round, oval, linear (following path of scratching).

Distribution   Easily reached areas such as neck, wrists, ankles, pretibial area, thighs, vulva, scrotum, and perianal area.

DIFFERENTIAL DIAGNOSIS

Lichen simplex chronicus can be confused with tinea corporis, psoriasis, contact or atopic dermatitis.

LABORATORY EXAMINATIONS

Hyperkeratosis, acanthosis, and elongated and broad rete ridges. Spongiosis is infrequent and vesiculation is absent. In the dermis, there is a chronic inflammatory infiltrate with fibrosis.

MANAGEMENT

Topical tar preparations and corticosteriods will decrease pruritus. Occlusive dressings can also prevent itching. Cordran tape is an adhesive impregnated with medium-potency steroid that is especially convenient for the treatment of LSC, however, it should be used judiciously and sparingly since all steroids under occlusion are much more potent. The side effects of prolonged or potent topical steroids should be reviewed. Continued use of topical steroids can lead to thinning of the skin, stretch marks, and accentuation of the blood vessels in the skin. For small-localized areas of LSC, intralesional corticosteroids are often highly effective.

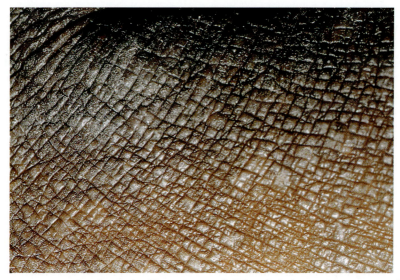

Figure 2-4 Lichen simplex chronicus *Hyperpigmented, lichenified plaque with accentuated skin lines caused by repeated rubbing of the area.*

DYSHIDROTIC ECZEMATOUS DERMATITIS

Dyshidrotic eczema is a special vesicular type of hand and foot eczema. It is an acute, chronic, or recurrent dermatosis of the fingers, palms, and soles characterized by a sudden onset of deep-seated pruritic, clear, "sago-like" vesicles; later, scaling, fissures, lichenification, and possibly, secondary bacterial infection may occur.

Synonym Pompholyx.

EPIDEMIOLOGY

Age 12 to 40 years old.

Gender M = F.

PATHOPHYSIOLOGY

The etiology is unclear and likely multifactorial. About half the patients have an atopic background. Emotional stress is possibly a precipitating factor. Hyperhidrosis may or may not be present.

HISTORY

Duration of Lesions Onset in a few days.

Skin Symptoms Pruritus and especially painful fissures that are incapacitating. Summer exacerbations are not infrequent.

PHYSICAL EXAMINATION

Skin Lesions

Type

    a. *Early* Vesicles, usually small (1 mm), deep-seated, appear like "tapioca" in clusters (Fig. 2-5), occasionally bullae, especially on the feet.

    b. *Later* Scaling, lichenification, painful fissures, and erosions.

Arrangement Vesicles grouped in clusters.

Distribution Regional [hands (80%) and feet] with sites of predilection bilaterally on the sides of fingers, palms, and soles.

Nails Dystrophic changes (transverse ridging, pitting, and thickening).

Other Hyperhidrosis is present in some patients.

DIFFERENTIAL DIAGNOSIS

Pomphylox can mimic a vesicular reaction to active dermatophytosis on the feet, an "id" reaction, or an acute contact dermatitis.

DERMATOPATHOLOGY

Intraepidermal vesicles with balloon cells and sparse inflammation.

COURSE AND PROGNOSIS

Recurrent attacks with intervals of weeks to months with spontaneous remissions in 2 to 3 weeks.

MANAGEMENT

1. Dry skin care with limited oil-in-water baths and good moisturization with water-in-oil ointments (hydrated petrolatum, petroleum jelly, or Aquaphor healing ointment) are preventative measures.
2. For the active vesicular stage (early): Burrow's wet dressings; large bullae should be drained but not unroofed.
3. For the more chronic eczematous stage (later): Topical corticosteroids are successful in a few patients.

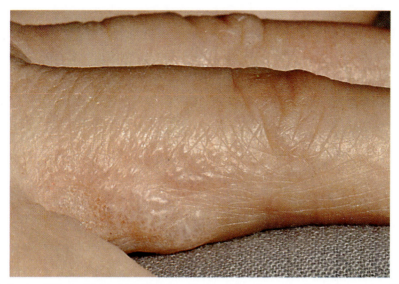

Figure 2-5 Atopic dermatitis, dyshidrotic type *Tapioca-like, deep-seated vesicles on the sides of the fingers.* (Reproduced with permission from IM Freedberg et al., Dermatology in General Medicine, 5th edition. New York: McGraw-Hill, 1999).

4. Bacterial infection may be present and topical or oral antibiotics may be helpful.
5. PUVA (oral or topical as "soaks" in psoralen with controlled UVA hand-foot light box treatment) is successful in older patients if given over prolonged periods of time and is worth trying, especially in severe cases.

NUMMULAR ECZEMA

Nummular eczema is a chronic, pruritic, inflammatory dermatitis occurring in the form of coin-shaped plaques. It is seen in individuals with dry skin and/or atopic dermatitis.

EPIDEMIOLOGY

Age Any age. Seen more commonly in older children and adolescents.

Gender M = F.

Incidence Common.

Etiology Unclear. Exacerbated by winter, excessive bathing, irritants.

PATHOPHYSIOLOGY

Unclear. A common eczematous reaction pattern, frequently occurring in atopics.

HISTORY

Duration of Lesions Weeks, with remissions and recurrences.

Skin Symptoms Pruritus, may be mild or severe.

PHYSICAL EXAMINATION

Skin Lesions

Type Closely grouped, small vesicles and papules that coalesce into lichenified plaques, often more than 4 to 5 cm. Dry scaly plaques that may be lichenified.

Color Dull red to hyperpigmented dark.

Shape Round or coin-shaped (Fig. 2-6), hence the adjective nummular (Latin *nummularis,* "like a coin").

Distribution Extensor surfaces of hands, arms, legs.

DIFFERENTIAL DIAGNOSIS

Nummular dermatitis can be confused with contact or atopic dermatitis, tinea corporis, or psoriasis.

LABORATORY EXAMINATIONS

Dermatopathology Subacute inflammation with acanthosis, intraepidermal vesicles, and spongiosis in the epidermis.

COURSE AND PROGNOSIS

Remissions with treatment but frequent recurrences unless the skin is kept hydrated and lubricated.

MANAGEMENT

1. Preventative measures include good dry skin care with limited oil-in-water baths followed by application of water-in-oil ointments (hydrated petrolatum, Vaseline, or Aquaphor healing ointment).
2. Topical corticosteroids can be applied for a limited time to the more moderate to severely affected areas. (See Topical corticosteroids, page 48.)

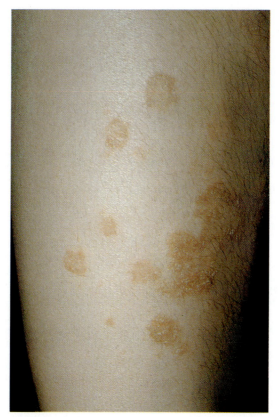

Figure 2-6   Nummular eczema   *Round coin-shaped lesions of eczema on the legs of a child.*

CONTACT DERMATITIS

There are 2 types of contact dermatitis.

1. Allergic contact: caused by sensitization of the skin to a topical allergen.
2. Irritant contact: caused by irritation of chemical against skin.

Both reactions are characterized by pruritus or burning of the skin.

EPIDEMIOLOGY

Age Irritant dermatitis can occur at any age, whereas allergic contact dermatitis is unusual in < 1 year of age given time needed to sensitize/expose skin to allergen/irritant.

Gender M = F.

Incidence Only seen in 1.5% of children.

Etiology Clinical syndrome usually *delayed-hypersensitivity reaction* (type IV), with a latent period of a few days or years from the first exposure and the reexposure that precipitates the allergic contact dermatitis, *or* a primary irritant that produces inflammation on first or repeated contact in irritant contact dermatitis.

PATHOPHYSIOLOGY

Allergic contact dermatitis is the classic example of type IV hypersensitivity reaction (cellular, cell-mediated, delayed, or tuberculin type) caused by sensitized lymphocytes (T cells) after contact with antigen. The antigen processing occurs via Langerhans cells. The tissue damage results from cytotoxicity by T cells or from release of lymphokines. Irritant contact dermatitis causes immediate physical damage to the localized area of skin to which it is exposed.

HISTORY

Duration of Lesion(s) Acute contact—days, weeks; chronic contact—months, years.

Skin Symptoms Pruritus, mild to moderate. Extensive acute lesions may be painful.

PHYSICAL EXAMINATION

Skin Findings

Type a. *Acute* Inflammatory papules and vesicles coalescing into plaques.

b. *Subacute* Patches of mild erythema showing small, dry scales or superficial desquamation, sometimes associated with small, red, pointed or rounded, firm papules.

c. *Chronic* Patches of lichenification (thickening of the epidermis with deepening of the skin lines in parallel or rhomboidal pattern), with satellite, small, firm, rounded or flat-topped papules, excoriations, and pigmentation.

Arrangement Well-demarcated patterns suggestive of an external cause or "outside job." Plant allergic contact dermatitis often results in linear lesions Fig. 2-7A and 2-7B).

Distribution In exposed areas that come into contact with irritant or allergen.

LABORATORY EXAMINATIONS

Dermatopathology Inflammation with intraepidermal intercellular edema (spongiosis) and monocyte and histiocyte infiltration in the dermis suggest allergic contact dermatitis, whereas more superficial vesicles containing polymorphonuclear leukocytes suggest a primary irritant dermatitis. In chronic contact dermatitis, there is lichenification (hyperkeratosis, acanthosis, elongation of rete ridges, and elongation and broadening of papillae).

Patch Tests Sensitization is present on every part of the skin; therefore application of the allergen to any area of normal skin will provoke inflammation. A positive patch test shows erythema *and* papules, possibly vesicles confined to the test site.

MANAGEMENT

Prompt identification and removal of the etiologic agent is recommended.

Acute Wet dressings using cloths soaked in Burrow's solution and changed every 2 to 3 h

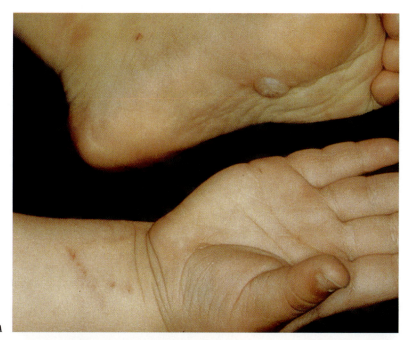

Figure 2-7 Allergic contact dermatitis *(A) Linear arrangement of vesicles on the wrist and bulla on the foot of a child exposed to poison ivy. (B) Plant: poison ivy with characteristic shiny, red, 3-leaf configuration.*

is recommended. More extensive cases can gain symptomatic relief with Aveeno oatmeal baths. Medium- to strong-potency topical corticosteroid creams can be used bid for 2 weeks on involved areas. In severe cases, systemic corticosteroids may be indicated.

Subacute and Chronic Short courses of potent topical corticosteroid preparations (Ultravate, Psorcon, or Diprolene) can be used limitedly bid for up to 2 weeks, but should quickly be replaced by weaker steroid preparations.

Subsequent avoidance of the irritant or allergenic agent is recommended.

SEBORRHEIC DERMATITIS

Seborrheic dermatitis occurs on the areas of the skin in which the sebaceous glands are most active, such as the face and scalp, and in the diaper area.

Synonym Cradle cap.

EPIDEMIOLOGY

Age Infancy (within the first 10 weeks) and adolescence (puberty).

Gender More common in males.

Incidence Two to 5% of the population.

Etiology Unknown. May be related to *Pityrosporum ovale* overgrowth on the skin since topical ketoconazole improves the condition.

PATHOPHYSIOLOGY

Pityrosporum ovale overgrowth may play a role in the pathogenesis, but no etiologic agent has been proved.

HISTORY

Duration of Lesions Gradual onset, commonly in infancy.

Skin Symptoms Typically asymptomatic or mildly pruritic.

PHYSICAL EXAMINATION

Skin Lesions

Type Yellowish-red, often greasy, scaling macules and papules of varying size (5 to 20 mm), coalescing into plaques.

Color Salmon erythematous.

Arrangement Scattered, discrete on the face (Fig. 2-8) and trunk; diffuse involvement of scalp and diaper area.

Distribution Scalp, face, diaper area.

DIFFERENTIAL DIAGNOSIS

Differential includes dermatophytosis, candidiasis (KOH examination and cultures will help), and atopic dermatitis (much more pruritic than seborrheic dermatitis). There may be an overlap seen in patients with psoriasis, so-called "sebo-psoriasis."

DERMATOPATHOLOGY

Site Epidermis.

Process Focal parakeratosis, with few pyknotic neutrophils, moderate acanthosis, spongiosis (intercellular edema), nonspecific inflammation of the dermis.

COURSE AND PROGNOSIS

Infantile seborrhea usually is asymptomatic and clears spontaneously within months. Childhood and adolescent seborrheic dermatitis can clear spontaneously but may have a recurrent course.

TREATMENT

Scalp (Cradle Cap) Removal of the thick scale with mineral oil and fine tooth comb lifting off of scale can provide symptomatic and/or cosmetic relief. For older children and adolescents, shampoos containing selenium sulfide (Selsun), zinc pyrithione (Head and Shoulders), tar (T-gel), or ketoconazole (Nizoral) used intermittently 2 to 3 times a week can control the eruption. It is important to instruct the patient or parent to lather the shampoo and let it sit on the scalp for 5 to 10 min before rinsing.

Face and Diaper Area Creams containing ketoconazole are helpful and can be used bid on a regular basis. Weak topical steroid preparations (Desowen, Aclovate, 1 to 2.5% hydrocortisone cream) can be used bid sparingly for 2 to 3 days for acute flares.

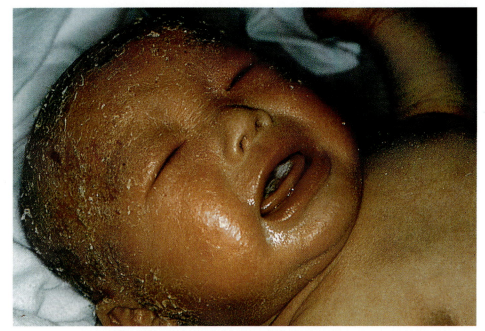

Figure 2-8 Seborrheic dermatitis *Greasy scale and erythema involving the scalp and face of an infant.* (Reproduced with permission from Lisa Cohen).

DIAPER DERMATITIS AND RASHES IN THE DIAPER AREA

DIAPER DERMATITIS

Diaper dermatitis is a broad term that describes a multifactorial cutaneous eruption located in the diaper area.

Synonym Diaper rash.

EPIDEMIOLOGY

Age Most babies develop some form of diaper dermatitis during their diaper wearing years. The prevalence reaches a maximum between 6 to 12 months of age.

Gender M = F.

Prevalence At any one point in time, up to one-third of infants may have diaper dermatitis. The prevalence of severe diaper dermatitis (defined as extreme erythema with ulcerations, oozing papules, and pustules) is 5%.

Etiology Excessive hydration of the skin and frictional injury leads to a compromised skin barrier and irritation from ammonia, feces, cleansing products, fragrances, and possible superinfection with *Candida albicans* or bacteria.

Season Reportedly highest during winter months, perhaps due to less frequent diaper changing.

PATHOPHYSIOLOGY

The warm moist environment inside the diaper and frictional damage decreases the protective barrier function of the skin in the diaper area. Then predisposing factors such as seborrhea, atopic dermatitis, and systemic disease, as well as activating factors such as allergens (in detergents, rubbers, and plastic), primary irritants (ammonia from urine and feces), and infection (by yeast of bacteria) lead to a rash in the diaper area.

PHYSICAL EXAMINATION

Skin Findings

Type of Lesion Ranges from macular erythema (Fig. 3-1) to papules, plaques, vesicles, erosions, and ulcerated nodules.

Color Ranges from mild erythema to diffuse beefy redness.

Palpation Ranges from nonindurated to prominently elevated lesions.

Distribution Diaper area, convex surfaces involved, folds spared. Severe cases may involve folds and have characteristic *C. albicans* satellite pustules.

DIFFERENTIAL DIAGNOSIS

Diagnosis The diagnosis of diaper dermatitis should be made clinically, although, refractory response to conventional treatments should raise the suspicion of less common rashes in the diaper area.

Differential Diagnosis Diaper dermatitis must be differentiated from psoriasis, granuloma gluteal infantum (foreign body reaction, typically to baby powder or topical steroids), primary candidiasis (perianal involvement with satellite lesions), seborrheic dermatitis, acro-

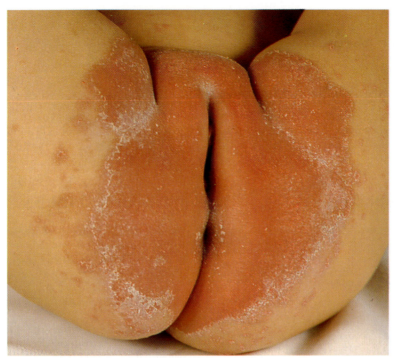

Figure 3-1 Diaper dermatitis *Red, macerated areas in the diaper region of an infant.* (Reproduced with permission from IM Freedberg et al., Dermatology in General Medicine, 5th edition. New York: McGraw-Hill, 1999).

dermatitis enteropathica (due to zinc deficiency), and histiocytosis X.

COURSE AND PROGNOSIS

Most episodes of diaper dermatitis are self-limited with a duration of 3 d or less. Severe cases of diaper dermatitis are usually due to candidiasis or bacterial superinfection and may require appropriate antifungal or antibacterial regimens to clear.

MANAGEMENT

Rashes in the diaper area can be minimized by:

1. Keeping the diaper area clean and dry with gentle cleansing of the area (cotton balls dipped in warm water are least irritating) and frequent diaper changes promptly after defecation and urination.
2. Remove any irritating agent or allergen from the diaper environment.
3. Exposing the skin to air will help keep it dry.

4. Powders (talc, cornstarch, baby powder, magnesium stearate, zinc stearate, and baking soda) can be used to absorb moisture and reduce friction between the skin and other surfaces.
5. Protective creams and ointments such as zinc oxide (Desitin), petrolatum (Vaseline), mineral oils, baby oils, lanolin, or vitamins A and D (A&D ointment) may protect the skin from moisture or help heal the infant's skin.
6. For severe inflammation, weak topical steroids (Desowen, 1 or 2.5% hydrocortisone) may be used sparingly. Since the diaper area is always under occlusion, the steroid effects will be augmented, and baby skin in the groin area is already very sensitive.
7. Cutaneous candidiasis requires topical antifungal treatment with topical nystatin or clotrimazole creams. Be careful to avoid anticandidal preparations that are mixed with cortisone to prevent steroid side effects in the occluded diaper area.
8. Bacterial infections are treated with topical [mupirocin (Bactroban), bacitracin, or polysporin] or oral antibiotics.

RASHES IN THE DIAPER AREA

PSORIASIS IN DIAPER AREA

Psoriasis can first manifest itself as a recalcitrant diaper rash, and should be considered if conventional diaper rash remedies are not effective. Other stigmata of early psoriasis include seborrhea, nail pitting, intergluteal erythema, and a family history of psoriasis.

EPIDEMIOLOGY

Age Any age, typically seen first in the diaper area of children under the age of 2 years.

Gender F > M.

Incidence Uncommon.

Etiology Unclear.

Genetics Possible autosomal dominant inheritance with incomplete penetrance. Associated with HLA B13, HLA B17, HLA Bw16, HLA B37, and HLA Cw6.

PATHOPHYSIOLOGY

In normal skin, the cells mature, shed and are replaced every 3 to 4 weeks. In psoriasis, there is a defective inhibitor of epidermal proliferation with shortening of the cell cycle to 3 to 4 d. This leads to increased epidermal cell turnover with decreased shedding and, hence, the accumulation of dead cells as layers of silvery-white scale.

PHYSICAL EXAMINATION

Skin Findings

Type Scattered eythematous papules, may coalesce into a well-delineated erythematous plaque.

Color Dark red plaques, may have a silvery mica-like scale.

Size Pinpoint to several centimeters.

Distribution Anogenital area, may also involve intergluteal cleft, umbilicus, behind or inside the ears, scalp, extremities (Fig. 3-2).

Nails May have pinpoint pits indicative of psoriasis.

DIFFERENTIAL DIAGNOSIS

The well-delineated bright red plaque and silvery mica-like scale is characteristic of psoriasis. Removal of the scale causes bleeding points (Auspitz sign).

LABORATORY EXAMINATIONS

Dermatopathology Epidermal thickening with edema of dermal papillae, thinning of suprapapillary area.

COURSE AND PROGNOSIS

Chronic course with remissions and exacerbations, very unpredictable. Some children progress to mild disease with asymptomatic intermittent exacerbations. Other children have a more severe course with recurrent flares and 5% develop an associated arthritis.

MANAGEMENT

Treatment of psoriasis in the diaper area can be both refractory and/or recurrent.

1. Emollients such as petrolatum, moisturizers, or diaper creams can help minimize flares and reduce itching.
2. Allowing the diaper area to be exposed to air for short periods can also help reduce the chafing that can exacerbate psoriasis (Koebner phenomenon).
3. Sunlight exposure is thought to help psoriasis, but sunburns should be avoided.
4. Topical tar preparations are antiinflammatory and can be used in the bath water (Balnetar or Polytar) or in creams (MG217 or Elta tar creams). Prolonged use of these agents is not recommended.

5. More severe cases may require short courses of mild topical steroids (Desowen, 1 or 2.5% hydrocortisone creams). It is important to use steroid in the diaper area sparingly since the occlusive diaper increases the steroid potency as well as the risk of steroid side effects such as skin thinning and striae.

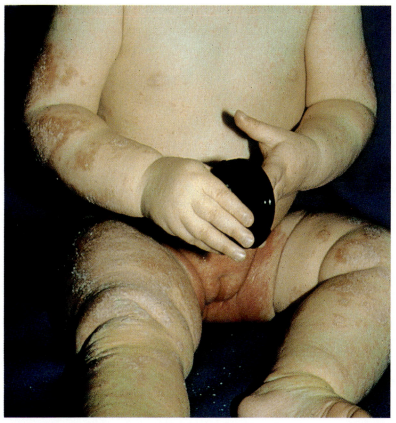

Figure 3-2   Psoriasis in the diaper area   *Well-delineated bright red erythematous plaques in the diaper area and on the extremities of a child.*

CANDIDAL INFECTION

Commonly overlooked, *Candida* diaper dermatitis should be suspected whenever a diaper rash fails to respond to conventional treatment, especially following a course of systemic antibiotic therapy. The infection is propagated by the chronic occlusive state of diapers worn during infancy.

Synonym   Monilial diaper dermatitis.

EPIDEMIOLOGY

Age   Any diaper wearing stage (approximately infancy to 3 years of age).

Gender   M = F.

Incidence   Common.

Etiology   *Candida albicans* organisms are harbored in the lower intestinal tract of the infant. Upon defecation, infected feces introduce yeast into area. The moist occlusive diaper environment favors candidal overgrowth and leads to a rash.

PATHOPHYSIOLOGY

Candida albicans in mouth or GI tract of infant can proliferate in moist diaper environment. Predisposing factors such as systemic antibiotics can also contribute to *Candida* overgrowth.

HISTORY

Candidal overgrowth is seen most frequently following systemic antibiotic therapy. Lesions appear first in the perianal area and then spread to perineum and inguinal creases. The diaper rash may occur in conjunction with oral thrush.

PHYSICAL EXAMINATION

Skin Findings

Type   Erythema with fragile satellite pustules (Fig. 3-3). Rash involving perineum is sharply demarcated with elevated rim and white scales along the border. Pinpoint satellite vesiculopustules often present.

Color   Beefy red erythematous base.

Distribution   Genitocrural area, buttocks, lower abdomen, and inner aspects of the thighs, does not spare folds.

DIAGNOSIS AND DIFFERENTIAL DIAGNOSIS

Diagnosis   Observation of beefy red rash with pustulo-vesicular satellite lesions is diagnostic. Scrapings and cultures can be confirmatory.

Differential Diagnosis   Primary candidal infection in the diaper area has characteristic satellite papules and pustules that are virtually diagnostic. It may be confused with other recalcitrant rashes in the diaper area such as psoriasis, acrodermatitis enteropathica, or histiocytosis X. Most commonly, it can be seen in conjunction with other diaper rashes as a secondary superinfection.

LABORATORY EXAMINATIONS

Microscopic examination of skin scrapings with potassium hydroxide, Gram's stain or periodic acid-Schiff, demonstrate budding yeasts and hyphae or pseudohyphae. Lesions may be cultured on Sabouraud's or Nickerson's medium. White mucoid colonies grow within 48 to 72 h.

COURSE AND PROGNOSIS

Rash progresses until *Candida* is treated. Area can become quite macerated and painful.

MANAGEMENT

1. Topical nystatin (Mycostatin) or clotrimazole (Lotrimin) creams tid to area will clear rash. Care should be taken to avoid anticandidal preparations that are mixed with cortisones since these may be too strong and yield unwanted steroid side effects in the occluded diaper area against baby skin.

2. Oral nystatin suspension (nystatin swish and swallow, 1 to 3 mL PO qid) can be applied to the affected mouth areas to treat oral thrush or gastrointestinal candidal overgrowth. This will also reduce chance of candidal recurrence in the diaper area.

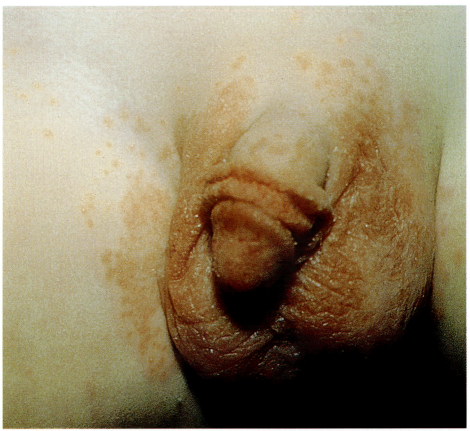

Figure 3-3 Primary candidal infection in the diaper area *Beefy red plaque in the diaper area surrounded by characteristic satellite pustules.*

ACRODERMATITIS ENTEROPATHICA

Acrodermatitis enteropathica (AE) is a hereditary or acquired clinical syndrome caused by zinc deficiency. It is characterized by an acral, vesiculobullous eczematous dermatitis characteristically distributed on the face, hands, feet, and anogenital area.

EPIDEMIOLOGY

Age

Hereditary   In infants given bovine milk: days to few weeks after birth. In breast-fed infants: soon after weaning.

Acquired   Older children and adults with illness that depletes zinc supply.

Gender   M = F.

Etiology   Hereditary or acquired deficiency in zinc.

Hereditary   Autosomal recessively inherited disorder in zinc absorption thought to be secondary to abnormal zinc-binding ligands. Zinc in human milk appears to be more bioavailable to infants than zinc from bovine milk.

Acquired   Long-term zinc deficiency can be seen in patients with parenteral nutrition lacking zinc, bowel bypass syndrome, Crohn's disease, HIV, cystic fibrosis, alcoholism, vegetarian diets, essential fatty acid deficiencies, and other syndromes.

PATHOPHYSIOLOGY

Low serum zinc levels in infancy or childhood leads to acrodermatitis enteropathica (AE). The basic defect is a GI malabsorption of zinc. Hereditary AE may be secondary to an abnormal zinc-binding ligand. Acquired AE can be seen with any systemic disease with GI malabsorption of zinc. The major function of zinc is to be incorporated into enzymes and there are over 200 zinc metalloenzymes in the body.

HISTORY

Review of systems includes diarrhea, weight loss, listlessness, mental changes (irritability, crying, restlessness).

PHYSICAL EXAMINATION

Skin Findings

Type of Lesion   Eczematous or psoriasiform plaques may progress to vesiculobullae or erosions that crust and dry out (Fig. 3-4A).

Color   Erythematous base.

Arrangement   Acral and periorificial (mouth, nose, ears, eyes, perineum).

Distribution   Perioral with perleche (Fig. 3-4B), aphthous-like lesions, symmetrically located on buttocks, extensor surfaces (elbows, knees), and acral areas (fingers and toes).

General Findings

Diarrhea, cachexia, alopecia, nail dystrophy, glossitis, stomatitis, hypogeusia (decreased sense of taste), photophobia, drooling, and growth retardation. Hypogonadism in males (more evident in adolescence). Emotional mental disturbances.

LABORATORY EXAMINATIONS

Low serum zinc ($< 50 \mu$g/DL) or alkaline phosphatase levels. "Zebra striped" light banding of hair can be seen with polarized light microscopy. However, zinc levels can fluctuate with stress or infection.

DIFFERENTIAL DIAGNOSIS

Based on clinical features. Differential diagnosis includes other bullous diseases (linear IgA, chronic bullous disease of childhood, psoriasis, histiocytosis X, and candidal infection). Other causes of diaper dermatitis that are refractory to treatment or associated with periorificial and acral findings should lead the clinician to suspect AE.

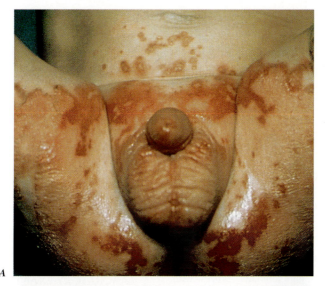

A

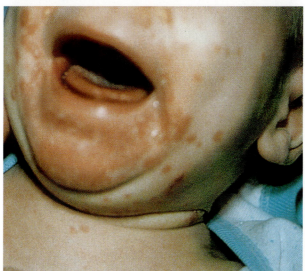

B

Figure 3-4 Acrodermatitis enteropathica *(A) Refractory erythematous, scaly macerated plaque in the diaper area. (B) Periorificial rash in the same child with erythematous papules and confluent plaques.*

COURSE AND PROGNOSIS

If unrecognized, AE has a relentlessly progressive course leading to infection and disability. Once recognized and treated, AE manifestations are quickly corrected and reversed.

TREATMENT

1. Topical zinc creams (Desitin, A&D ointment, zinc oxide paste) can begin to improve the rash.
2. Dietary supplement of zinc gluconate, acetate, or sulfate (5 mg/kg/d divided bid/tid) is usually curative. The RDA (recommended daily allowance) of zinc is 15 mg/d.
3. In severe cases, $ZnCl_2$ can be used intravenously.

GRANULOMA GLUTEALE INFANTUM

Granuloma gluteale infantum is a benign rash in the diaper area characterized by reddish-purple granulomatous nodules. The disorder represents a cutaneous response to a foreign body (talc or zirconium), topical steroids, infection (*Candida*), or inflammation.

Synonyms   Kaposi sarcoma-like granuloma and granuloma intertriginosum infantum.

EPIDEMIOLOGY

Age   Any diaper wearing age, typically birth to 3 years.

Gender   M = F.

Incidence   Rare.

Etiology   Initiating inflammatory process with maceration and secondary infection leads to a granulomatous response.

PATHOPHYSIOLOGY

Lesions believed to be a unique benign granulomatous response to a foreign body, inflammtion, maceration and/or secondary infection.

HISTORY

Lesions appear in the diaper area several months after treatment of inciting factors. The rash symptoms can range from being asymptomatic to very painful.

PHYSICAL EXAMINATION

Skin Findings

Type   Granulomatous papules and nodules (Fig. 3-5).

Color   Reddish-purple.

Size   0.5 to 4.0 cm in diameter.

Distribution   Groin, buttocks, lower aspect of abdomen, penis, rarely intertriginous areas of axillae, and/or neck.

DIFFERENTIAL DIAGNOSIS

The papular and nodular lesions of granuloma gluteale infantum can appear very worrisome despite their benign nature because nodular lesions can also be seen in sarcomatous and lymphomatous processes. Granulomas are found in Kaposi sarcoma, tuberculosis, syphilis, and deep fungal infections. The diagnosis of granuloma gluteale infantum is often made clinically and can be confirmed by skin biopsy.

LABORATORY EXAMINATIONS

Light and Electron Microscopy (EM)   Hyperplastic epidermis with inflammatory cells (mostly neutrophils), a parakeratotic stratum corneum, and a dense inflammatory infiltrate throughout the depth of the cutis with hemorrhage, neutrophils, lymphocytes, histiocytes, plasma cells, eosinophils, newly formed capillaries, and giant cells. Lesions of granuloma gluteale infantum lack the masses of patchy accumulations of lymphoma cells seen in lymphomatous disorders. Granuloma gluteale infantum may be differentiated from more severe granulomatous processes by its lack of fibrous proliferative features, spindle cell formations, and mitoses.

COURSE AND PROGNOSIS

Benign. Lesions resolve completely and spontaneously several months after treatment of the primary inciting inflammatory process and/or infection.

MANAGEMENT

Treatment begins with the identification and elimination of the primary inciting inflammatory process and/or infection.
For the nodular lesions:

1. If topical steroids are being used, discontinuing them often leads to resolution of the nodules.
2. Conversely, if topical steroids are not being used, a short 2-week trial of topical,

intralesional, or impregnated steroid tape (Cordran tape) may hasten resolution of these nodules. Close follow-up is necessary because steroids often worsen the condition.

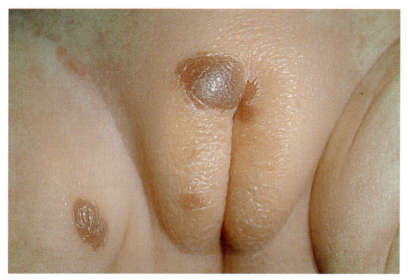

Figure 3-5   **Granuloma gluteale infantum**   *Nodular granulomatous response in the diaper area to topical steroids.*

HISTIOCYTOSIS X IN DIAPER AREA

Histiocytosis X is a rare disorder of the phagocyte system. Although the disease is rare, it frequently presents in infancy as a rash in the diaper area. Histiocytosis X should be considered if a diaper rash is particularly recalcitrant to usual remedies, especially if systemic symptoms are present.

EPIDEMIOLOGY

Age Usually in first year of life. Can be seen up to 3 years of age.

Gender F = M.

Incidence Extremely rare.

Etiology Unclear.

Genetics Possibly autosomal recessive with reduced penetrance.

PATHOPHYSIOLOGY

Unclear. Several proposed mechanisms include a disturbance of intracellular lipid metabolism, a reactive histiocytic response to infection, or a neoplastic process. All theories somehow implicate the Langerhans cell as a primary component.

PHYSICAL EXAMINATION

Skin Findings

Type Begins as erythema and scale and progresses to purpuric papules and nodules (Fig. 3-6).

Color Reddish-brown or purple.

Size Pinpoint to 1 cm.

Distribution Inguinal and perineal areas, axilla, behind ears and scalp.

General Findings

Decreased immunity and thus increased susceptibility to infections.

LABORATORY EXAMINATIONS

Dermatopathology Skin biopsy will reveal characteristic Langerhans cells, which are diagnostic of a histiocyte proliferative disorder. Langerhans cells can be identified with S-100 stains, which will be positive, or electron microscopy demonstration of Birbeck granules in the cytoplasm of the histiocytes.

DIFFERENTIAL DIAGNOSIS

The initial presentation of histiocytosis X is similar to seborrhea, with a red brown scaly rash, but histiocytosis X becomes more extensive cutaneously and can have associated systemic disease. A skin biopsy is usually needed to confirm the diagnosis.

COURSE AND PROGNOSIS

Histiocytosis X can have three clinical forms. The highest mortality rate is seen in the most severe form: Letterer–Siwe disease (associated with fever, anemia, thrombocytopenia, lymphadenopathy, hepatosplenomegaly, and skeletal tumors). Less severe clinical courses are seen with Hand–Schuller–Christian disease (associated with osteolytic defects, diabetes mellitus, and exophthalmos), and eosinophilic granuloma (associated with osteolytic defects and spontaneous fractures).

MANAGEMENT

The diagnosis of histiocytosis X is important to recognize when a sick infant appears with a refractory or recurrent diaper rash. The diagnosis should be entertained and confirmed by skin biopsy at an early age. Treatment with corticosteroids, immunosuppressive agents, and supportive measures may help the disease go into remission (see Section 19-1, "Langerhans Cell Histiocytosis" for more details).

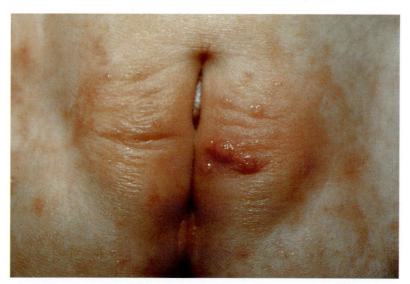

Figure 3-6 Histiocytosis X in the diaper area *Refractory diaper rash with scattered erythematous papules and a petechial component. Skin biopsy revealed Langerhans cells, diagnostic of histiocytosis X.*

SECTION 4

DISORDERS OF EPIDERMAL PROLIFERATION

PSORIASIS

Psoriasis is a hereditary disorder of skin characterized by chronic scaling papules and plaques in a characteristic distribution, largely at sites of repeated minor trauma. The HLA types most frequently associated with psoriasis are HLA-B13, -B17, -Bw16, -B37, and -Cw6.

EPIDEMIOLOGY

Age Before 20 years of age 37% of patients develop skin lesions, and 10% have onset of lesions before age 10.

Gender F > M, 2:1.

Prevalence Affects 1 to 3% of the population in western countries.

Race Low incidence in West Africans, American Indians, and Japanese.

Other Features Multifactorial inheritance. Minor trauma is a major factor (45% of patients) in eliciting lesions (Koebner's phenomenon). Infection also plays a major role. Many episodes of psoriasis follow sore throats or upper respiratory infections. Stress, cold weather, and lack of sunlight exposure aggravate the condition. Certain drugs (lithium, alcohol, chloroquine, corticosteroid withdrawal) can also precipitate psoriasis.

PATHOPHYSIOLOGY

In normal skin, the cells mature, shed, and are replaced every 3 to 4 weeks. In psoriasis, there is a defective inhibitor of epidermal cell proliferation with shortening of the cell cycle to 3 to 4 d. This leads to increased epidermal cell turnover with decreased shedding and the accumulation of dead cells appear clinically as stuck-on silvery-white scale.

HISTORY

Onset of Lesions Usually months but may be sudden as in acute guttate psoriasis and generalized pustular psoriasis (von Zumbusch).

Skin Symptoms Pruritus is reasonably common, especially in scalp and anogenital psoriasis.

Constitutional Symptoms In 5% of cases, psoriasis can be associated with arthritis, fever, and/or an "acute illness" syndrome (weakness, chills, fever) with generalized erythroderma.

PHYSICAL EXAMINATION

Skin Lesions

Type Well-delineated plaques with a characteristic silvery-white scale (Fig. 4-1A). Removal of scale results in the appearance of miniscule blood droplets (Auspitz phenomenon).

Color Salmon pink to red.

Shape Round, oval, polycyclic, or annular.

Arrangement Localized (e.g., elbows), regional (e.g., scalp), generalized (e.g., guttate psoriasis or erythroderma).

Distribution Bilateral, rarely symmetrical; predominantly in unexposed or traumatized areas.

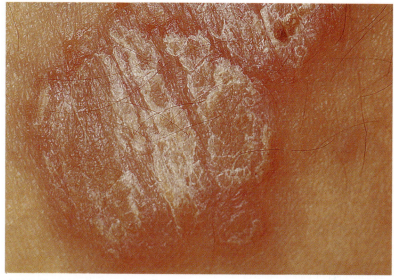

A

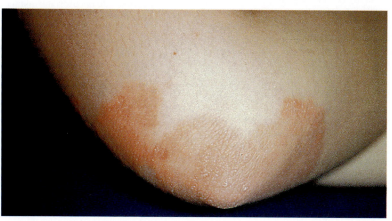

B

Figure 4-1   Psoriasis vulgaris, Koebner phenomenon   *(A) Well-delineated erythematous plaque with a silvery-white scale characterisitic of psoriasis. (B) Well-delineated erythematous plaque located on the elbow of a child with psoriasis.*

Sites of Predilection Favors elbows (Fig. 4-1B), knees, facial region, scalp, and intertriginous areas.

Other Scalp involvement is common (Fig. 4-1C). Hair loss (alopecia) is not a common feature even with severe scalp involvement. Fingernails and toenails are frequently (25%) involved. Nail changes include pitting (frequent but nonspecific), subungual hyperkeratosis, onycholysis (also nonspecific), and yellow spots under the nail plate "oil spot" (Fig. 4-1D).

General Findings

Psoriatic arthritis is rare before age 20 and the incidence is uncertain (estimated to be about 5%).
There are two types:

1. "Distal"—seronegative and without subcutaneous nodules, involving terminal interphalangeal joints of hands and feet.
2. Mutilating psoriatic arthritis with bone erosion, osteolysis, and, ultimately, ankylosis, especially involving the sacroiliac, hip, and cervical areas with ankylosing spondylitis. This type is seen especially in erythrodermic and pustular psoriasis and associated with HLA-B28.

DIFFERENTIAL DIAGNOSIS

Psoriasis may be confused with seborrheic dermatitis. The two entities may be indistinguishable and often an overlap, so-called sebopsoriasis presentation can be seen. Psoriasis must also be distinguished from atopic dermatitis, lichen simplex chronicus, pityriasis rosea, contact dermatitis, and psoriasiform drug eruptions (from beta-blockers, gold, and methyldopa).

LABORATORY EXAMINATIONS

Dermatopathology Skin biopsy reveals (1) epidermal hyperplasia with thinning of the suprapapillary plates and elongation of the rete ridges; (2) increased mitosis of keratinocytes, fibroblasts, and endothelial cells; (3) parakeratotic hyperkeratosis (nuclei retained in the stratum corneum); and (4) inflammatory cells in the dermis (usually lymphocytes and monocytes) and in the epidermis (polymorphonuclear cells), forming microabscesses of Munro in the stratum corneum.

Throat Culture Throat culture for beta-hemolytic streptococcus is indicated in cases of guttate psoriasis or in cases that are precipitated by a sore throat. If positive, antibiotic may be needed to clear both the infection and the psoriasis.

COURSE AND PROGNOSIS

Psoriasis typically has a chronic course with numerous remissions and exacerbations. Some children progress to mild disease with intermittent asymptomatic flares. Other children have a more severe course with recurrent extensive flares, and 5% may develop an associated arthritis in adulthood.

MANAGEMENT

The treatment of psoriasis depends upon the extent and severity of the disease, as well as the site involved. For all areas, patients should be instructed never to rub or scratch the areas since trauma can stimulate psoriatic plaques (Koebner's phenomenon).

1. Emollients such as petrolatum, mineral oil, vaseline, or moisturizers (Lubriderm, Eucerin, Moisturel, and Aquaphor creams) should be used to keep the skin well hydrated.
2. Sunlight exposure helps psoriasis (hence the refractory and recurrent nature of scalp psoriasis, which is covered by the hair), and children should be encouraged to expose the affected areas to the sun for short periods during the day. Sunscreen should be used, and sunburning should be avoided because it will aggravate psoriasis.
3. Baths are helpful in soothing the itching and removing the scale. They should be lukewarm and limited to 10 min in duration. For some, it may be helpful to add bath oil or tar (Balnetar, Robinol bath oil) to the water.
4. Tar preparations can be suggested to reduce the skin inflammation. Bath emulsions, creams (Elta tar) and ointments (MG217) can be used twice daily, but are not recommended for prolonged periods of time.
5. Topical steroid creams are effective if used in appropriate strengths:
   a. Low-potency steroids (Desowen, 1% or 2.5% hydrocortisone) can be used on the face and groin area, no more than bid × 2 weeks.

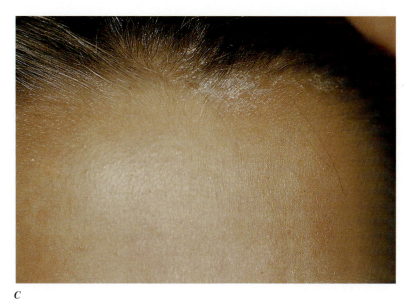

C

Figure 4-1 (continued)   Psoriasis vulgaris, scalp and nail findings   *(C) Diffuse erythema and scale in the scalp of a child with psoriasis. Hair loss is minimal.*

b. Medium-potency steroids (Elocon, Dermatop, Cutivate) can be used on the extremities or body no more than bid × 2 weeks.

c. Strong steroids (Ultravate, Psorcon, Diprolene) should be reserved for older children/adults on severely affected areas bid for no more than 2 weeks. (See page 48.)

6. Oral antibiotics are effective, especially in psoriasis flares precipitated by upper respiratory illnesses such as strep throat and subsequent guttate psoriasis. Oral antibiotics are also anti-inflammatory and can help if there are signs of infection—open moist areas that weep or become crusted. The most commonly prescibed antibiotics include Penicillin VK (25 to 50 mg/kg/d divided qid, not to exceed 3 g/d), Keflex (25 to 50 mg/kg/d divided qid, not to exceed 4 g/d), dicloxacillin (25 to 50 mg/kg/d divided qid, not to exceed 2 g/d), Duricef (30 mg/kg/d divided bid), and erythromycin (30 to 50 mg/kg/d divided qid, not to exceed 2 g/d).

7. Steroid-sparing topical creams include:
   a. Vitamin D analogs (Dovonex) typically used bid to affected areas. Can also be used in conjunction with topical steroids. Current recommendations suggest that Dovonex should be used bid to affected areas Monday through Friday and a topical steroid should be used bid Saturday and Sunday.

   b. Retinoids (Retin A, Tazorac) can be used qd to bid to affected areas. The retinoids typically help reduce the psoriatic scale, but often are too irritating for use in younger children.

   c. Anthralin (Drithrocreme) can be used qd to affected areas, but often is too irritating for use in younger children.

8. In severe refractory cases, UVB light treatments may be necessary.

9. For the scalp, tar (T-gel) selenium sulfide (Selsun), zinc pyrithione (Head & Shoulders), or ketoconazole (Nizoral) shampoos used 2 or 3 × week can help reduce scaling. Topical steroid solutions (Cormax scalp solution) can be applied qAM sparingly to the affected areas to help decrease erythema and itching.

10. Other treatments include intralesional steroids, oral steroids, PUVA, methotrexate, cyclosporin, and oral retinoids, all of which are not generally recommended for children.

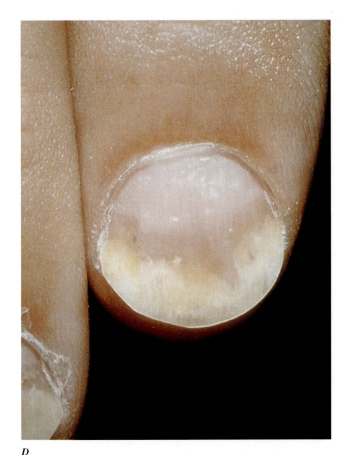

D

Figure 4-1 (continued)   Psoriasis vulgaris, scalp and nail findings   *(D) Pinpoint pits and distal ony-cholysis (so-called "oil-spot" discoloration) seen in the fingernails of a child with psoriasis.*

PSORIASIS VULGARIS, GUTTATE TYPE

This type of psoriasis, which is relatively rare (less than 2.0% of all psoriasis), is like an exanthem: a shower of lesions appearing rather rapidly in children and often following streptococcal pharyngitis. Guttate psoriasis may, however, be chronic and unrelated to streptococcal infection.

PHYSICAL EXAMINATION

Skin Lesions

Type   Papules 2.0 mm to 1.0 cm.

Color   Salmon pink.

Shape   Guttate (Latin, "spots that resemble drops").

Arrangement   Scattered discrete lesions (Fig. 4-2).

Distribution   Generalized, usually sparing the palms and soles and concentrating on the trunk, less on the face, scalp, and nails.

DIFFERENTIAL DIAGNOSIS

Guttate psoriasis needs to be differentiated from pityriasis rosea, a viral exanthem, a psoriasiform drug eruption, and secondary syphilis.

LABORATORY EXAMINATION

Serologic   Increased antistreptolysin titer in those patients with antecedent streptococcal infection.

Throat culture   May be positive for beta-hemolytic streptococcus A.

COURSE AND PROGNOSIS

Often, but not always, this type of psoriasis spontaneously disappears in a few weeks, especially with antibiotic treatment.

MANAGEMENT

The resolution of lesions can be accelerated by judicious exposure to sunlight. For persistent lesions, treatment same as for generalized plaque psoriasis. Penicillin VK (25 to 50 mg/kg/d divided qid, not to exceed 3 g/d) if group A beta-hemolytic streptococcus is cultured from throat.

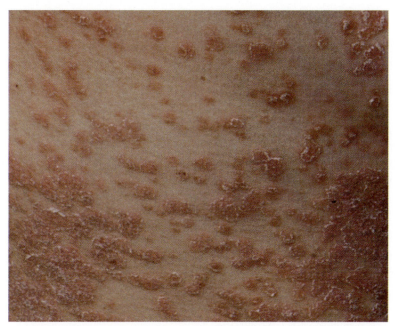

Figure 4-2 Psoriasis vulgaris, guttate type *Erythematous scaling papules coalescing into plaques on the trunk of a child after streptococcal pharyngitis.* (Reproduced with permission from TB Fitzpatrick et al., Color Atlas and Synopsis of Clinical Dermatology, 3rd edition. New York: McGraw-Hill, 1997).

PALMOPLANTAR PUSTULOSIS

Palmoplantar pustulosis is a rare, relapsing eruption limited to the palms and the soles characterized by numerous yellow, deep-seated pustules that evolve into crusts and scales.

PHYSICAL EXAMINATION

Skin Lesions

Type Pustules that evolve into crusts and scaling.

Color Dusky red base, yellow pustules.

Size 2 to 5 mm.

Distribution Localized to palms (Fig. 4-3A) and soles (Fig. 4-3B).

DIFFERENTIAL DIAGNOSIS

Palmoplantar pustulosis needs to be differentiated from tinea manuum, tinea pedis, dyshydrotic eczema, or a contact dermatitis.

LABORATORY EXAMINATION

Dermatopathology Skin biopsy would reveal edema and exocytosis of mononuclear cells forming a vesicle. Later neutrophils form a pustule.

COURSE AND PROGNOSIS

Palmoplantar pustulosis can recur for years and is difficult to treat. Rarely, psoriasis vulgaris may develop elsewhere.

MANAGEMENT

The resolution of lesions can be accelerated by judicious exposure to sunlight. Steroids under occlusion at night can hasten resolution.

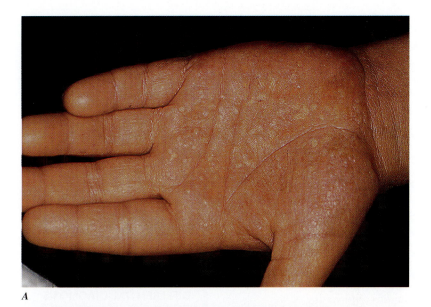

A

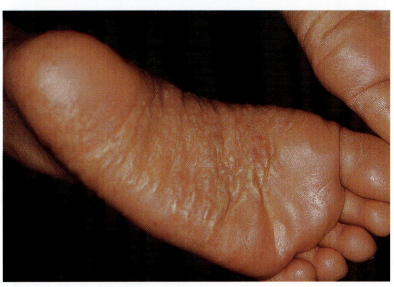

B

Figure 4-3   Palmoplantar pustulosis, palms and soles   *(A) Deep-seated yellow vesicles on the palms which progress to crusts and scales. (B) The soles of the same individual with similar deep-seated pustular lesions.*

PSORIASIS VULGARIS, ERYTHRODERMIC

Erythrodermic psoriasis is a serious, often life-threatening condition in patients with psoriasis, characterized by full-body erythroderma and scaling. A preexisting dermatosis can be identified in 50% of patients and psoriasis is the second most common cause of erythroderma after atopic dermatitis.

Synonyms   Dermatitis exfoliativa, erythroderma of Wilson – Brocq.

EPIDEMIOLOGY

Age   Any age.

Gender   M > F.

Incidence   Rare.

Etiology   In childhood, erythroderma is more likely due to preexisting dermatitis such as atopic dermatitis or psoriasis.

Classification   Acute phase with generalized scaly erythema with fever, lymphadenopathy. Chronic form characterized by nail dystrophy but no loss of scalp and body hair (compared to other forms of erythroderma, e.g., drugs, mycosis fungoides).

HISTORY

Duration of Lesions   Acute onset of systemic symptoms and red swollen patches that evolve into a widespread exfoliative erythema in the setting of previous psoriasis.

Skin Symptoms   Generalized pruritus.

Generalized Symptoms   Chills, malaise, fatigue, anorexia, weight loss.

PHYSICAL EXAMINATION

Skin Findings

Type of Lesions   Confluent diffuse erythema covered by laminated scales. Skin becomes dull, scarlet, swollen, with areas of oozing (Fig. 4-4). Desquamation usually occurs after a few days. The palms and soles are covered by thick scales and have deep fissures. Secondary infections by bacteria can develop.

Color   Bright red.

Arrangement   Confluent.

Distribution   Generalized.

Hair   Normal.

Nails   Onycholysis, shedding of nails with dystrophy.

General Findings

Generalized lymphadenopathy.

DIAGNOSIS AND DIFFERENTIAL DIAGNOSIS

Diagnosis   Clinical diagnosis of psoriatic erythroderma is not always easy, especially in the absence of previous history of psoriasis. Cutaneous signs of psoriasis are helpful, such as pitting of the nails, psoriasiform plaques on the scalp, or intergluteal erythema.

Differential Diagnosis   Other causes of erythroderma include pityriasis rubra pilaris, seborrheic dermatitis, drug hypersensitivity, atopic dermatitis, cutaneous T-cell lymphoma, lichen planus, pemphigus foliaceus, epidermolytic hyperkeratosis, and acute graft-versus-host disease.

LABORATORY EXAMINATIONS

Hematology   Elevated sedimentation rate.

Chemistry   Low serum albumin and increased gammaglobulins.

Microbiology   Blood cultures will be negative (usually obtained to rule out infection in the setting of high fever).

Dermatopathology   Psoriasiform dermatitis with elongated and thickened ridges, marked parakeratosis, absent granular layer, intra- and intercellular edema, epidermal invasion by leukocytes, and a dermal perivascular inflammatory infiltrate.

COURSE AND PROGNOSIS

Variable. Can be very prolonged and recurrent.

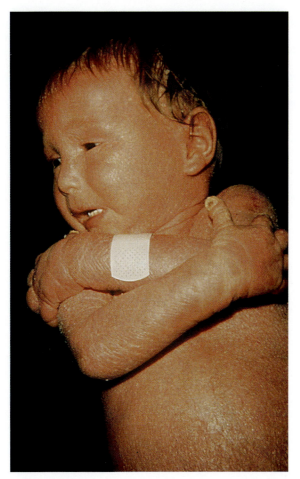

Figure 4-4   Psoriasis vulgaris: erythrodermic   *Entire skin surface is dull-red in color with diffuse swelling and oozing.*

MANAGEMENT

Supportive care often requiring hospitalization is necessary to maintain fluid–electrolyte homeostasis and body temperature. Skin biopsy should be performed if the cause of the erythroderma is not known (no known predisposition to psoriasis). Topical treatment includes emollients and steroids under wraps. Systemic steroids, retinoids, or immunosuppressives (methotrexate or cyclosporin) may be necessary. In older children, light treatment with PUVA or UVB may be pursued.

ICHTHYOSIFORM DERMATOSES

The ichthyosiform dermatoses are a group of hereditary disorders, characterized by an excess accumulation of cutaneous scale. The clinical severity varies from very mild and asymptomatic to life-threatening.

CLASSIFICATION

Ichthyosis vulgaris: Autosomal dominant.
X-linked ichthyosis (XLI): Recessive X-linked, only expressed in males.
Epidermolytic hyperkeratosis: Autosomal dominant.
Lamellar ichthyosis (LI): Autosomal recessive.

PATHOPHYSIOLOGY

Lamellar ichthyosis shows increased germinative cell hyperplasia and increased transit rate through the epidermis. In ichthyosis vulgaris and X-linked ichthyosis, the formation of thickened stratum corneum is caused by increased adhesiveness of the stratum corneum cells and/or failure of normal cell–cell separation. Epidermolytic hyperkeratosis shows increased epidermal cell turnover with vacuolization (due to intracellular edema).

HISTORY

All types of ichthyosis tend to be worse during the dry, cold winter months and improve during the hot, humid summer. Patients living in tropical climates may remain symptom free, but may experience symptomatic appearance or worsening on moving to a more temperate climate.

DIAGNOSIS

Usually can be made based on clinical findings.

MANAGEMENT

Hydration of Stratum Corneum   Pliability of stratum corneum is a function of its water content. Hydration is best accomplished by immersion in bath followed by the application of petrolatum (vaseline petoleum jelly, hydrated petrolatum, or Aquaphor).

Keratolytic Agents   Propylene glycol with lactic acid (Epilyt) is effective without occlusion. Combinations of salicylic acid and propylene glycol (Keralyt) can be used alone or under plastic occlusion. Alpha-hydroxy acids such as lactic acid bind water or control scaling. Urea-containing preparations (2 to 20%) (Aquacare, Carmol) help to bind water in the stratum corneum. Lac-hydrin contains buffered lactic acid.

Systemic Retinoids   Retinoids such as isotretinoin (Accutane) and acitretin (Psoriatane) are reserved for severe cases of lamellar ichthyosis, but careful monitoring for toxicity is required. Severe cases may require intermittent therapy over long periods of time. Continuous long-term use in children is contraindicated.

COLLODION BABY

Ichthyosis in the newborn often presents as a collodion baby (Fig. 4-5A). The newborn is encased in a clear, parchment-like membrane, which impairs respiration and sucking. When the membrane is shed 2 to 3 weeks later, the infant may have difficulties with thermal regulation and an increased susceptibility to infections. After healing the skin will appear normal (Fig. 4-5B). Sixty to 70% of these babies will go on to develop some form of ichthyosis later in life.

EPIDEMIOLOGY

Age   Newborn.

Gender   M = F.

Incidence   Rare.

Etiology   Unclear.

HISTORY

Onset   Membrane is present at birth.

Duration of Lesions   Desquamation of the membrane is usually complete by 2 to 3 weeks of life.

PHYSICAL EXAMINATION

Skin Findings

Type   Transparent, parchment-like membrane encasing the newborn.

Color   Clear.

Distribution   Membrane covers the entire body surface.

General Findings

Impaired respiration, sucking, and mobility due to thick membrane encasement present at birth. Temperature and fluid–electrolyte instability when membrane sheds.

DIFFERENTIAL DIAGNOSIS

Clinical findings are diagnostic. A collodion baby needs to be clinically differentiated from a harlequin fetus: a more severe, usually lethal condition. The skin in a harlequin fetus has a thickened stratum corneum with deep cracks and fissures (see Fig. 4-6).

COURSE AND PROGNOSIS

The collodion membrane breaks up and peels during the first 2 weeks of life predisposing the infant to difficulties in thermal regulation and an increased risk of infection. The final appearance of the skin depends on the etiology of the condition. In 60% of cases, the collodion baby may be the initial presentation of lamellar ichthyosis or some rare ichthyosiform syndromes such as Netherton's or Conradi's that ultimately manifest neurologic, metabolic, orthopedic, otologic, and ocular symptoms.

MANAGEMENT

The management and treatment of the collodion baby are primarily supportive. Collodion babies require hospitalization and incubation at birth. The infant should be kept in a high-humidity environment to maximize membrane hydration and pliability. Clear fluids or IV hydration may be needed until the infant's ability to eat has been ascertained. Respiratory efforts may also need external support. As the membrane begins to shed 2 to 3 weeks later, the infant should be frequently monitored for temperature, and electrolyte instability. Throughout the molting process, careful monitoring for skin and lung infections is also recommended.

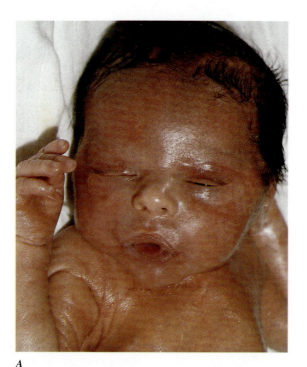

A

Figure 4-5   Collodion baby at birth   (*A*) *A baby soon after birth with a clear parchment-like membrane covering the entire skin.* (Reprinted with permission from TB Fitzpatrick et al., Color Atlas and Synopsis of Clinical Dermatology, 4th edition. New York: McGraw-Hill, 2001).

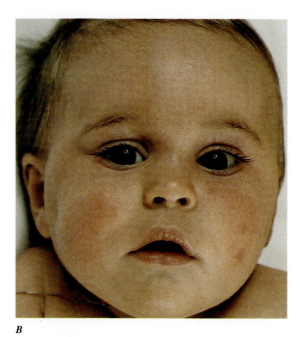

B

Figure 4-5 (continued)   Collodion baby at 6 months old   (*B*) *The skin of the same infant at age 6 months is entirely normal.* (Reprinted with permission from TB Fitzpatrick et al., Color Atlas and Synopsis of Clinical Dermatology, 4th edition. New York: McGraw-Hill, 2001).

HARLEQUIN FETUS

A harlequin fetus is a rare, severe form of congenital ichthyosis. The severe skin findings at birth correlate with a poor prognosis.

EPIDEMIOLOGY

Age   Newborn.

Gender   M = F.

Incidence   Fewer than 100 case reports.

Etiology   Defective keratin and possibly presence of an abnormal fibrous protein.

Genetics   Possibly autosomal recessive.

PATHOPHYSIOLOGY

The stratum corneum exhibits excess cross-B-fibrous protein and a defect in lipid metabolism is postulated.

HISTORY

Onset   Thickened fissured skin is present at birth and is permanent.

Skin Symptoms   Skin is rigid.

PHYSICAL EXAMINATION

Skin Findings

Type   Polygonal/triangular/diamond-shaped plaques due to skin fissuring.

Color   Red/brown skin with gray/yellow cracked scale.

Distribution   Whole-body is involved with a marked ectropion (turning out of the eyelids), eclabium (fish-mouth deformity), and distorted flat ears (Fig. 4-6).

General Findings

Most infants are stillborn or die in the neonatal period. Newborns exhibit poor feeding and difficulties with temperature and electrolyte regulation. The rigidity of the skin impairs movement.

DIFFERENTIAL DIAGNOSIS

The clinical presentation of a harlequin fetus is diagnostic. It should be differentiated from the less severe form of congenital ichthyosis—a collodion baby.

LABORATORY EXAMINATIONS

Histopathology   Skin biopsy reveals hyperkeratosis, absent granular layer, plugged sweat ducts, and sebaceous follicles filled with hyperkeratotic debris.

COURSE AND PROGNOSIS

The course and prognosis for a harlequin fetus is very poor. Most infants die early of prematurity, infection, or thermal or electrolyte imbalance.

MANAGEMENT

Intensive supportive measures and systemic isotretinoin (Accutane) and acetretin (Psoriatane) can increase survival, but the harlequin skin is permanent and the resultant quality of life is poor.

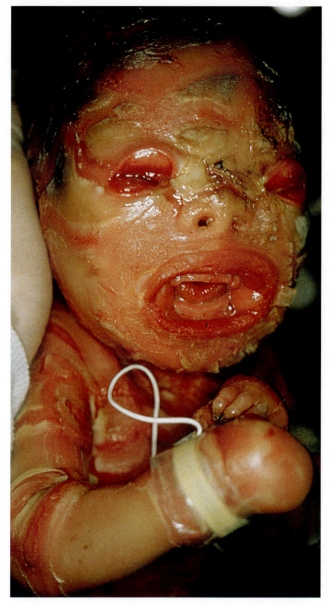

Figure 4-6 Harlequin fetus *Newborn with rigid skin, marked ectropion, fishmouth deformity, and distorted flat ears.*

ICHTHYOSIS VULGARIS

Ichthyosis vulgaris (IV) is characterized by mild generalized hyperkeratosis with xerosis (dry skin) most pronounced on the lower legs. It is frequently associated with atopy.

EPIDEMIOLOGY

Age of Onset   Childhood.

Gender   M = F.

Mode of Inheritance   Autosomal dominant.

Incidence   Common, 1/300 people.

Etiology   Reduction in cellular component, filaggrin, results in decreased hydration of the stratum corneum.

HISTORY

Very commonly associated with atopy (atopic dermatitis, allergies, hay fever, asthma). Xerosis and pruritus worse in winter months. Hyperkeratosis and less commonly xerosis are of cosmetic concern to many patients.

PHYSICAL EXAMINATION

Skin Findings

Type   Xerosis (dry skin) with fine powdery scale (Fig. 4-7). Increased accentuation of the palmar and plantar creases.

Color   Normal skin color, white powdery scale.

Distribution   Diffuse involvement, accentuated on the shins, arms, and back, but sparing the body folds (axillae, antecubital and popliteal fossae); face is also usually spared.

General Findings

Ichthyosis vulgaris may be seen with other signs of atopy: atopic dermatitis, asthma, allergies, hay fever, and keratosis pilaris.

DIFFERENTIAL DIAGNOSIS

Ichthyosis vulgaris needs to be differentiated from X-linked ichthyosis, lamellar ichthyrosis and drug-induced ichthyoses.

LABORATORY EXAMINATIONS

Dermatopathology   Hyperkeratosis with a thickened stratum corneum; reduced or absent granular layer.

COURSE AND PROGNOSIS

May show improvement in the summer and in adulthood.

MANAGEMENT

1. Emollients such as petrolatum, mineral oil, vaseline, or moisturizers (Lubriderm, Eucerin, Moisturel, and Aquaphor creams) should be used to keep the skin well hydrated.
2. Keratolytic agents such as Epilyt, Keralyt, Lac-Hydrin, and Carmol can be used bid to the affected areas to help exfoliate the diffuse scale, but should be avoided in young children because the stinging sensation is usually not well tolerated. The face and groin areas should also be avoided.

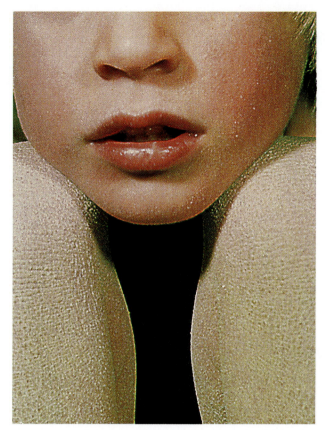

Figure 4-7 Ichthyosis vulgaris *Fine powdery scale on the shins of a child with ichthyosis vulgaris. The face is spared.*

X-LINKED ICHTHYOSIS

X-linked ichthyosis occurs in males and is characterized by prominent dirty brown scales occurring on the face, back, and extensor surfaces with onset soon after birth. Female carriers may exhibit mild skin findings.

Synonym   Ichthyosis nigricans.

EPIDEMIOLOGY

Age of Onset   Usually appears in the first 3 to 12 months of life.

Gender   Males only. Female carriers may exhibit partial abnormalities.

Incidence   1/6000 males.

Mode of Inheritance   X-linked recessive. Gene has been cloned; prenatal diagnosis is possible.

Genetic Defect   Steroid sulfatase deficiency.

PATHOPHYSIOLOGY

X-linked ichthyosis is caused by a deficiency of steroid sulfatase, which leads to an increased accumulation of cholesterol sulfate. This, in turns, leads to increased cellular adhesion and clinically apparent hyperkeratosis.

HISTORY

In addition to the discomfort due to xerosis, the dirty brown scales on the neck, ears, scalp, and arms are a major cosmetic disfigurement, causing the patient to appear "dirty" all the time.

PHYSICAL EXAMINATION

Skin Findings

Type   Large firmly adherent scales separated by zones of normal-appearing skin gives the area a cracked appearance (Fig. 4-8).

Color   Scales are light to dark brown.

Shape   Fish-scale pattern.

Distribution   Lateral neck, back, upper arms, chest and abdomen; prominent scalp scaling may occur. Palms and soles are normal.

General Findings

During the second or third decades, deep corneal opacities develop in almost all individuals with X-linked ichthyosis. These opacities may also be present in female carriers but are asymptomatic.

LABORATORY EXAMINATIONS

Dermatopathology   Skin biopsy will show hyperkeratosis with a moderately increased stratum corneum and a granular layer present in contrast to ichthyosis vulgaris.

Laboratory Findings   High levels of cholesterol sulfate can be measured in the serum, stratum corneum, or nails.

COURSE AND PROGNOSIS

X-linked ichthyosis is chronic and persistent but may wax and wane with the seasonal variation in humidity. The skin findings do not cause physical limitations, but can be cosmetically distressing.

MANAGEMENT

1. Emollients such as petrolatum, mineral oil, vaseline, or moisturizers (Lubriderm, Eucerin, Moisturel, and Aquaphor creams) should be used to keep the skin well hydrated.
2. Keratolytic agents such as Epilyt, Keralyt, Lac-Hydrin, and Carmol can be used bid to the affected areas to help exfoliate the diffuse scale, but should be avoided in young children because the stinging sensation is usually not well tolerated. The face and groin areas should also be avoided.

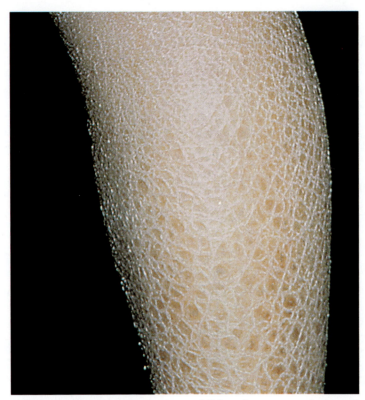

Figure 4-8 **X-linked ichthyosis** *More pronounced fish-scale pattern on the legs of a child with X-linked ichthyosis. The diffuse brown scale gives the child a "dirty" appearance.*

EPIDERMOLYTIC HYPERKERATOSIS

Epidermolytic hyperkeratosis is an autosomal dominant disorder that initially presents with blistering. Gradually the skin changes to a more diffuse, hyperkeratotic, almost verrucous appearance. Two forms have been described: (1) Brocq (most common) and (2) Siemens; they are not easy to separate by clinical criteria.

Synonym   Bullous congenital ichthyosiform erythroderma.

EPIDEMIOLOGY

Onset   The disease is present at or shortly after birth.

Gender   M = F.

Prevalence   1/300,000.

Etiology   Genetic mutation of keratin 1, 10, or 2e.

Inheritance   The disease has a autosomal dominant inheritance, but 50% of patients exhibit new mutations.

PATHOPHYSIOLOGY

Mutations in keratins 1 and 10 have been found in a number of families of the Brocq type, while mutations of keratin 2e have been found in the Siemens type. These are responsible for filament aggregation and the genetic mutations result in skin blistering.

HISTORY

The major complaint early in life is blistering, which is painful and can cause widespread denudation. Later the hyperkeratosis is a problem because of the disfigurement, malodor from secondary infection, and discomfort from limitation of motion.

PHYSICAL EXAMINATION

Skin Findings

Type   Early flaccid blisters (Fig. 4-9A) can lead to large denuded areas. Later there is erythematous hyperkeratosis with verrucous plaques.

Color   Early, skin is red color (Fig. 4-9B). Later, skin is brown or black.

Distribution   All surfaces of the body can be involved, and flexural areas are accentuated.

General Findings

Hair, nails, and teeth are normal.

DIFFERENTIAL DIAGNOSIS

The clinical appearance may be confused with lamellar ichthyosis but the pathology is usually diagnostic.

LABORATORY EXAMINATIONS

Skin biopsy reveals hyperkeratosis and vacuolar degeneration of the upper epidermis, which can lead to cell lysis. Electron microscopy reveals clumping of the tonofilaments.

COURSE AND PROGNOSIS

The blistering ceases during the second decade, but hyperkeratosis persists for life.

MANAGEMENT

1. Keratolytic agents can be used bid to the affected areas to help exfoliate the diffuse scale, but should be avoided in young children because the stinging sensation is usually not well tolerated. The face and groin areas should also be avoided.
2. Systemic retinoids such as isotretinoin (Accutane) and acitretin (Psoriatane) are useful in controlling the hyperkeratosis, but they may cause flares of the blistering. The side effects of the drugs on bones and tendons are a concern and long-term use is not recommended.

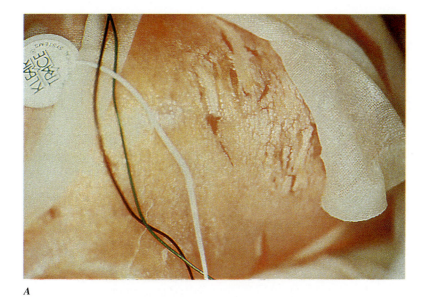

A

B

Figure 4-9   Epidermolytic hyperkeratosis   *(A) Born with diffuse flaccid blistering of the skin later diagnosed to have epidermolytic hyperkeratosis. (B) Extensive verrucous brown plaques in a child with epidermolytic hyperkeratosis.*

LAMELLAR ICHTHYOSIS

Lamellar ichthyosis often presents at birth with the infant encased in a collodion-like membrane (see Collodion baby, Fig. 4-5A), which is soon shed with subsequent formation of large, coarse scales involving all flexural areas as well as palms and soles. It can be divided into two categories: (1) classic lamellar ichthyosis (LI, the more severe form), or (2) congenital ichthyosiform erythroderma (CIE, the more mild form).

Synonym   Nonbullous congenital ichthyosiform erythroderma.

EPIDEMIOLOGY

Age of Onset   A collodion baby at birth is usually the initial presentation (see Fig. 4-5A). In some cases, the disease is not evident until 3 months of age.

Gender   M = F.

Incidence   Classic LI: 1/200,000. CIE: 1/100,000.

Mode of Inheritance   Autosomal recessive.

PATHOPHYSIOLOGY

Mutation of transglutaminase has been found in a number of patients, but at least two other genetic loci have been identified.

HISTORY

Lamellar ichthyosis typically presents at birth as a collodion baby. After 2 to 3 weeks the collodion membrane is shed and replaced by large gray scales. During exercise and hot weather, high fevers may occur due to a decreased ability to sweat. Fissuring of stratum corneum may result in excess water loss and dehydration. Young children have increased nutritional requirements due to excessive shedding of stratum corneum. Fissures on hands and feet are painful.

PHYSICAL EXAMINATION

Skin Lesions

Type   At birth, infant typically presents as a collodion baby, encased in a collodion-like membrane, which is shed in 2 to 3 weeks. Subsequently, large parchment-like scales develop over the entire body (Fig. 4-10A and B). Scales are large and very thick. Fissuring of hands and feet is common.

Distribution   Generalized.   Hyperkeratosis around joints may be verrucous. Involvement of eyelids results in ectropion (eyelids are turned outward).

Hair and Nails   Hair bound down by scales; frequent infections result in scarring alopecia. Nails show ridges and grooves.

Mucous Membranes   Usually spared.

General Findings

Hyperkeratosis results in obstruction of eccrine sweat glands with resultant impairment of sweating. Patient is at an increased risk of overheating and also infections.

LABORATORY EXAMINATIONS

Dermatopathology   Skin biopsy shows hyperkeratosis, patchy parakeratosis, increased granular layer (in contrast to ichthyosis vulgaris), acanthosis, and papillomatosis.

COURSE AND PROGNOSIS

For lamellar ichthyosis, the collodion membrane present at birth is shed. However, plate-like diffuse scales persist throughout life and there is no improvement with age. For congenital ichthyosiform erythroderma, the course is more mild and the patient is more erythrodermic than scaly.

DISORDERS OF EPIDERMAL PROLIFERATION

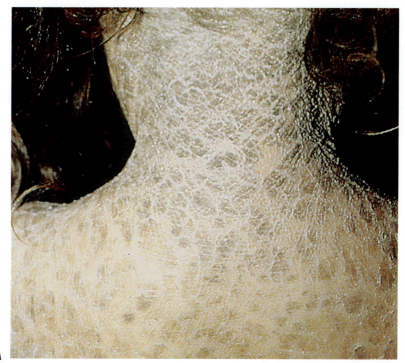

A

Figure 4-10   Lamellar ichthyosis   *(A) Plate-like scale on the posterior neck of a child with lamellar ichthyosis.*

MANAGEMENT

Patients with lamellar ichthyosis should avoid situations that may lead to overheating. Their skin appearance can be improved with:

1. Keratolytic agents such as Epilyt, Keralyt, Lac-Hydrin, and Carmol can be used bid to the affected areas to help exfoliate the diffuse scale. In young children, they may cause a stinging sensation and only emollients can be used. The face and groin areas should also be avoided.

2. Systemic retinoids such as isotretinoin (Accutane) and acitretin (Psoriatane) are useful in controlling the hyperkeratosis. The side effects of the retinoids on bones and tendons are a concern and long-term use is not recommended.

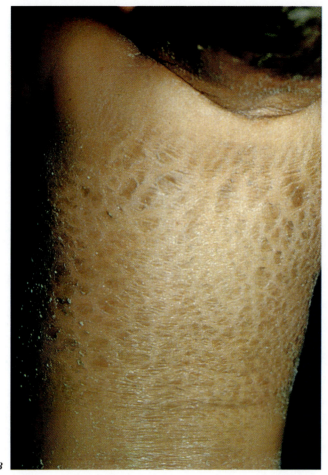

B

Figure 4-10 (continued)   Lamellar ichthyosis   (B) *The back of the same child with lamellar ichthyosis.*

OTHER

KERATOSIS PILARIS

Keratosis pilaris (KP) is a common benign skin condition characterized by follicular-based hyperkeratosis most prominent on the lateral upper arms and thighs. It is commonly seen in individuals with a personal or family history of atopy.

EPIDEMIOLOGY

Age Appears in early childhood.

Gender M = F.

Incidence Common.

Etiology Abnormal follicular cornification.

Genetics Autosomal dominant inheritance.

Season Worse during cold seasons.

PHYSICAL EXAMINATION

Skin Findings

Type of Lesion Discrete follicular papules often with superimposed keratotic plug (Fig. 4-11A).

Color Red or brown.

Distribution Lesions are prominent on the outer aspects of upper arms and thighs.

Palpation Skin has a rough texture reminiscent of gooseflesh or plucked chicken skin.

General Findings

Often associated with other signs of atopy: atopic dermatitis, asthma, allergies, hay fever, or ichthyosis vulgaris.

DIFFERENTIAL DIAGNOSIS

The diagnosis of keratosis pilaris is made clinically. KP is common, but there are rare KP-like variants:

1. Ulerythema ophryogenes (keratosis pilaris atrophicans faciei). X-linked condition notable for widespread KP that begins with follicular-based keratotic papules on the lateral eyebrows that resolve with depressed pits and alopecia.
2. Keratosis rubra faciei. Similar to ulerythema ophryogenes, except that the le-

sions begin on the cheeks and temples (Fig. 4-11B).
3. Atrophoderma vermiculata (folliculitis ulerythema reticulata). Characterized by symmetric atrophic pits on the cheeks, forehead, and eyebrows.

LABORATORY EXAMINATIONS

Dermatopathology Skin biopsy reveals follicular hyperkeratosis and a sparse inflammatory infiltrate in the dermis.

COURSE AND PROGNOSIS

Keratosis pilaris is benign but persistent and chronic. Occasionally it subsides after the age of 20 years. Patients are most distressed by its rough texture and cosmetic appearance.

MANAGEMENT

1. Emollients such as petrolatum, mineral oil, vaseline, or moisturizers (Lubriderm, Eucerin, Moisturel, and Aquaphor creams) should be used to keep the skin well hydrated.
2. Keratolytic agents such as Epilyt, Keralyt, Lac-Hydrin, and Carmol can be used bid to the affected areas to help exfoliate the diffuse scale, but should be avoided in young children because the stinging sensation is usually not well tolerated. The face and groin areas should also be avoided.
3. Topical steroid creams can be used intermittently to decrease the erythematous appearance of the rash:
   a. Low-potency steroids (Desowen, 1% or 2.5% hydrocortisone) can be used on the face or body no more than bid × 2 weeks.
   b. Medium-potency steroids (Elocon, Dermatop, Cutivate) can be used on the extremities or body no more than bid × 2 weeks. (See page 48).

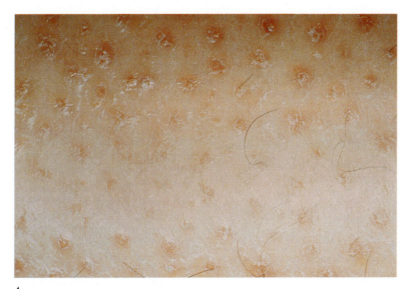

A

Figure 4-11 Keratosis pilaris *(A) Erythematous follicular-based papules with keratotis plugs on the shin of an adolescent.*

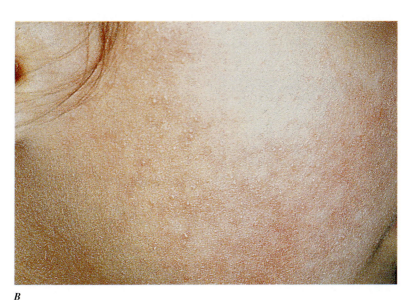

B

Figure 4-11 (continued) Keratosis rubra faciei *(B) Follicular-based erythematous papules on the cheek of a child.*

POROKERATOSIS OF MIBELLI

Porokeratosis of Mibelli is an uncommon skin disorder characterized by scattered erythematous patches with a characteristic double-edged scale for a border.

EPIDEMIOLOGY

Age   Onset may be in childhood, more common in adolescence or adulthood.

Gender   M > F, 2:1.

Incidence   Uncommon.

Genetics   Autosomal dominant inheritance.

Etiology   May be inherited or secondary to immunosuppression (chemotherapy or immunosuppressed transplant patients)

PATHOPHYSIOLOGY

It has been hypothetized that porokeratosis is caused by an abnormal clone of keratinocytes with disordered metabolism and/or an increased growth rate.

PHYSICAL EXAMINATION

Skin Findings

Type of Lesion   Keratotic papule that spreads centifugally, and forms a plaque with an atrophic, center and a serpiginous hyperkeratotic ridge (Fig. 4-12).

Color   Skin-colored.

Shape   Annular, oval, or irregular.

Distribution   Predominantly on the dorsal aspects of hands and fingers, ankles and feet. They can also involve the face and scalp (resulting in bald patches), oral and genital mucosa, and nail matrix (causing dystrophic changes).

DIAGNOSIS AND DIFFERENTIAL DIAGNOSIS

Diagnosis   Based on clinical and histopathological findings.

Variants of porokeratosis include disseminated superficial actinic porokeratoses (seen on the shins of older people), porokeratosis palmaris et plantaris disseminata, and linear porokeratosis.

Differential Diagnosis   Porokeratosis needs to be differentiated from tinea corporis, granuloma annulare, annular erythemas, lichen planus, lichen sclerosus et atrophicans, and morphea.

LABORATORY EXAMINATIONS

Dermatopathology   Skin biopsy of the double-edged periphery showing hyperkeratosis, parakeratosis, and invagination of epidermis containing a thick column of keratin (cornoid lamellae) is pathognomonic for porokeratosis.

COURSE AND PROGNOSIS

Lesions of porokeratosis are chronic and persistent. In adulthood, occasional malignant degeneration into squamous cell or basal cell carcinoma has been reported (especially in the linear type).

MANAGEMENT

Lesions are usually treated to avoid possibility of malignant degeneration. Lesions can be excised or destroyed with topical 5-FU cream, cryotherapy, or CO_2 laser treatment.

DISORDERS OF EPIDERMAL PROLIFERATION

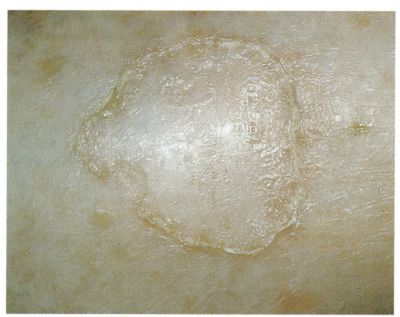

Figure 4-12   Porokeratosis of Mibelli   *Plaque on the shin with a characteristic serpiginous hyperkeratotic ridge.*

PITYRIASIS RUBRA PILARIS

Pityriasis rubra pilaris (PRP) is a chronic disease characterized by follicular papules, yellow to pink scaly plaques, and a palmoplantar keratoderma.

EPIDEMIOLOGY

Classification   (1) Familial, an autosomal disorder presenting at birth or with onset during infancy or childhood, and (2) Acquired type, seen in individuals older than 15 years old.

Gender   M = F.

Incidence   Uncommon.

PATHOPHYSIOLOGY

Inherited abnormal cornification of unclear pathogenesis.

HISTORY

Skin Symptoms   Mild to moderate pruritus. Pain in areas of fissured skin.

PHYSICAL EXAMINATION

Skin Findings

Scaling of the scalp and erythema of the face and ears (often initial sign). Punctate firm, keratotic, reddish-brown papules with central keratotic plug. Symmetric and diffuse orange or salmon-colored psoriasiform plaques with characteristic islands of normal skin (Fig. 4-13). Thickened hyperkeratotic palms and soles (forming "sandal"). Nail dystrophy (thickening, opacification, subungual hyperkeratosis; pitting not common).

Distribution   Psoriasiform plaques on the trunk and extremities. Punctate keratoses on the dorsal aspects of first and second phalanges, hands, wrists, knees, ankles, feet, sides of neck, and trunk.

General Findings

Disease can rarely progress into an exfoliative erythroderma associated with fever, chill, malaise, and diarrhea.

DIFFERENTIAL DIAGNOSIS

The diagnosis of PRP is made clinically, but often confirmed by skin biopsy. The differential diagnosis includes psoriaisis, lichen planus, lichen nitidis, atopic dermatitis, and viral exanthem.

LABORATORY EXAMINATIONS

Dermatopathology   Skin biopsy reveals psoriasiform hyperplasia, follicular plugging, parakeratosis at the follicular orifice, and a mononuclear cell infiltrate in the dermis.

COURSE AND PROGNOSIS

Childhood PRP has a persistent course characterized by spontaneous remissions and exacerbations.

MANAGEMENT

1. Emollients such as petrolatum, mineral oil, vaseline, or moisturizers (Lubriderm, Eucerin, Moisturel, and Aquaphor creams) should be used to keep the skin well hydrated.
2. Keratolytic agents such as Epilyt, Keralyt, Lac-Hydrin, and Carmol can be used bid to the affected areas to help exfoliate the diffuse scale, but should be avoided in young children because the stinging sensation is usually not well tolerated. The face and groin areas should also be avoided.
3. Topical steroids creams can be used intermittently to decrease the erythematous appearance of the rash:
   a. Low potency steroids (Desowen, 1% or 2.5% hydrocortisone) can be used on the face or body no more than bid × 2 weeks.
   b. Medium potency steroids (Elocon, Dermatop, Cutivate) can be used on the

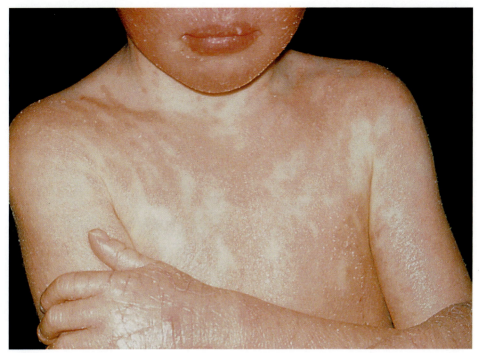

Figure 4-13 Pityriasis rubra pilaris *Diffuse salmon-colored plaques with characteristic islands of sparing on the chest of a child.*

extremities or body no more than bid × 2 weeks.

c. Strong steroids (Ultravate, Psorcon, Diprolene) are reserved for older children/adults on severely affected areas bid for no more than 2 weeks. (See page 48.)

4. Retinoids such as isotretinoin (Accutane) and acetretin (Psoriatane) may be helpful for hyperkeratosis.

5. Systemic steroids can be cautiously tried in recalcitrant cases of PRP.

DARIER'S DISEASE

Darier's disease is an autosomal dominant disorder that presents with keratotic crusted papules on the scalp, face, neck, and trunk.

Synonyms   Keratosis follicularis, Darier–White disease.

EPIDEMIOLOGY

Age   Onset between 8 and 15 years.

Gender   M > F.

Incidence   1:55,000 to 100,000 live births.

Genetics   Autosomal dominant disease. Genetic mutation localized to the ATP2A2 gene on chromosome 12q.

Season   Exacerbation during summer months/sun exposure (photo-Koebner phenomenon).

PATHOPHYSIOLOGY

The disease has been localized to the ATP2A2 gene suggesting a role for the SERCA2 pump in cell adhesion.

PHYSICAL EXAMINATION

Skin Lesions

Type   Small keratotic crusted papules with greasy scale coalescing into warty plaques (Fig. 4-14A).

Color   Flesh colored to yellow-brown.

Palpation   Rough.

Distribution   Follicular distribution on face, scalp, chest.

Sites of Predilection   Sebhorrheic areas are sites of predilection (Fig. 4-14B). Keratotic papules on dorsal surface of hands and feet and punctate lesions on palms/soles.

Nail Findings   Red, gray, or white longitudinal streaks with V-shaped notch at end and subungal hyperkeratosis.

Mucous Membranes   White cobblestone papules coalescing into plaques. Oropharynx, larynx, or anorectal mucosa may be involved.

General Findings

Increased susceptibility to infections. Rarely mental deficiency, schizophrenia, epilepsy, small stature reported.

DIFFERENTIAL DIAGNOSIS

Lesion of Darier's disease developing later in life may be confused with transient acantholytic dermatosis, pemphigus foliaceous, and Hailey–Hailey disease. These can be differentiated clinically or histopathologically.

LABORATORY EXAMINATIONS

Dermatopathology   Skin biopsy shows suprabasal acantholysis and dyskeratotic cells indicating premature keratinization. Hyperkeratosis is present and can be quite thick. Characteristic corps ronds and corp grains (dyskeratotic cells) can be seen in the stratum corneum.

COURSE AND PROGNOSIS

Darier's disease persists throughout life, but does have periods of exacerbation and partial remission. This rare disorder is usually worse in the summer months and is aggravated by sun exposure, heat, sweat, and humidity. Additionally, individuals are more susceptible to infections.

MANAGEMENT

1. Emollients such as petrolatum, mineral oil, vaseline, or moisturizers (Lubriderm, Eucerin, Moisturel, and Aquaphor creams) should be used to keep the skin well-hydrated.
2. Keratolytic agents such as Epilyt, Keralyt, Lac-Hydrin, and Carmol can be used bid to the affected areas to help exfoliate the diffuse scale, but should be avoided in young

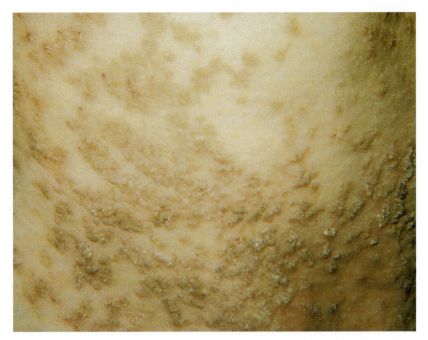

A

Figure 4-14 Darier's disease *(A) Keratotic crusted papules coalescing into plaques.*

children because the stinging sensation is usually not well tolerated. The face and groin areas should also be avoided.

3. Topical steroid creams can be used intermittently to decrease the erythematous appearance of the rash:
   a. Low-potency steroids (Desowen, 1% or 2.5% hydrocortisone) can be used on the face or body no more than bid × 2 weeks.
   b. Medium-potency steroids (Elocon, Dermatop, Cutivate) can be used on the extremities or body no more than bid × 2 weeks.
   c. Strong steroids (Ultravate, Psorcon, Diprolene) are reserved for older children/adults on severely affected areas bid for no more than 2 weeks.

Patients need to be cautioned about topical steroid side effects. Continued use can cause thinning of the skin, striae formation, and systemic absorption, especially in younger children and infants. Prolonged steroid use can also lead to tachyphylaxis (the skin becomes used to the medication and it no longer works as well). Steroids used around the eye area for prolonged periods can lead to glaucoma and/or cataract formation.

4. Retinoid creams may also be helpful (Retin A, Differin, Azelex, Tazorac) but are limited by their irritating side effects.

5. Systemic retinoids such as isotretinoin (Accutane) and acitretin (Psoriatane) are effective at smoothing the keratotic surface; however, long-term use of these agents is not recommended.

6. Darier's disease can flare from secondary bacterial infection and responds to antibiotics. The most common antibiotic include Keflex (25 to 50 mg/kg/d divided qid, not to exceed 4 g/d), dicloxacillin (25 to 50 mg/kg/d divided qid, not to exceed 2 g/d), Duricef (30 mg/kg/d divided bid), and erythromycin (30 to 50 mg/kg/d divided qid, not to exceed 2 g/d).

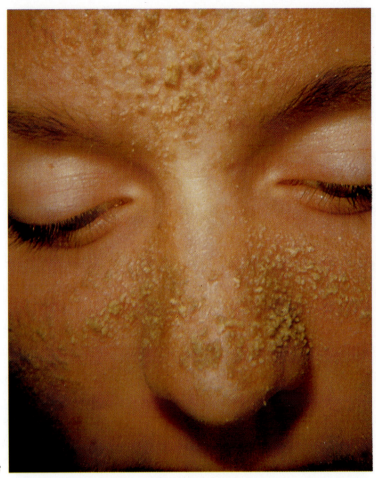

B

Figure 4-14 (continued)   Darier's disease   (B) *Keratotic papules in a seborrheic distribution on the face.*

PRIMARY BULLOUS DERMATOSES

EPIDERMOLYSIS BULLOSA

Epidermolysis bullosa (EB) defines a group of rare mechanobullous skin disorders that include over 23 distinctive diseases. They are characterized by skin fragility, bullae formation, and varying degrees of mucous membrane and nail involvement.

CLASSIFICATION

A recent revised classification of inherited epidermolysis bullosa (EB) based on phenotype and genotype has been proposed by a year 2000 international consensus meeting. It subdivided EB as follows:

1. Epidermolysis bullosa simplex (EBS) (intraepidermal bullae):
   a. EBS Weber–Cockayne (abnormal keratins 5 or 14).
   b. EBS Koebner (abnormal keratins 5 or 14).
   c. EBS Dowling–Meara (abnormal keratins 5 or 14).
   d. EBS with muscular dystrophy (abnormal plectin)

2. Junctional epidermolysis bullosa (JEB) (lamina lucida bullae):
   a. JEB Herlitz (abnormal laminin 5).
   b. JEB nonHerlitz (abnormal laminin 5 or type XVII collagen).
   c. JEB with pyloric atresia (abnormal α6β4 integrin).

3. Dystrophic epidermolysis bullosa (DEB) (sub-basal lamina bullae):
   a. Dominant DEB (abnormal type VII collagen).
   b. Recessive DEB Hallopeau–Siemens (abnormal type VII collagen).
   c. Recessive DEB non-Hallopeau–Siemens (abnormal type VII collagen).

EPIDERMOLYSIS BULLOSA SIMPLEX

Epidermolysis bullosa simplex (EBS) is an autosomal dominantly inherited, nonscarring, blistering disorder caused by a defective keratin that leads to cleavage at the basal cell layer of the epidermis. There are at least four subtypes recognized:

1. Weber–Cockayne (localized EBS).
2. Koebner (generalized EBS).
3. Dowling–Meara (EBS herpetiformis).
4. EBS with muscular dystrophy.

Synonym   Epidermolytic EB.

EPIDEMIOLOGY

Age

1. Weber–Cockayne: Blisters may appear in first 2 years of life. Can also begin in adolescence.
2. Koebner: Bullae at birth, at areas of friction; improves in adolescence.
3. Dowling–Meara: Bullae at birth; widespread, severe, and extensive spontaneous blisters; improves in adolescence.
4. EBS with muscular dystrophy (MD) bullae at birth.

Incidence   Weber–Cockayne variant is most common, estimated at 1/50,000 live births.

Gender   M = F.

Etiology   Abnormal keratin 5 or 14 in first 3 types. Abnormal plectin in EBS associated with muscular dystrophy.

Genetics   Autosomal dominant (rare cases of autosomal recessive inheritance reported).

Precipitating Factors   Bullae are mechanically induced by friction and can be exacerbated by warm temperatures, running, prolonged walking, and other sources of trauma. Only the Dowling–Meara variant seems not to be aggravated by heat.

PATHOPHYSIOLOGY

Mutations in the genes encoding keratin 5 (chromosome 12q) or 14 (chromosome 17q) or plectin cause abnormal keratinocyte formation in basal cell layer of the skin. Trauma leads to intraepidermal cleavage at the level of the basal cell layer with resultant blister formation. Because the split is so superficial, the bullae heal without scarring.

HISTORY

Healthy infants are born with seemingly fragile skin. Blisters form in areas of greatest friction, but blistering tendency usually improves with age.

PHYSICAL EXAMINATION

Skin Findings

Type and Distribution

1. Weber–Cockayne: Flaccid bullae on hands and feet (Fig. 5-1).
2. Koebner: Generalized bullae with milia formation on heeling areas. Little to no mucosal involvement, 20% with nail dystrophy.
3. Dowling–Meara: Widespread bullae with "herpetiform" grouping, can be acute with an associated palmoplantar keratoderma.
4. EBS with muscular dystrophy: localized bullae.

LABORATORY EXAMINATION

Dermatopathology   Light microscopy reveals an intraepidermal split consistent with basal cell cytolysis. Electron microscopy is more sensitive and can demonstrate the cleavage through the basal layer and basal cell cytolysis. In Dowling–Meara, EM will show clumping of tonofilaments in addition to basal cell cytolysis. Immunofluorescence staining shows the BP antigen, laminin, and collagen IV to be located beneath the level of cleavage. Immunofluorescent antigenic mapping with monoclonal antibodies can demonstrate absent keratins 5 or 14 or plectin.

Molecular Testing Can be performed based on keratin gene mutations and/or abnormal production of keratins 5 or 14 or plectin.

DIAGNOSIS

Bullae formation in an otherwise seemingly healthy newborn should lead one to suspect mechanobullous disorders, but specific disease entities require histologic and molecular testing.

COURSE AND PROGNOSIS

Most forms of EBS improve with age, and blister formation can be limited by decreasing traumatic activities. Only the Dowling–Meara variant can be severe and extensive enough to cause morbidity and mortality.

MANAGEMENT

The treatment of epidermolysis bullosa is palliative:

1. Bullae formation can be minimized by limiting traumatic activities; using soft, well-fitted shoes; and avoiding warm temperatures.
2. When blisters occur, extensive blisters may be avoided by careful aseptic aspiration of the blister fluid with a sterile pin or needle. The roofs of the blisters may be carefully trimmed with sterile scissors.
3. Daily baths, gentle cleansers (Aquanil or Cetaphil liquid cleansers), and topical petrolatum-impregnated gauze (Xeroform) can help reduce chance of secondary infection and will also help healing of the blistered area.
4. Topical emollients (Vaseline petroleum jelly, hydrated petrolatum, or Aquaphor healing ointment) can reduce friction on the healing area.
5. Topical antibiotics (Bactroban, bacitracin, neosporin, or polysporin) can be used if evidence of bacterial superinfection is present (yellow exudate, frank pus, crusting).
6. A water mattress with fleece covering may be necessary to limit extensive blistering.
7. Widespread denudation of the skin requires hospitalization with IV fluids, IV antibiotics if appropriate, and burn-unit wound care.
8. Genetic counseling to the family is important and prenatal testing should be offered if available.
9. A national epidermolysis registry has been established and can be used as a support and informational system for families who have children with epidermolysis bullosa.

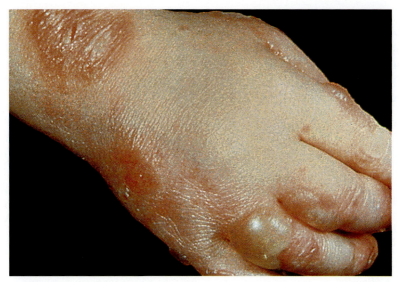

Figure 5-1 Epidermolysis bullosa simplex *Localized flaccid bullae on the hand of an infant.*

JUNCTIONAL EPIDERMOLYSIS BULLOSA

Junctional epidermolysis bullosa (JEB) is an autosomal recessive inherited mechanobullous disease. Bullae are caused by cleavage at the lamina lucida level (at the junction of the epidermis and dermis).

Several subtypes have been described:
1. Herlitz type, letalis.
2. Non-Herlitz type, mitis (generalized atrophic EB).
3. JEB with pyloric atresia.

EPIDEMIOLOGY

Age   Onset of blisters at birth or early infancy (Fig. 5-2A).

Gender   M = F.

Incidence   Rare.

Etiology   Abnormal hemidesmosomes in lamina lucida.

Genetics   Autosomal recessive.

PATHOPHYSIOLOGY

Abnormal hemidesmosome formation leads to skin fragility at the lamina lucida level. Mole-cular defects identified include abnormalities in hemidesmosome components: laminin 5, 19-DEJ-1, integrin $\beta4$, collagen XVII, and integrin $\alpha6$.

HISTORY

Blistering onset occurs during infancy for all types of JEB. The spectrum of disease (depending on subtype) can range from mild blistering tendencies to severe widespread blistering with a poor prognosis (Herlitz variant). Mucosal/esophageal/laryngeal blistering and scarring can lead to death in infancy.

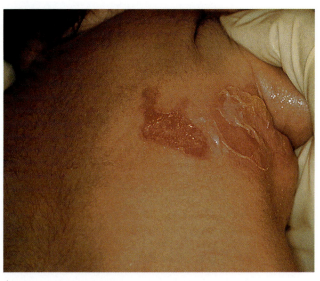

A

Figure 5-2   Junctional epidermolysis bullosa, newborn   *(A) Blister formation noted at areas of mild friction on the right chest wall of an otherwise healthy 7-day-old infant.*

PRIMARY BULLOUS DERMATOSES

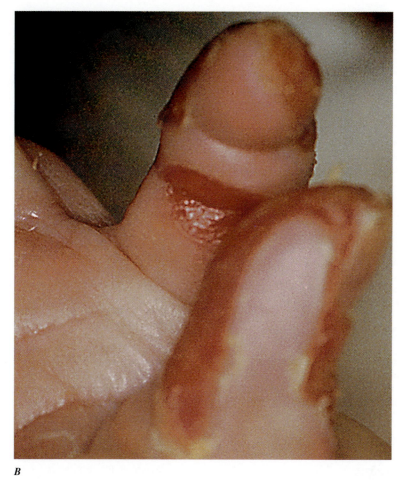

B

Figure 5-2 (continued)   Junctional epidermolysis bullosa, age 1 month   *(B) Same infant at age 1 month with severe blistering of the entire skin surface.*

PHYSICAL EXAMINATION

Skin Findings

Type and Distribution

1. Herlitz type, letalis: Extensive bullae formation (Fig. 5-2B) with perioral involvement (Fig. 5-2C). Nails may have paronychial inflammation, teeth may be dysplastic.
2. Non-Herlitz type, mitis: Serosanguinous blisters, atrophic scarring, dystrophic or absent nails, mild mucous membrane involvement.

General Findings

1. Herlitz type, letalis: Laryngeal involvement leads to 50% mortality within first 2 years of life. Survivors have severe growth retardation and anemia.
2. Non-Herlitz type, mitis (generalized atrophic EB): Scarring alopecia.

LABORATORY EXAMINATIONS

Dermatopathology   Light microscopy reveals subepidermal cleavage. Electron microscopy shows split in the lamina lucida and abnormal or reduced hemidesmosomes. Immunofluorescent antigenic mapping with monoclonal antibodies can demonstrate absent laminin 5, type XVII collagen, or $\alpha 6\beta 4$ integrin.

DIAGNOSIS

Blister formation tendencies in the newborn implicate a mechanobullous disease but histologic and molecular studies are needed for definitive diagnosis to differentiate junctional EB from other blistering disorders.

COURSE AND PROGNOSIS

1. Herlitz type, letalis: Severe blistering at birth and laryngeal lesions lead to a 50% mortality before age 2. Pyloric atresia can also be seen. The patients who survive heal with atrophic changes of the skin. Attempts at laminin 5 replacement and gene therapy are in progress.
2. Non-Herlitz type, mitis: Affected patients have normal growth and lifespan.

MANAGEMENT

The treatment of epidermolysis bullosa is palliative:

1. Bullae formation can be minimized by limiting traumatic activities; using soft, well-fitted shoes; and avoiding warm temperatures.
2. When blisters occur, extensive bullae may be avoided by careful aseptic aspiration of the blister fluid with a sterile pin or needle. The roofs of the blisters may be carefully trimmed with sterile scissors.
3. Daily baths, gentle cleansers (Aquanil or Cetaphil liquid cleansers), and topical petrolatum-impregnated gauze (Xeroform) can help reduce chance of secondary infection and will also help healing of the blistered area.
4. Topical emollients (Vaseline petroleum jelly, hydrated petrolatum, or Aquaphor healing ointment) can reduce friction on the healing area.
5. Topical antibiotics (Bactroban, bacitracin, neosporin, or polysporin) can be used if evidence of bacterial superinfection is present (yellow exudate, frank pus, crusting).
6. A water mattress with fleece covering may be necessary to limit extensive blistering.
7. Widespread denudation of the skin requires hospitalization with IV fluids, IV antibiotics if appropriate, and burn-unit wound care.
8. Watching for respiratory or GI involvement is also important. Soft food and liquid diets may help symptoms. Ultimately, corrective surgical intervention may be needed.
9. For severe disease, systemic steroids, hyperbaric chambers, laminin 5 replacement, and other therapeutic attempts have been reported, with limited success.
10. Genetic counseling to the family is important and prenatal testing should be offered if available.
11. A national epidermolysis registry has been established and can be used as a support and informational system for families who have children with epidermolysis bullosa.

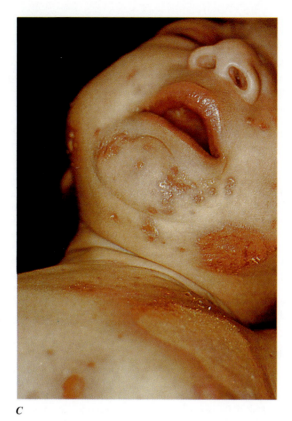

C

Figure 5-2 (continued)   Junctional epidermolysis bullosa, age 1 month   *(C) Severe perioral, oral and GI involvement. Infant was subsequently hospitalized and despite burn-unit supportive measures, eventually passed away from sepsis.*

DYSTROPHIC EPIDERMOLYSIS BULLOSA

Dystrophic epidermolysis bullosa (DEB) is a scarring mechanobullous disease that has two subtypes based on inheritance patients: (1) dominant DEB (AD) and (2) recessive DEB (AR). Bullae are caused by cleavage at the subepidermal level of the skin. These deeper bullae cause permanent disfiguring scarring.

Synonyms Dermolytic bullous dermatosis, dysplastic epidermolysis bullosa.

EPIDEMIOLOGY

Age Blistering in both forms appears at birth.

Gender M = F.

Incidence Rare.

Etiology Abnormal anchoring fibrils (collagen type VII).

Genetics Autosomal dominant and autosomal recessive forms.

PATHOPHYSIOLOGY

Abnormal collagen VII leads to abnormal, decreased, or absent anchoring fibrils between the epidermis and dermis. A spilt in the dermal–epidermal junction results in deep blisters that heal with scarring, fusion, and flexion deformities.

HISTORY

Blistering onset at infancy (Fig. 5-3A), then:

1. Dominant DEB: Intermittent blistering episodes that improve with age. Mild hair and teeth involvement.
2. Recessive DEB: Widespread dystrophy and scarring leading to incapacity and nail and mucous membrane involvement leading to poor growth, poor development.

PHYSICAL EXAMINATION

Skin Findings

Type and Distribution

1. Dominant DEB: Bullae on dorsal aspect of extremities result in either hypertrophic (Cockayne–Touraine variant) or atrophic (Pacini variant) scars and milia. Mucous membrane involvement in 20%; 80% have thickened nails. Typically no hair or teeth abnormalities.

2. Recessive DEB: In the more severe form (Hallopeau–Siemens variant) there is widespread dystrophic scarring, severe involvement of the mucous membranes, and severe nail dystrophy. Bullae heal with atrophic scarring and milia resetting in mitten deformities of the hands and feet, extremities become contracted with scars (Fig. 5-3B). In the more mild form (the mitis variant), blistering is less severe.

General Findings

1. Dominant DEB: Generally healthy and of normal stature.
2. Recessive DEB: In the more severe form (Hallopeau–Siemens variant) progressive deformity of the extremities leads to increasing incapacity. Eye involvement leads to blepharitis, symblepharon, conjunctivitis, keratitis, and corneal opacities. Laryngeal and pharyngeal involvement leads to hoarseness and aphonia (inability to speak). Esophageal strictures can occur leading to failure to thrive. Teeth are malformed and susceptible to caries. Scalp and body hair is sparse or absent. In the more mild form (the mitis variant), internal involvement in minimal.

LABORATORY EXAMINATIONS

Dermatopathology Light microscopy reveals a split at the dermal–epidermal junction. Electron microscopy shows a cleavage beneath the basal lamina and decreased or absent anchoring fibrils. Immunofluorescent antigenic mapping using monoclonal antibodies can demonstrate an absence of type VI collagen.

DIAGNOSIS

Blistering at infancy would suggest a mechanobullous disorder, but a definitive diagnosis of recessive dystrophic epidermolysis bul-

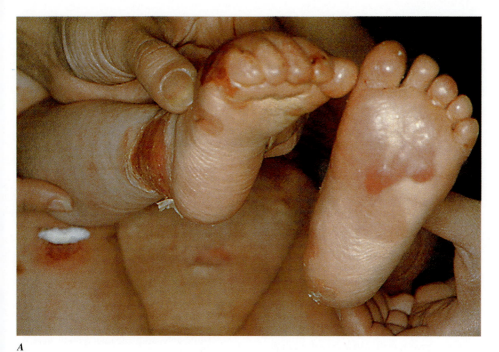

A

Figure 5-3   Recessive dystrophic epidermolysis bullosa, newborn   *(A) Bullae occur at areas of minimal trauma at or near birth.*

losa is based on histopathologic and molecular findings.

COURSE AND PROGNOSIS

1. Dominant DEB: After blisters at birth, intermittent episodes of less severe blistering occur, but lifespan and growth/development are normal. The blistering episodes are worse than epidermolysis bullosa simplex, but milder than recessive DEB.
2. Recessive DEB: In more severely affected individuals (the Hallopeau–Siemens variant), the extensive blistering may result in scarring, fusion, and flexion deformities that are functionally incapacitating. Recessive DEB blistering may result in death secondary to septicemia, fluid loss, or malnutrition. Surviving patients are chronically susceptible to infection and repeated blistering leads to further and further disabilities. These patients tend to have difficulties with laryngeal complications, esophageal strictures, and scarring of the anal area, and have a predisposition to basal cell and squamous cell carcinomas in the scarred skin areas. In the more mild cases (the mitis variant), life expectancy is normal and there is little to no increased risk of carcinoma formation.

MANAGEMENT

The treatment of dystrophic epidermolysis bullosa is palliative:

1. Bullae formation can be minimized by limiting traumatic activities; using soft, well-fitted shoes; and avoiding warm temperatures.
2. When blisters occur, extensive bullae may be avoided by careful aseptic aspiration of the blister fluid with a sterile pin or needle. The roofs of the blisters may be carefully trimmed with sterile scissors.
3. Daily baths, gentle cleansers (Aquanil or Cetaphil liquid cleansers), and topical petrolatum-impregnated gauze (Xeroform) can help reduce chance of secondary infection and will also help healing of the blistered area.
4. Topical emollients (Vaseline petroleum jelly, hydrated petrolatum, or Aquaphor healing ointment) can reduce friction on the healing area.
5. Topical antibiotics (Bactroban, bacitracin, neosporin, or polysporin) can be used if evidence of bacterial superinfection is present (yellow exudate, frank pus, crusting).
6. A water mattress with fleece covering may be necessary to limit extensive blistering.
7. Widespread denudation of the skin requires hospitalization with IV fluids, IV antibiotics if appropriate, and burn-unit wound care.
8. Oral and GI complications lead to aphonia and aphasia. A liquid or soft food diet may help symptoms. Aggressive oral, dental, and nutritional care should be given. Ultimately, surgical intervention may be needed.
9. Occupational and physical therapy for the fusion and flexion deformities is recommended, and repeated plastic surgical reconstruction may be needed to prolong functional use of the hands and feet.
10. Other reported treatments include systemic steroids, phenytoin (Dilantin), and FK506, which all have anecdotal limited success.
11. Genetic counseling to the family is important and prenatal testing should be offered if available.
12. An international support group, Dystrophic Epidermolysis Bullosa Research Association (DEBRA), is available for the families of patients with DEB.

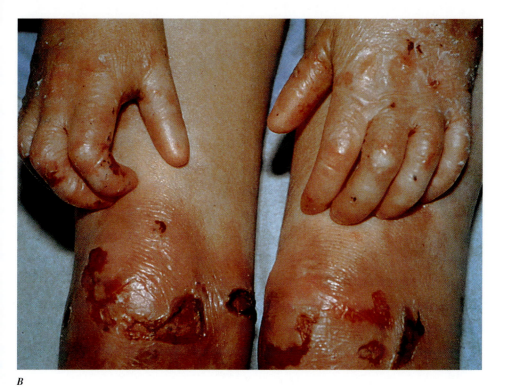

B

Figure 5-3 (continued)   Recessive dystrophic epidermolysis bullosa, child   (*B*) *Scarring leading to flexion contractures of the hands in a child with RDEB. The child eventually progressed to have mitten deformities of the hands and feet with significant physical impairment.* (Slide courtesy of Lisa Cohen).

OTHER

LINEAR IGA BULLOUS DISEASE OF CHILDHOOD

Linear IgA bullous disease of childhood is a rare, benign, self-limited bullous eruption thought to be caused by IgA autoantibodies targeting antigens at the basement membrane zone of the skin.

Synonyms Chronic bullous disease of childhood, benign chronic bullous dermatitis of childhood, bullous disease of childhood.

EPIDEMIOLOGY

Age Between 6 months and years (mean age, 4.5 years).

Gender F:M 3:2.

Incidence Rare.

Etiology IgA autoantibodies to antigens in the basement membrane zone.

PATHOPHYSIOLOGY

Circulating IgA autoantibodies target antigens (both 97 kDa and a 285 kDa antigen have been implicated) in the basement membrane zone, leading to cleavage of the skin at that level and blister formation.

HISTORY

Onset Preschool years.

Duration of Lesions Several months to 3 years.

Skin Symptoms Mild to severe pruritus.

Review of Symptoms Negative.

PHYSICAL EXAMINATION

Skin Findings

Type Large tense bullae, central crusting (Fig. 5-4A).

Color Clear or hemorrhagic bullae on erythematous base.

Size Bullae 1 to 2 cm.

Shape Bullae are sausage-shaped.

Arrangement Annular or rosette configuration like "a string of pearls" (Fig. 5-4B).

Distribution Widespread.

Sites of Predilection Face (Fig. 5-4C) scalp, lower trunk, buttocks, inner thighs, dorsa of feet.

General Findings

Blistering can occur in the mouth in 50% of cases.

DIFFERENTIAL DIAGNOSIS

Linear IgA bullous disease of childhood needs to be distinguished from other blistering diseases such as mechanobullous disorders, dermatitis herpetiformis, or bullous pemphigoid. The diagnosis is made on the basis of clinical findings and usually confirmed by skin biopsy.

LABORATORY EXAMINATIONS

Dermatopathology Subepidermal blister with dermal papillary edema and mixed cell infiltrate. Immunofluorescence reveals linear deposits of IgA in the basement membrane zone. Indirect immunofluorescence may detect circulating IgA autoantibodies against antigens in the lamina lucida and sublamina densa.

COURSE AND PROGNOSIS

Most cases of linear IgA bullous disease of childhood are self-limited. Affected children have disease-free remissions and then spontaneously clear within 2 to 4 years, typically before puberty. Only a small subset of patients experience episodic recurrences that persist into adulthood.

MANAGEMENT

Treatment of linear IgA chronic bullous diseases is directed at reducing the frequency and severity of outbreaks.

1. The disease is very responsive to sulfapyridine (100 to 200 mg/kg/d divided qid, not to exceed 4 g/d). Once the existing lesions have improved, the dosage may be tapered to the least amount needed to keep the skin under control (usually less than 0.5g PO qd). Signs of sulfapyridine toxicity include nausea, vomiting, headache, fever, leukopenia, agranulocytosis, hemolytic anemia, serum sickness, hepatitis, dermatitis, and renal crystallinuria. A screening test for glucose-6-phosphate dehydrogenase deficiency should be performed, and pretreatment as well as monthly blood work should be followed.

2. Dapsone (25 to 50 mg/kg/d, not to exceed 400 mg/d) can also be used; however the side effects are more prevalent and severe. Once the existing lesions have improved, the dosage may be tapered to the least amount required to keep the skin under control (usually less than 5 mg PO tid). Side effects of dapsone include hemolysis, methemoglobinemia, nausea, vomiting, headache, tachycardia, psychoses, fever, dermatitis, liver necrosis, lymphadenitis, and neuropathy. As with sulfapyridine, a screening test for glucose-6-phosphate dehydrogenase deficiency should be performed and monthly blood work as well as a urinalysis is recommended.

3. Patients who fail to respond to sulfonamides alone may improve with the addition of systemic steroids. Medication may be required anywhere from several months to 3 years.

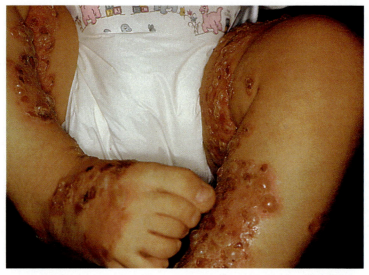

A

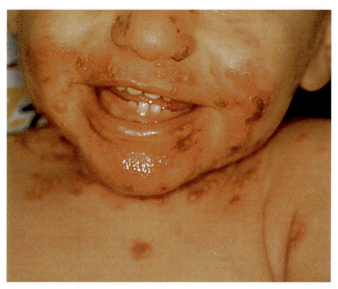

B

Figure 5-4   Linear IgA bullous disease of childhood   *(A) Legs of a 13-month old infant with characteristic annular plaques with a peripheral "string of pearls" configuration of bullae. (B) Blistering on the face on the same infant.*

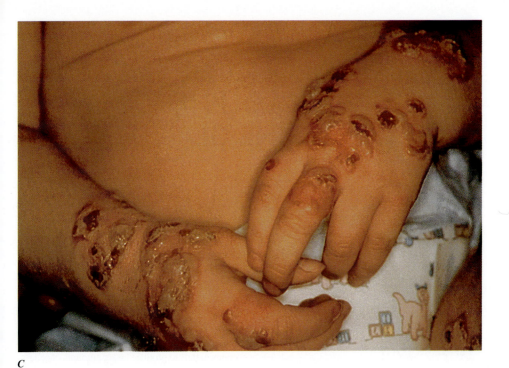

C

Figure 5-4 (continued)   Linear IgA bullous disease of childhood   *(C)* *Large tense bullae with central crusting on the hands of the same infant.*

DISORDERS OF THE SEBACEOUS AND APOCRINE GLANDS

ACNE VULGARIS

Acne vulgaris is the most common skin disorder in the second and third decades of life. It is a multifactorial disease characterized by chronic inflammation of the pilosebaceous units of certain areas (face and trunk) that manifests as comedones, papules, nodules, cysts, or papulopustules, often but not always followed by pitted or hypertrophic scars.

EPIDEMIOLOGY

Age   Begins at puberty; may appear first at 25 years.

Gender   M > F, and males tend to be more severely affected.

Incidence   Most common adolescent skin problem.

Prevalence   Approximately 85% of 15 to 18-year-olds have some form of acne.

Drugs   Systemic corticosteroids, iodides, bromides, anticonvulsants (phenytoin and trimethadione), and antidepressants (lithium) can exacerbate acne in susceptible patients.

Genetic Aspects   Family history may be a predictor of acne severity.

Other Factors   Emotional stress (school, social problems, lack of sleep, menses) can definitely cause exacerbations. Pressure on skin by leaning face on the hands is a very important factor causing exacerbation. Androgen excess can also lead to severe refractory cases.

PATHOPHYSIOLOGY

The lesions of acne (comedones) are the result of complex effects of hormones (androgens) and bacteria (*Propionibacterium acnes*) in the pilosebaceous unit. Androgens stimulate sebaceous glands to produce larger amounts of sebum; bacteria contain lipase that converts lipids into fatty acids. Both excess sebum and fatty acids block the pilosebaceous unit and comedones (whiteheads) are formed. If the comedo is open to the skin surface, the oxidized keratin protrudes (the blackhead). Closed comedones may break under the skin and the contents (sebum, lipid, fatty acids, keratin) enter the dermis, provoking inflammation (papule, pustule, nodule). Rupture plus intense inflammation may lead to scarring.

HISTORY

Duration of Lesions   Months.

Season   Worse in fall and winter.

Symptoms   Itching or pain in lesions (especially nodulocystic type).

PHYSICAL EXAMINATION

Skin Lesions

Type

Comedo. Open comedones are "blackheads." Closed comedones are "whiteheads" (Fig. 6-1A).
Papules with or without inflammation, pustules (Fig. 6-1B).

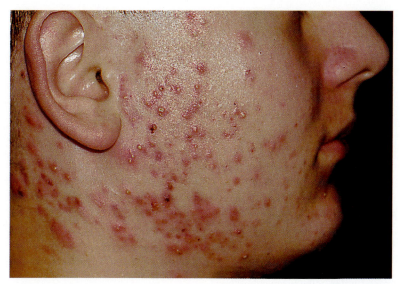

A

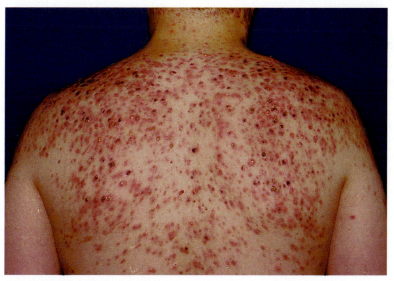

B

Figure 6-1   Acne vulgaris   *(A) Scattered inflammatory papules and pustules on the cheek of an adolescent. (B) Scattered inflammatory papules, pustules, and nodules on the back of the same individual.*

Nodules, noduloulcerative lesions, 2 to 5 cm in diameter.

Postinflammatory hyperpigmentation.

Scars. Atrophic depressed (often pitted) or hypertrophic (keloid) scars.

Shape   Round; nodules may coalesce to form linear mounds.

Arrangement   Isolated single lesion (e.g., nodule) or scattered discrete lesions (papules; cysts, nodules).

Sites of Predilection   Face, chest, back, shoulders.

DIFFERENTIAL DIAGNOSIS

Persistent acne in a hirsute female with irregular or no menses is an indication for a search for hypersecretion of androgens, plasma testosterone, and/or dihydroepiandrosterone (e.g., polycystic ovarian syndrome). Also, recalcitrant acne can be related to partial 11- or 12-hydroxylase block.

COURSE AND PROGNOSIS

Acne can have a mild self-limited course or a protracted recurrent course that may persist up to age 35.

MANAGEMENT

Patients and parents should be educated on factors that may aggravate acne:

1. Repeated pressure, leaning, touching, or scrubbing acne-prone areas.
2. Occlusive garments such as headband, helmets, and hats.
3. Oil and grease in moisturizers, face creams, makeup, or hair products.
4. Greasy-air-filled environments in fast-food kitchens.
5. Squeezing or popping pimples can lead to worse acne and/or scarring.
6. Certain medications taken for other problems (e.g., oral contraceptives, lithium, hydantoin, topical and systemic steroids).
7. Emotional stress.
8. Hormonal changes with menses.
9. Foods typically do not play a major role, but some people find specific foods trigger their acne and are helped by avoiding them.

Mild

1. Topical antibiotics such as clindamycin (Cleocin) or erythromycin (Emgel, Erycette, or Akne-mycin) help decrease bacterial load and inflammation.
2. Topical benzoyl peroxide (Benzac, Brevoxyl, or Desquam-E) also suppresses *P. acnes.*
3. Topical salicylic acid (SalAc, Stridex) or hydroxy acid preparations (Aqua Glycolic) help slough the outer layer of skin preventing follicular blockage.
4. Topical retinoids (Retin A, Differin, Renova) are effective, but require detailed instructions and gradual increases in concentration. Retinoids help the skin turn over more rapidly to decrease possible follicular blockage and rupture.
5. Topical sulfur (Sulfacet) is antimicrobial and keratolytic.

Severe

1. Oral antibiotics such as tetracycline (25 to 50 mg/kg/d divided bid not to exceed 3 g/d), erythromycin (30 to 50 mg/kg/d divided bid, not to exceed 2 g/d), doxycycline (5 mg/kg/d divided qd–bid, not to exceed 200 mg/d), or minocycline (2 mg/kg/d, not to exceed 200 mg/d) is probably the most effective and can be tapered to low doses qd once the acne is under good control. Minocycline, tetracycline, and doxycyline should only be used in children >8 years old because of potential permanent staining of growing teeth. Erythromycin should not be taken with astemizole, terfenadine, or cisapride, and can also increase theophylline levels. All oral antibiotics also theoretically interfere with the efficacy of oral contraceptives and backup contraceptive methods should be used.
2. In females only, acne can be controlled with oral contraceptives (currently orthotricyclin is the only FDA-approved OCP for acne treatment).
3. Oral 13-*cis*-retinoic acid (Accutane) is highly effective for cystic acne. This treatment requires experience. As retinoids are teratogenic in females, it is necessary that female patients have a pretreatment pregnancy test and they must be on two forms of birth control at least 1 month prior to beginning treatment, throughout treatment,

and for 1 month after treatment is discontinued. Furthermore, a patient must have a negative serum pregnancy test within the 2 weeks prior to beginning treatment. Dosage: 0.5 to 1 mg/kg/d with meals for a 15- to 20-week course, which is usually adequate. About 30% of patients require a second course. Careful monitoring of the blood is necessary during therapy, especially in patients with elevated blood triglycerides before therapy is begun.

INFANTILE ACNE

Infantile acne is acne that appears when the infant is 3 to 4 months or older. Unlike neonatal acne, which is short-lived and self-resolving, infantile acne can be more long-standing, refractory to treatment, and predictive of a more severe resurgence of acne at puberty.

EPIDEMIOLOGY

Age 3 to 4 months or < 8 years.

Gender M > F.

Genetics More common in children with parents who have a history of acne.

PHYSICAL EXAMINATION

Skin Findings

Type Comedos (closed and open), papules, pustules, and occasional nodules (Fig. 6-2).

Distribution Face predominantly.

COURSE AND PROGNOSIS

Infantile acne has a variable course. In some individuals, it clears spontaneously after a few weeks. In others, especially cases with earlier onset and a family history of acne, the course is more protracted and severe resurgence at puberty is likely. Persistent severe infantile acne should be worked up for an endocrine abnormality, and an elevated level (> 0.5 μg) of 17-ketosteroids in a 24-hour urine collection is suggestive of gonadal and adrenal hyperactivity.

MANAGEMENT

Infant skin is usually quite sensitive, and mild cases of infantile acne can be managed with gentle cleansing. More severe cases may require topical medications, but they should be used sparingly and in low doses to the affected areas qd-bid to avoid overdrying and irritating the skin. Topical medications include the following.

1. Topical antibiotics such as clindamycin or erythromycin (Emgel, Erycette, or Aknemycin) help decrease bacterial load and inflammation.
2. Topical benzoyl peroxide (Benzac, Brevoxyl, Desquam-E, or Triaz) also suppresses *P. acnes*.
3. Topical salicylic acid (SalAc, Stridex) or hydroxy acid preparations (Aqua Glycolic) help slough the outer layer of skin, preventing follicular blockage.
4. Topical retinoids (Retin A, Differin, or Renova) are effective, but require detailed instructions and gradual increases in concentration. Retinoids help the skin turn over more rapidly to decrease possible follicular blockage and rupture.
5. Topical sulfur (Sulfacet) is antimicrobial and keratolytic.

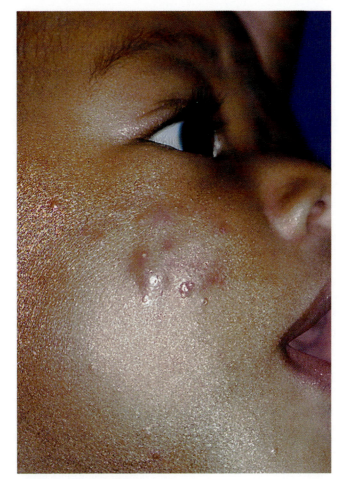

Figure 6-2 **Infantile acne** *Scattered inflammatory papules and pustules on the cheek of a 5-month-old child.*

PERIORAL DERMATITIS

Perioral dermatitis is a variant of acne on the perioral skin characterized by discrete erythematous papules that often coalesce, forming inflammatory plaques.

EPIDEMIOLOGY

Age   Any age. Seen in both young children and adults, ages 15 to 40 years.

Gender   F > M.

Etiology   Unknown.

Other Factors   May be markedly aggravated by potent topical (fluorinated) corticosteroids and/or cosmetics.

HISTORY

Duration of Lesions   Weeks to months.

Skin Symptoms   Occasional itching or burning.

PHYSICAL EXAMINATION

Skin Lesions

Type   Initial lesions are erythematous papules. Confluent plaques may appear eczematous with erythema and scale (Fig. 6-3).

Color   Pink to red.

Size   1 to 2-mm papules coalescing into larger plaques.

Arrangement   Papules are irregularly grouped.

Distribution   Initial lesions usually around mouth and nasolabial folds with sparing around the vermilion border of lips.

DIFFERENTIAL DIAGNOSIS

The diagnosis of perioral dermatitis is made clinically and needs to be differentiated from contact dermatitis, atopic dermatitis, seborrheic dermatitis, rosacea, acne vulgaris, and sarcoidosis.

COURSE AND PROGNOSIS

Appearance of lesions is usually subacute over weeks to months. Perioral dermatitis is, at times, misdiagnosed as an eczematous or a seborrheic dermatitis and treated with a potent topical corticosteroid preparation, which worsens the condition. Untreated, perioral dermatitis fluctuates in activity over months to years. With treatment for several months, mild recurrences can occur but clear easily.

MANAGEMENT

Treatment should begin by eliminating any topical agents that may be aggravating or precipitating the condition, such as topical corticosteroids, toothpaste with fluoride, or cosmetics. Often, just by eliminating the offending agent, the rash will clear. More refractory cases may require topical medications qid to bid sparingly to the affected areas, such as:

1. Topical antibiotics such as clindamycin (Cleocin), erythromycin (Emgel, Erycette, or Akne-mycin), or metronidazole (Metrocream) can help decrease inflammation.
2. Topical benzoyl peroxide (Benzac, Brevoxyl, Desquam-E, or Triaz).
3. Topical salicylic acid (SalAc, Stridex) or hydroxy acid preparations (Aqua Glycolic) help slough the outer layer of skin preventing follicular blockage.
4. Topical retinoids (Retin A, Differin), are effective, but require detailed instructions and gradual increases in concentration. Retinoids help the skin turn over more rapidly to decrease possible follicular blockage and rupture.
5. Topical sulfur (Sulfacet) is antimicrobial and keratolytic.
6. Many cases require a course of oral antibiotics (See page 134).

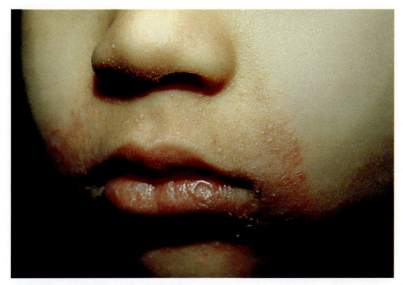

Figure 6-3 Perioral dermatitis *Scattered inflammatory papules, erythema, and scale in a child who has been applying topical steroids to the area.*

HIDRADENITIS SUPPURATIVA

Hidradenitis suppurativa is a chronic disease of apocrine-gland-bearing skin (typically the axillae and inguinal folds) that results in suppurative nodules and cribriform scarring of the involved areas.

Synonyms Apocrinitis, hidradenitis axillaris, abscess of the apocrine sweat glands; sometimes associated with severe cystic acne.

EPIDEMIOLOGY

Age Develops after puberty.

Gender F > M.

Race Affects blacks more than whites.

Etiology Predisposing factors: Obesity, genetic predisposition to acne, apocrine duct obstruction, secondary bacterial infection.

PATHOPHYSIOLOGY

Sequence of changes: (1) keratinous plugging of the apocrine duct, (2) dilatation of apocrine duct and hair follicle, (3) severe inflammatory changes limited to a simple apocrine gland, (4) bacterial growth in dilated duct, (5) ruptured duct/gland results in extension of inflammation/infection, (6) extension of suppuration/tissue destruction, (7) ulceration and fibrosis, sinus tract formation.

HISTORY

Intermittent pain, abscess formation in axilla(e) and/or inguinal area. The area under the breast may also be affected, and associated severe cystic acne of the face, chest, and back is also seen.

PHYSICAL EXAMINATION

Skin Findings

Type of Lesion Inflammatory nodule or abscess that drains purulent or seropurulent material. Eventually sinus tracts form and result in fibrosis and "bridge," hypertrophic, and keloidal scars (Fig. 6-4).

Size 0.5 to 1.5 cm nodules.

Color Erythematous nodules.

Palpation Lesions moderately to exquisitely tender. Pus emitted from opening of abscess.

Distribution of Lesions Axillae, under breasts, inguinal folds, anogenital areas (Fig. 6-5).

General

Often obesity. Associated with severe cystic acne of the face (acne conglobata), chest, or back.

DIFFERENTIAL DIAGNOSIS

The diagnosis of hidradenitis suppurativa is made clinically by the characteristic distribution of the rash and by the resultant cribiform scarring. Early disease may be confused with furuncles, carbuncles, lymphadenitis, ruptured tricholemmal cysts, cat-scratch disease, or tularemia. Late disease can resemble lymphogranuloma venereum, donovanosis, scrofuloderma, actinomycosis, or the sinus tracts and fistulae associated with ulcerative colitis and regional enteritis.

LABORATORY EXAMINATIONS

Bacteriology *Staphylococcus aureus* or streptococci are organisms that commonly secondarily infect skin lesions.

Dermatopathology Early: keratin occlusion of apocrine duct and hair follicle, ductal/tubular dilatation, and inflammatory changes. Late: destruction of apocrine/eccrine/pilosebaceous apparatus, fibrosis, and scarring.

COURSE AND PROGNOSIS

Spectrum of disease is very broad. Many patients have mild involvement. The disease usually undergoes a spontaneous remission with age (over 35 years). In some individuals, the course can be relentlessly progressive, with marked morbidity related to chronic pain, draining sinuses, and scarring.

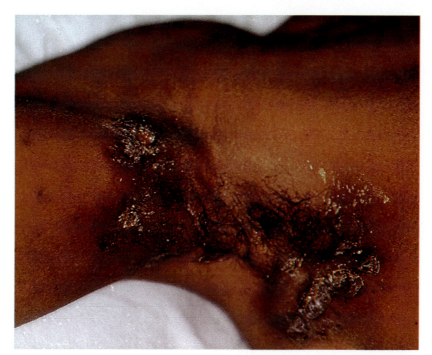

Figure 6-4 Hidradenitis suppurativa *Axillae with inflammatory cysts, siuns tract formation, and keloids.*

TREATMENT

Mild disease can be controlled with topical antibiotics, benzoyl peroxide, hydroxy acids, or retinoids. Severe cases may require oral antibiotics, oral contraceptives, or systemic retinoids (See page 134).

Intralesional triamcinolone (3 to 5 mg/mL) into early inflammatory lesions can hasten resolution and decrease pain.

Systemic steroids may also be given concurrently if pain and inflammation are severe.

With extensive, chronic disease, complete excision of involved axillary tissue or inguinal area may be required.

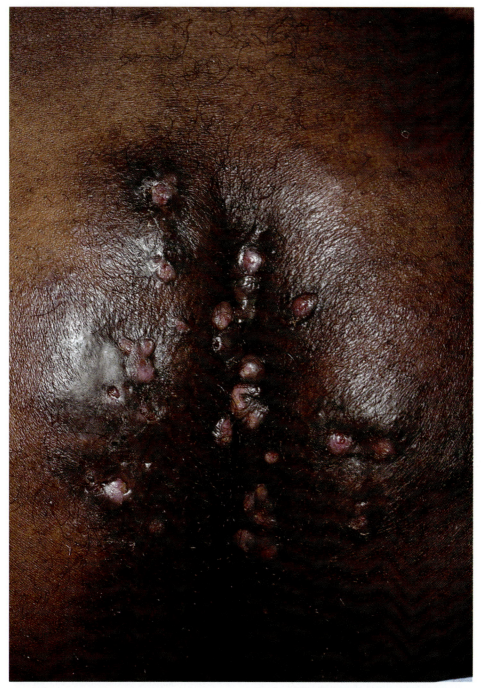

Figure 6-5 Hidradenitis suppurativa *A 15-year-old female with undiagnosed hidradenitis suppurativa of the buttocks treated with oral and IV antibiotics. Definitive treatment was excision and grafting of the involved sites.* (Reproduced with permission from TB Fitzpatrick et al., Color Atlas and Synopsis of Clinical Dermatology, 4th edition. New York: McGraw-Hill, 2001).

DISORDERS OF MELANOCYTES

INTRODUCTION:

ACQUIRED MELANOCYTIC NEVOCELLULAR NEVI (MOLES)

Acquired melanocytic nevocellular nevi are small (< 1.0 cm), benign, well-circumscribed, pigmented lesions comprised of groups of melanocytes or melanocytic nevus cells. They can be classified into three groups:

1. Junctional nevi (cells grouped at the dermal–epidermal junction, above basement membrane).
2. Dermal nevi (cells grouped in the dermis).
3. Compound nevi (combination of histologic features of junctional and dermal).

Synonym Pigmented nevi.

EPIDEMIOLOGY

Age Appears after 6 to 12 months of age, and reach a maximum number in adolescence.

Incidence Common, by age 25, most Caucasians will have 20 to 40 moles.

Gender M = F.

HISTORY

Duration of Lesions Commonly called *moles,* lesions appear after age 6 to 12 months and reach a maximum number in adolescence. By age 60, most moles fade and/or disappear.

Skin Symptoms Nevocellular nevi are asymptomatic. If a mole is symptomatic, it should be evaluated and/or removed.

MANAGEMENT

Indications for removal of acquired melanocytic nevi are:

1. *Asymmetry in shape.* One half is different from the other.

2. *Border.* Irregular borders are present.
3. *Color.* Color is or becomes variegated. Shades of gray, black, white are worrisome.
4. *Diameter.* Greater than 6 mm (may be congenital mole, but should be evaluated).
5. *Symptoms.* Lesion begins to persistently itch, hurt, or bleed.
6. *Site.* If lesion is constantly traumatized in any given location (e.g., waistline, neck) or if lesion is in a high-risk/difficult-to-monitor site such as the mucous membranes or anogenital area, it may warrant removal.

These criteria are based on anatomic sites at risk for change of acquired nevi to malignant melanoma *or* on changes in individual lesions (color, border) that indicate the development of a focus of cells with *dysplasia,* the precursor of malignant melanoma. Dysplastic nevi are *usually* > 6 mm, and darker, with a variegation of color (tan, brown), and irregular borders.

Melanocytic nevi, if treated, should always be excised for histologic diagnosis and for definitive treatment. Destruction by electrocautery, laser, or other means is not recommended.

JUNCTIONAL NEVUS

PHYSICAL EXAMINATION

Skin Lesions

Type   Macule.

Size   Less than 1.0 cm.

Color   Uniform tan, brown, or dark brown.

Shape   Round or oval with smooth regular borders (Fig. 7-1).

Arrangement   Scattered discrete lesions.

Distribution   Random.

Sites of Predilection   Trunk, upper extremities, face, lower extremities; may be located on palms, soles, and genitalia.

DERMATOPATHOLOGY

In junctional nevi, the cells and/or nest of nevus cells are located in the lower epidermis.

Figure 7-1 Junctional nevus *Two uniformly brown small macules, round in shape with smooth regular borders.* (Reproduced with permission from TB Fitzpatrick et al., Color Atlas and Synopsis of Clinical Dermatology, 4th edition. New York: McGraw-Hill, 2001).

DERMAL NEVUS

Synonym   Intradermal nevus.

PHYSICAL EXAMINATION

Skin Lesions

Type   Papule, nodule, polypoid, or papillomatous lesion.

Color   Skin-colored, tan, brown, or flecks of brown.

Shape   Round, dome-shaped (Fig. 7-2).

Distribution   More common on the face and neck, but can occur on the trunk or extremities.

Other Features   Coarse hairs may be present within the lesion. Dermal nevi usually appear in late adolescence, 20s, and 30s.

DIFFERENTIAL DIAGNOSIS

Dermal nevi are sometimes difficult to distinguish from junctional nevi; and on the face, from basal cell carcinoma.

DERMATOPATHOLOGY

Dermal nevi have nevus cells and/or nests in the dermis.

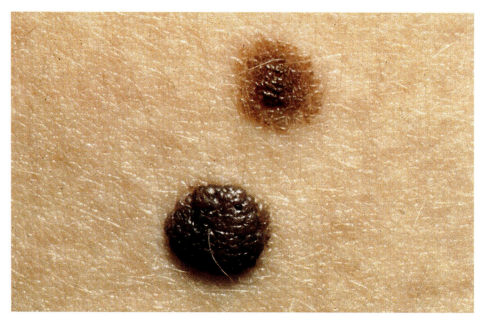

Figure 7-2   Dermal nevus   *Raised brown dome-shaped papule with regular borders and uniform pigment.* (Reproduced with permission from TB Fitzpatrick et al., Color Atlas and Synopsis of Clinical Dermatology, 4th edition. New York: McGraw-Hill, 2001).

COMPOUND NEVUS

PHYSICAL EXAMINATION

Skin Lesions

Type Macular lesion or slightly elevated, may have a central raised papule, or nodule (Fig. 7-3).

Color Skin-colored, tan, or brown.

Shape Round.

Distribution Any site.

Other Features In late childhood, compound nevi can increase in darkness and become more elevated.

DERMATOPATHOLOGY

In compound nevi, nevus cells and/or nests are seen in both the epidermis and dermis.

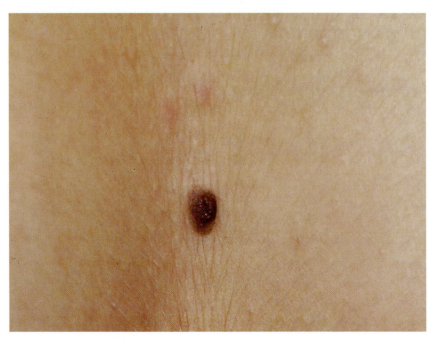

Figure 7-3　Compound nevus　*Slightly raised nevus with regular borders and pigment.*

CONGENITAL NEVOMELANOCYTIC NEVUS

Congenital nevomelanocytic nevi (CNN) are pigmented lesions of the skin usually present at birth. CNN may be any size from very small to very large. CNN are benign neoplasms comprised of cells called *nevomelanocytes,* which are derived from melanoblasts. All CNN, regardless of size, have an increased incidence of malignant melanoma.

Synonym Giant pigmented nevi.

EPIDEMIOLOGY

Age Present at birth (congenital). Rarely, some CNN become visible after birth ("tardive"), usually within the first 3 to 12 months of life.

Gender M = F.

Race All races.

Prevalence Small congenital nevi ($<$ 1.5 to 2 cm) are present in 2.5% of newborns. Medium congenital nevi (presently defined as 1.5 to 20 cm) are present in 1/2000 newborns. Large/giant congenital nevi ($>$ 20 cm) have a prevalence of 1/20,000 newborns.

Etiology Likely multifactorial. Rare familial cases have been reported.

PATHOPHYSIOLOGY

Congenital and acquired nevomelanocytic nevi are thought to occur as the result of a developmental defect in neural crest-derived melanoblasts. This defect probably occurs embryologically after 10 weeks in utero but before the sixth uterine month.

HISTORY

Congenital nevi are present at or soon after birth. They begin as pale brown to tan macules, which become darker more elevated during infancy. Most are benign and grow proportionately with the child and are asymptomatic for life. As the child grows older, the lesions develop coarse terminal hairs and may become more verrucous in appearance.

PHYSICAL EXAMINATION

Skin Lesions

Type Well-circumscribed macules, papules, or plaques with or without coarse terminal hairs (Fig. 7-4).

Borders Sharply demarcated; regular contours.

Surface May or may not have altered skin surface ("pebbly," mammillated, rugose, cerebriform, bulbous, tuberous, or lobular).

Color Light or dark brown.

Size Congenital nevi range in size from 1 mm (small CNN) to $>$ 20 cm (large/giant CNN).

Shape Oval or round.

Distribution Isolated, discrete lesions on any site.

DIFFERENTIAL DIAGNOSIS

Without a good birth history, a CNN may be confused with a common acquired nevomelanocytic nevus, dysplastic nevus, Mongolian spot, nevus of Ota, congenital blue nevus, nevus spilus, Becker's nevus, a pigmented epidermal nevus, and café-au-lait macules.

LABORATORY EXAMINATIONS

Histopathology In congenital nevi, the nevomelanocytes occur as well-ordered clusters in the epidermis, and in the dermis as sheets, nests, or cords. Unlike the common acquired nevomelanocytic nevus, the nevomelanocytes in CNN tend to occur in the skin appendages

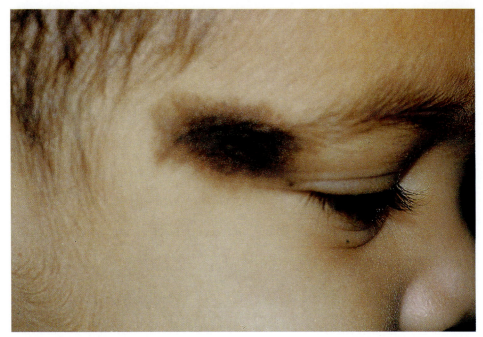

Figure 7-4 Congenital nevus *Small nevus present since birth on the face of a 2-year-old. Note the terminal hairs in the center of the lesion.*

DISORDERS OF MELANOCYTES

(eccrine ducts, hair follicles, sebaceous glands) and in nerve fascicles and/or arrectores pilorum muscles, blood vessels (especially veins), and lymphatic vessels, and extend into the lower two-thirds of the reticular dermis and deeper. Large/giant CNN may have nevus cells extend into the muscle, bone, and dura mater.

COURSE AND PROGNOSIS

By definition CNN appear at birth but varieties of CNN may arise during infancy (so-called tardive CNN). The lifetime risk for development of melanoma in small CNN is smaller than 5%, and large CNN have been estimated to have a lifetime risk of at least 6.3%. Giant CNN of the head and neck may be associated with involvement of the leptomeninges with the same pathologic process; this presentation may be asymptomatic or be manifested by seizures, focal neurologic defects, or obstructive hydrocephalus. Giant CNN of the trunk (so called bathing-trunk nevi) that overlie the vertebral column may be associated with spina bifida or a meningomyelocele.

MANAGEMENT

There is no consensus regarding treatment for CNN. Small (<1.5 cm) and benign-appearing congenital nevi can be monitored until puberty, when excision under local anesthesia is more feasible if warranted. There is insufficient data to warrant removal of all congenital nevi; thus patients should be instructed about signs of malignant transformation:

1. *Changes in shape.* One half is different from the other.
2. *Irregular or fuzzy borders.* Irregular borders are present.
3. *Color variegation.* Shades of gray, black, white are worrisome.
4. *Symptoms.* Lesion begins to persistently itch, hurt, or bleed.

Large CNN can become malignant before puberty. It is important to follow these lesions clinically with measurements and/or photographs. Complete surgical removal lesions is difficult and often requires multiple surgeries with tissue expansion, skin grafting, and/or artificial skin replacement.

For the management of large CNN on the head or neck, neurologic evaluation is recommended. An MRI with contrast may be indicated if signs of increased intracranial pressure are present.

Dermabrasion, laser removal, cryosurgery, electrocautery, and curettage destruction of congenital nevi of any size are *not* recommended.

DYSPLASTIC MELANOCYTIC NEVUS

Dysplastic nevi are irregular-appearing, acquired nevi associated with an increased life-time risk of developing melanoma.

Synonyms Atypical nevus, Clark's nevus.

EPIDEMIOLOGY

Age May appear at any age.

Gender M = F.

Race White > black.

Incidence 2 to 5% of white population.

Etiology Familial tendency.

Genetics Autosomal dominant.

PATHOPHYSIOLOGY

Genetic loci (1p36 and 9p21) have been implicated in familial cases of dysplastic nevi/melanoma. Sunlight can also be a factor. Immunosuppression also is associated with an increased risk of dysplastic nevi.

HISTORY

Dysplastic nevi typically appear later in childhood (puberty) than benign nevi, and are more numerous in sun-exposed areas.

Skin Symptoms Typically asymptomatic. Itching or bleeding may be indicators of malignant change.

PHYSICAL EXAMINATION

Skin Findings

Type Macules, papules, or poorly circumscribed nodules.

Size 6 to 15 mm.

Color Asymmetrically brown, tan, pink, or variegated.

Shape Round to oval with irregular or angulated borders (Fig. 7-5).

Distribution Back > chest > arms/legs.

DIAGNOSIS

Dysplastic nevi can be confused with acquired nevomelanocytic nevi, melanoma, Spitz nevi, and other pigmented lesions.

LABORATORY EXAMINATIONS

Dermatopathology The histologic criteria for a dysplastic nevus include the following:

1. Architectural disorder with asymmetry of the lesion.
2. Intraepidermal melanocytes in a single file or in nests beyond the dermal component.
3. Lentiginous hyperplasia with elongation of the rete ridges (may be "bridging").
4. +/− Fibrotic changes around the rete ridges.
5. +/− Vascular changes.
6. +/− Inflammation.

MANAGEMENT

Patients with dysplastic nevi should have regular skin examinations with excision and histologic evaluation of any changing or worrisome lesions. Patients should be educated and instructed on worrisome signs in moles:

1. *Asymmetry in shape.* One half is different from the other.
2. *Border.* Irregular borders are present.
3. *Color.* Color is or becomes variegated. Shades of gray, black, white are worrisome.
4. *Diameter.* Greater than 6 mm (may be congenital mole, but should be evaluated).
5. *Symptoms.* Lesion begins to persistently itch, hurt, or bleed.
6. *Site.* If lesion is constantly traumatized in any given location (e.g., waistline, neck) or if lesion is in a high-risk/difficult-to-monitor site such as the mucous membranes or anogenital area, it may warrant removal.

First-degree relatives should also be examined for atypical nevi/melanoma. Sun avoidance and protection are recommended.

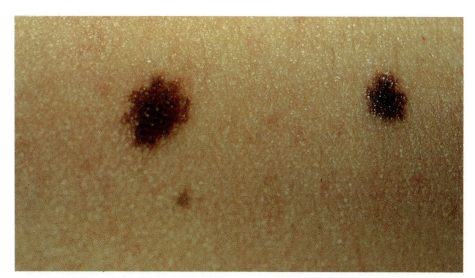

Figure 7-5 Dysplastic nevus *A 6 × 8 mm nevus with irregular notched borders.*

BLUE NEVUS

A blue nevus is an acquired, benign, small, dark blue to blue-black, sharply defined papule or nodule of melanin-producing dermal melanocytes.

Synonyms Blue neuronevus, dermal melanocytoma, common blue nevus.

EPIDEMIOLOGY

Age May appear at any age; 18% are present at birth.

Gender F: M 2:1.

Rare Variants Cellular blue nevus, combined blue nevus-nevomelanocytic nevus, plaque-type blue nevi.

PATHOPHYSIOLOGY

It is thought that a blue nevus arises from ectopic dermal melanocytes that represent arrested embryonal migration of the melanocytes.

HISTORY

Blue nevi are benign growths that appear at any age, remain stable in size, and persist for life.

In contrast, cellular blue nevi are generally > 1 cm in size and have a low but distinct danger of malignant transformation.

PHYSICAL EXAMINATION

Skin Lesions

Type Small macule or papule. Normal skin markings evident (in contrast to malignant melanoma, where the normal skin markings over a blue-black lesion would be disrupted).

Size 2 to 10 mm.

Color Blue, blue-gray, blue-black (Fig. 7-6). Occasionally has target-like pattern of pigmentation.

Shape Usually round to oval.

Distribution Scalp or the face (34%), arms (17%), hands (17%), feet (11%), or buttocks (6%).

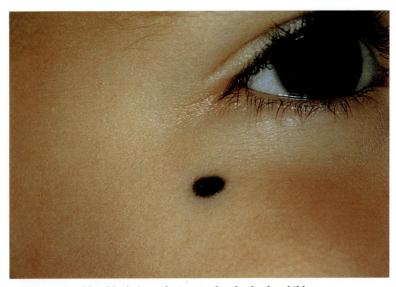

Figure 7-6 Blue nevus *Blue-black 4-mm lesion on the cheek of a child.*

DISORDERS OF MELANOCYTES

DIFFERENTIAL DIAGNOSIS

The diagnosis of a blue nevus is usually made on clinical findings. Although worrisome in color, blue nevi can be diagnosed by their normal skin markings. At times, the diagnosis is confirmed by excision and dermatopathologic examination. The differential diagnosis includes a radiation tattoo, traumatic tattoo (e.g., pencil lead tip), dermatofibroma, glomus tumor, primary or metastatic melanoma, and a pigmented spindle cell (Spitz) nevus.

DERMATOPATHOLOGY

Skin biopsy reveals spindle-shaped melanocytes grouped in bundles in the middle and lower third of the dermis.

COURSE AND PROGNOSIS

Blue nevi appear and persist throughout life. They may flatten and fade in color over time. Malignant degeneration is rare.

MANAGEMENT

Blue nevi smaller than 10 mm in diameter and stable for many years usually do not need excision. Those larger than 10 mm are more likely to be the cellular blue nevus variant, which does have a low risk of malignant degeneration, and surgical removal is recommended. The sudden appearance or change of an apparent blue nevus also warrants surgical excision.

HALO NEVUS

A halo nevus is a nevus (usually compound or dermal nevus) which becomes surrounded by a halo of depigmentation. The nevus then typically undergoes spontaneous involution and regression followed by repigmentation of the depigmented area.

Synonyms Sutton's nevus, leukoderma acquisitum centrifugum.

EPIDEMIOLOGY

Age Seen in ages 3 to 45. Typically appears in late adolescence.

Gender M = F.

Family History Halo nevi occur in siblings and with history of vitiligo in family.

Associated Disorders 30% of patients with halo nevi have vitiligo. Very rarely, metastatic melanoma (around lesions and around nevus cell nevi) can be seen.

Halo Depigmentation Around Other Lesions Typically halo nevi are compound or dermal nevi at the outset. However, halos have also been reported with blue nevi, congenital nevi, Spitz nevi, and melanomas.

PATHOPHYSIOLOGY

It is thought that a halo nevus represents an autoimmune response against melanocytes and nevus cells. The triggering mechanism is unclear.

HISTORY

Three Stages

1. Development (in months) of halo around preexisting nevus.
2. Disappearance (months to years) of nevus.
3. Repigmentation (months to years) of halo.

PHYSICAL EXAMINATION

Skin Lesions

Type Papular brown nevus (5 to 10 mm) with 1 to 5-mm halo of depigmentation (Fig. 7-7).

Shape Round to oval.

Arrangement Scattered discrete lesions (1 to 90).

Distribution Trunk (especially the back).

LABORATORY EXAMINATIONS

Dermatopathology Dermal or compound nevus surrounded by lymphocytic infiltrate (lymphocytes and histiocytes) around and between nevus cells. In the halo areas, there is a decrease or absence of melanin and melanocytes (as shown by electron microscopy).

MANAGEMENT

Halo lesions undergo spontaneous resolution and the central regressing nevus must always be evaluated for clinical criteria of malignancy (variegation of pigment and irregular borders) as a halo can and does occasionally develop around a melanoma. Worrisome or atypical lesions should be excised and sent for histologic evaluation.

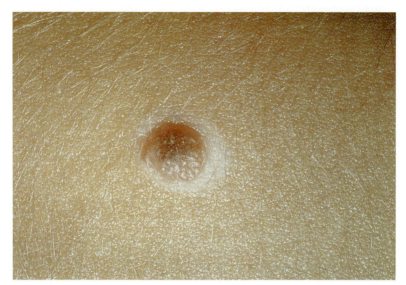

Figure 7-7 Halo nevus *Raised red-brown nevus with a depigmented halo surrounding it.*

NEVUS SPILUS

A nevus spilus is a flat brown macule dotted with superimposed smaller dark brown-to-black macules or papules.

Synonyms Speckled lentiginous nevus, spotty nevus, spotted grouped pigmented nevus, nevus-on-nevus.

EPIDEMIOLOGY

Age Usually present at birth. Can appear later in life.

Incidence Present in 1.7/1000 newborns, found in 2% of the adult population.

Etiology Presumed localized defect in neural crest melanoblasts. Genetic and environmental factors may play a role.

PATHOPHYSIOLOGY

Unclear.

HISTORY

A nevus spilus can be present at birth, but is more often acquired. They are asymptomatic and persist for life, growing proportionately with the child.

PHYSICAL EXAMINATION

Skin Findings

Type Well-delineated background macule studded with darker small macules or papules (Fig. 7-8).

Color Light brown to dark brown-black.

Size and Shape Macular background may be 1 to 20 cm in diameter. Smaller superimposed lesions range from 1 to 5 mm.

Distribution Any site.

Sites of Predilection Torso and extremities.

DIFFERENTIAL DIAGNOSIS

A nevus spilus can often be confused with a café-au-lait macule, Becker's nevus, compound nevus, congenital nevus, and/or junctional nevus.

LABORATORY EXAMINATIONS

Dermatopathology Skin biopsy of the background area shows epidermal hyperpigmentation with macromelanosomes or lentiginous melanocytic hyperplasia. The smaller speckled lesions show collections of junctional or dermal melanocytes.

COURSE AND PROGNOSIS

Nevus spilus rarely develop into malignant melanoma, and often persist throughout life asymptomatic and unchanging.

MANAGEMENT

Because nevus spilus does have nevus areas within it, it should be monitored clinically as with any other mole for signs of worrisome changes, which include:

1. *Asymmetry in shape.* One half is different from the other.
2. *Border.* Irregular borders are present.
3. *Color.* Color is or becomes variegated. Shades of gray, black, white are worrisome.
4. *Symptoms.* Lesion begins to persistently itch, hurt, or bleed.

Prophylactic surgical excision is not warranted.

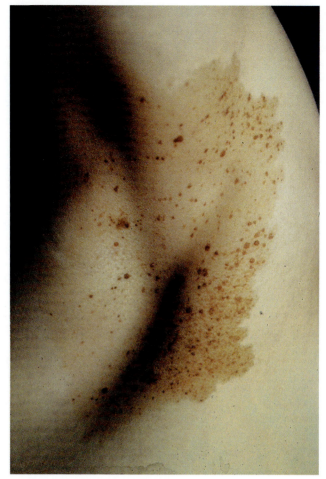

Figure 7-8 **Nevus spilus** *Large tan macule dotted with numerous superimposed small dark nevi.*

SPITZ NEVUS

A Spitz nevus is a benign small red-brown, dome-shaped nodule that appears suddenly on the face of a child. The pathology of the lesion is misleadingly worrisome, with spindle and epitheloid cells, some of which are atypical in appearance, resembling a melanoma.

Synonyms Spitz tumor, benign juvenile melanoma, epitheloid cell–spindle cell nevus.

EPIDEMIOLOGY

Age Usually appears between ages 3 and 13 years. Rare in persons > 40 years.

Gender M = F.

Incidence 1.4:100,000.

Etiology Unclear.

PATHOPHYSIOLOGY

Unclear.

HISTORY

Spitz nevi typically appear suddenly, rapidly grow and then are stable for years. They are typically asymptomatic and may persist for life or develop into a dermal nevus.

PHYSICAL EXAMINATION

Skin Findings

Type Papule or nodule.

Color Pink to red brown color (Fig. 7-9).

Size 6 mm–1.0 cm.

Shape Round, dome-shaped.

Distribution Cheek and face of children/adolescents.

DIAGNOSIS AND DIFFERENTIAL DIAGNOSIS

The diagnosis of a Spitz nevus is usually made clinically. The rapid onset and growth of the lesions helps to differentiate it from a dermal nevus, pyogenic granuloma, hemangioma, molluscum, juvenile xanthogranuloma, and nodular melanoma.

LABORATORY EXAMINATIONS

Dermatopathology Skin biopsy shows large epitheloid and spindle cells with abundant cytoplasm and occasional mitotic figures. The nests extend into the dermis in a characteristic "raining down" pattern. There are also coalescent eosinophilic globules (Kamino bodies) present in the basal layer in 80% of biopsies.

COURSE AND PROGNOSIS

Once a Spitz nevus appears, it rarely involutes. The majority are benign but there are case reports of "metastatic Spitz nevi" and in reported rare instances of progression to melanoma.

MANAGEMENT

Because Spitz nevi are benign, no treatment is needed. However, the rapid onset and growth of the lesion is often worrisome to clinicians and the lesions are removed by excisional biopsy. Once excised, good dermatopathologic examination is needed to distinguish the Spitz nevi from melanoma.

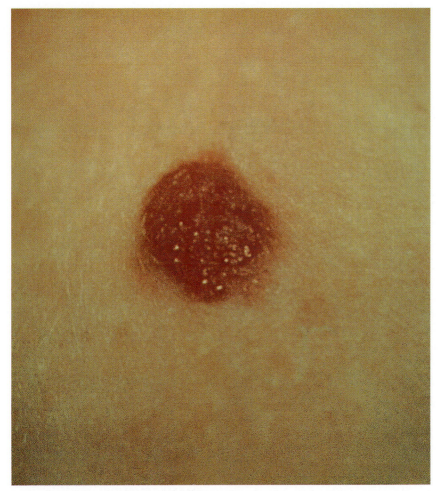

Figure 7-9 Spitz nevus *A 1-cm raised red dome-shaped nodule that suddenly appeared on the shoulder of a child.*

EPIDERMAL MELANOCYTIC DISORDERS

EPHELIDES

Ephelides (freckles) are light-brown macules that occur on sun-exposed skin most frequently observed in light-skinned individuals.

Synonym Freckles.

EPIDEMIOLOGY

Age Ephelides accumulate over childhood years of sun exposure and gradually fade with age.

Gender M = F.

Season Increase in size, number, and degree of pigmentation during summer Decrease in winter.

Etiology Related to sun exposure. May be autosomal dominantly inherited. Linked with light skin color and red or blond hair.

PATHOPHYSIOLOGY

It is thought that sun exposure stimulates the melanocytes to focally produce more melanin.

PHYSICAL EXAMINATION

Skin Findings

Type 3- to 5-mm macules.

Color Light-brown to brown.

Shape Round to stellate.

Distribution Sun-exposed skin.

Sites of Predilection Nose, cheeks, chest, shoulders, arms, and upper back (Fig. 7-10).

LABORATORY EXAMINATIONS

Dermatopathology Normal number of melanocytes but increased production of melanin.

Wood's Lamp May accentuate and reveal more freckling.

DIAGNOSIS

The diagnosis of ephelides is made clinically. When extensive ephelides are seen in persons with dark hair, xeroderma pigmentosum (XP), or a heterozygous carrier for XP should be considered. Ephelides (freckles) differ from lentigines in that lentigines do not darken with sun exposure.

COURSE AND PROGNOSIS

Mild sun-induced ephelides are benign (unless associated with XP) and tend to disappear with age. Severe sunburn-induced freckles (from a blistering sunburn) are typically more stellate in shape and permanent.

MANAGEMENT

Ephelides fade with time and do not require treatment. Avoidance of sun exposure or good sunscreen application will prevent further ephelides from developing. Cosmetically, ephelides can be masked by cover-up make-up, lightened with chemical peels and/or hydroquinone (Melanex). They can also be removed by laser.

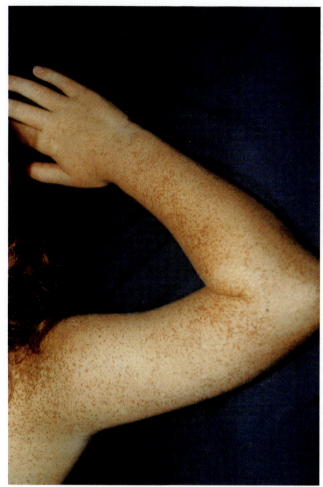

Figure 7-10   Ephelides   *Numerous red-brown freckles on the arms of a redheaded child.*

LENTIGO SIMPLEX AND LENTIGINES-ASSOCIATED SYNDROMES

Lentigines are small (< 1.0 cm) circumscribed brown macular lesions with increased numbers of melanocytes (which distinguishes them from ephelides). There are also several syndromes characterized by lentiginosis (Table 7-1).

EPIDEMIOLOGY

See Table 7-1.

PHYSICAL EXAMINATION

Skin Findings

Type   Macules < 1 cm (Fig. 7-11).

Color   Brown to dark-brown, variegated to uniformly colored.

Shape   Round to stellate.

Distribution   Isolated lesions may be found in sun-exposed areas or as multiple lesions on any cutaneous surface including palms and soles.

DIFFERENTIAL DIAGNOSIS

The diagnosis of lentigines is made by clinical exam. Lentigines can be difficult to distinguish from ephelides. Lentigines differ from ephelides (freckles) in that lentigines do not darken with sun exposure.

LABORATORY EXAMINATIONS

Dermatopathology   Increased number of melanocytes along the dermal–epidermal junction and elongation of the rete ridges.

Wood's Lamp   May accentuates and reveal more lentigines.

COURSE AND PROGNOSIS

Lentigines, as an isolated finding, are benign and asymptomatic. Their presence may be a marker of a more systemic lentiginosis syndrome. Typically, the pigmented macules are present at or near birth, increase in number during puberty, and may fade slightly in adulthood.

MANAGEMENT

Lentigines are benign and do not require treatment. Cosmetically, lentigines can be masked by cover-up makeup, lightened with chemical peels and/or hydroquinone (Melanex). They can also be removed by laser.

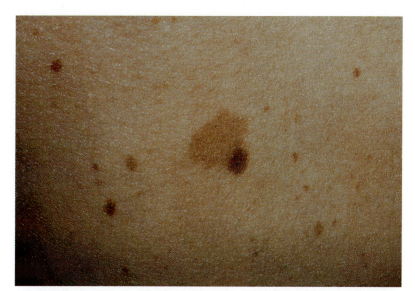

Figure 7-11 **Lentigines** *Scattered brown macular spots on the back of a child with multiple lentigines (LEOPARD) syndrome.*

Table 7-1 LENTIGINOUS SYNDROMES

Disorder	Synonyms	Age	Etiology	Cutaneous Findings	Associated Features
Eruptive lentiginosis		Adolescents and young adults		Widespread occurrence of several hundred lentigines over months to years	
Segmental lentiginosis				Lentigines confined to one side of the body	Dermatomal type: benign Nondermatomal type may be associated with CNS abnormality
Nevus spilus	Nevoid lentigo	Infancy or childhood		Macular café-au-lait background with overlying 1–3 mm more deeply pigmented spots	Typically benign. Rare malignant transformation into melanomas have been reported
PUVA lentigines			PUVA treatments	Disseminated hyperpigmented macules	Occur in 10–40% of PUVA patients
Inherited patterned lentiginosis in blacks		Infancy or early childhood	AD inherited	Lentiginosis of face, lips, extremities, buttocks, and palmoplantar surfaces	
Multiple lentigines syndrome	LEOPARD syndrome, Moynahan syndrome, Gorlin syndrome	Infancy and evolve until adulthood	AD inherited	Multiple lentigines especially on upper trunk and neck. Mucosal surfaces spared	L = Lentigines E = EKG abnormalities O = Ocular hypertelorism P = Pulmonary stenosis A = Abnormal genitalia R = Retardation of growth D = Deafness
LAMB and NAME syndromes	Syndrome myxoma, Carney syndrome	Childhood	AD inherited	Multiple lentigines; ephelides, blue nevi, mucocutaneous myxoma	L = Lentigines A = Atrial myxoma M = Mucocutaneous myxoma B = Blue nevi N = Nevi A = Atrial myxoma M = Mucocutaneous myxoma E = Ephelides

Table 7-1 (Continued)

Disorder	Synonyms	Age	Etiology	Cutaneous Findings	Associated Features
Peutz–Jeghers syndrome	Periorificial lentiginosis	Infancy and early childhood	AD inherited	Brown-black macules around mouth, lips, buccal mucosa, hands, and feet	Jejunal polyposis, increased risk of GI and non-GI malignancies
Cronkhite–Canada syndrome				Brown macules on face and extremities. Alopecia and dystrophic nail changes	GI polyposis
Tay's syndrome			AD inherited	Multiple lentigines, vitiligo, café-au-lait macules and canities	Growth retardation, MR, cirrhosis, hypersplenism, multiple skeletal defects
Soto's syndrome				Lentigines of the penile shaft and glans penis	Macrocephaly, unusual facies, skeletal abnormalities
Centrofacial neurodysraphic lentiginosis	Lentiginosis centrofaciale	Lesions appear at age 1–10	AD inherited	Closely clustered lentigines on the nose and infraorbital areas; mucous membranes spared	Status dysraphicus, neuropsychiatric disorder, epilepsy

PEUTZ–JEGHERS SYNDROME

Peutz–Jeghers syndrome is a rare autosomal dominantly inherited disorder characterized by familial polyposis and lentigines on the lips and oral mucous membranes. Polyps in the GI tract may occur, with abdominal symptoms manifesting in childhood or early adulthood.

EPIDEMIOLOGY

Age   Lentigines appear in infancy and early childhood. GI polyps appear in late childhood, before age 30.

Gender   M = F.

Genetics   Autosomal dominant with 100% penetrance and variable expressivity; > 40% of cases are due to spontaneous mutations.

Etiology   Unclear.

HISTORY

The lentigines can be congenital or may develop during infancy and early childhood. The pigmented macules may disappear over time on the lips, but the pigmentation of the mouth does not disappear and is therefore the sine qua non for the diagnosis. The lentigines occur in some patients who never have abdominal symptoms.

Systems Review   Abdominal pain can present anytime between ages 10 and 30. GI bleeding, melena, hematemesis, and anemia may also occur. The small bowel is most often affected, but large bowel, stomach, and esophageal polyps may also occur.

PHYSICAL EXAMINATION

Skin Findings

Type   Macule.

Color   Dark brown or black.

Size   2 to 5.0 mm. Lentigines on the face are smaller than those on the palms and soles and in the mouth.

Shape of Individual Lesion   Round or oval.

Arrangement of Multiple Lesions   Closely set clusters of lesions.

Distribution of Lesions   The lesions occur on the lips (especially the lower lip), around the mouth, bridge of the nose, palms, soles, and dorsa of hands.

General Findings

Intraoral lentigines are the sine qua non of Peutz–Jeghers syndrome; the lesions are dark brown, black, or bluish-black. They are irregularly distributed on the gums, buccal mucosa, and hard palate (Fig. 7-12).

Nails

May have pigmented streaks or diffuse involvement of the nail bed.

GI Tract

Polyps, which may lead to abdominal pain, GI bleeds, intussusception, and obstruction.

LABORATORY EXAMINATIONS

Dermatopathology   On skin biopsy, there is increased melanin in the melanocytes and basal cells.

Electron Microscopy   Numerous melanosomes with melanocytes, but few within the keratinocytes.

Pathology of GI Polyps   Hamartomas, with mixture of glands and smooth muscle.

Hematologic   Anemia from blood loss may be present.

Gastroenterology   Stool examinations may reveal occult bleeding.

Radiologic Studies   Imaging of the GI tract is important in patients with the clinical presentation of multiple lentigines of the type noted earlier.

DIFFERENTIAL DIAGNOSIS

In Peutz–Jeghers syndrome the mucosal pigmentation (intraorally) is the constant feature that remains throughout life. The differential diagnosis for mucosal hyperpigmentation includes normal mucosal pigmentation in darker skin types, amalgam tattoos, and staining from zidovudine therapy. The lentigines of Peutz–Jeghers can be differentiated from ephelides by

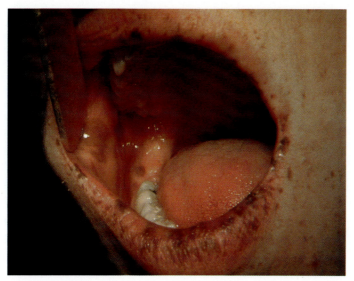

Figure 7-12   Peutz–Jeghers syndrome   *Scattered dark brown macules on the lips and buccal mucosa of a child with Peutz-Jeghers syndrome. The pigmented macules on the lips may fade with time, but the intraoral pigmentation persists for life.*

being much darker and occurring in areas not exposed to sunlight (e.g., palms, soles). Also the lentigines are not widely distributed as in the multiple lentigines syndrome (LEOPARD syndrome); they do not occur on the trunk or extremities, but are localized to the central areas of the face, palms and soles, and dorsa of the hands.

COURSE AND PROGNOSIS

There is a normal life expectancy. Symptomatic GI polyps are the most difficult aspect of this syndrome and may require multiple polypectomies to relieve the symptoms. There is also an increased risk of developing gastrointestinal and pancreatic carcinoma.

MANAGEMENT

Skin   Lentigines are benign and do not require treatment. Cosmetically, lentigines can be masked by cover-up makeup, lightened with chemical peels and/or hydroquinone (Melanex). They can also be removed by laser.

Other   It is recommended that patients with Peutz–Jeghers syndrome have:

1. Hematocrit checked every 6 months for anemia.
2. Stool exam annually looking for occult blood.
3. Routine examinations with a gastroenterologist and appropriate GI studies (for patients > 10 years old, small bowel follow-through examinations, upper endoscopies, and colonoscopies every 2 years).
4. Surgical polypectomies for symptomatic or large (> 1.5 cm) GI polyps.

MULTIPLE LENTIGINES SYNDROME

The multiple lentigines syndrome is a multiorgan genodermatosis commonly referred to by its mnemonic: LEOPARD syndrome. Its principal visible manifestation is generalized lentigines (dark brown macules). The seven features in the mnemonic are L (lentigines), E (EKG abnormalities), O (ocular hypertelorism), P (pulmonary stenosis), A (abnormal genitalia), R (retardation of growth or dwarfism), D (deafness).

Synonyms Multiple lentigines syndrome, cardiocutaneous syndrome, hypertrophic obstructive cardiomyopathy and lentiginosis, lentiginosis profusa syndrome, progressive cardiomyopathic lentiginosis, Moynahan syndrome, Gorlin syndrome.

EPIDEMIOLOGY

Age Lentigines usually present at birth. Extracutanous features do not appear until puberty. Mean age of diagnosis: 14 years.

Gender M > F.

Incidence Rare.

Genetics Autosomal dominant inheritance with variable expressivity.

Etiology Unclear.

HISTORY

The lentigines are often congenital and increase in number, size, and darkness around puberty. They then begin to fade slowly throughout adulthood. Extracutaneous feature are usually not manifested until puberty and include pulmonary stenosis, obstructive cardiomyopathy, atrial septal defects, primary pulmonary hypertension, pectus deformities, kyphoscoliosis, hypospadias, cryptorchidism, mental retardation, and sensorineural hearing loss. Cardiac abnormalities result in the greatest morbidity associated with the syndrome.

PHYSICAL EXAMINATION

Skin Findings

Type Numerous well-demarcated macules.

Size 1 to 5 mm.

Color Tan, brown, or black.

Shape Round or oval.

Distribution Lentigines are concentrated on the face (Fig. 7-13A), neck, and upper trunk

(Fig. 7-13B) but may also involve the arms, palms, soles, and genitalia. Mucous membranes are spared.

General Findings

Skeletal Growth retardation (< 25th percentile), hypertelorism, pectus deformities, kyphoscoliosis, and winged scapulae.

Cardiopulmonary Includes pulmonary stenosis and conduction defects.

Genitourinary Gonad hypoplasia, renal agenesis.

Neurologic Sensorineural deafness, abnormal EEG, slowed peripheral nerve conduction.

LABORATORY EXAMINATIONS

Dermatopathology On skin biopsy, there is increased melanin in the melanocytes and basal cells.

DIFFERENTIAL DIAGNOSIS

Other lentiginous syndromes such as Peutz–Jeghers should be considered. The multiple lentigines syndrome typically has facial lentigines with sparing of the mucous membranes whereas Peutz-Jeghers syndrome has marked intraoral involvement. Other lentigines syndromes and their features are listed in Table 7-1.

COURSE AND PROGNOSIS

The skeletal, cardiac, and endocrine abnormalities are the most problematic. The lentigines are only of cosmetic concern and can get darker, larger, and more numerous with age.

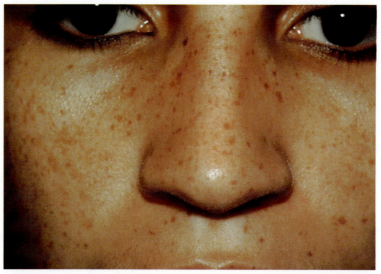

A

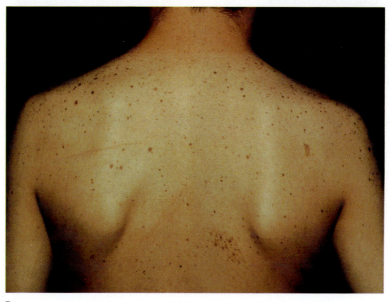

B

Figure 7-13 Multiple lentigines syndrome *(A) Scattered brown macules on the face of an individual with the multiple lentigines syndrome. (B) Scattered brown macules on the back of an individual with multiple lentigines syndrome.*

MANAGEMENT

Lentigines do not require treatment. Cosmetically, lentigines can be masked by cover-up makeup, lightened with chemical peels and/or hydroquinone (Melanex). They can also be removed by laser.

CAFÉ AU LAIT MACULES AND ASSOCIATED SYNDROMES

Café au lait macules (CALM) are large, round, well-circumscribed, light-brown patches that range in size from 1.0 to 2.0 cm. One to three CALM are seen in 10 to 28% of normal individuals, but more than three CALM may be a sign of more severe disease such as neurofibromatosis (Table 7-2).

EPIDEMIOLOGY

Age Present at birth or soon after. Can increase in size and number with age.

Gender M = F.

Prevalence Very common. Present in 10 to 28% of the normal population.

Etilogy Unclear.

PHYSICAL EXAMINATION

Skin Findings

Type Macule to patch.

Color 1.0 cm (sometimes smaller) to 15 to 20 cm (Fig. 7-14).

Shape Round to oval.

Distribution May occur anywhere on the body.

General Findings

One to three CALM are common in normal individuals, but more than three CALM can be a sign of a neurocutaneous disease such as neurofibromatosis, tuberous sclerosis, Albright's syndrome (polyostotic fibrous dysplasia), ataxia telangiectasia, Silver's syndrome, basal cell nevus syndrome, Turner's syndrome, or Cowden's disease.

LABORATORY EXAMINATIONS

Dermatopathology Increase in basal layer pigmentation with giant pigment granules in both the melanocytes and keratinocytes. Giant macromelanosomes (up to 5 µl in diameter) are usually present.

Wood's Lamp May accentuate and reveal CALM unapparent to visible light.

MANAGEMENT

CALM are asymptomatic and do not require treatment. Cosmetically, CALM can be masked by cover-up makeup, lightened with chemical peels and/or hydroquinone (Melanex). They can also be removed by laser.

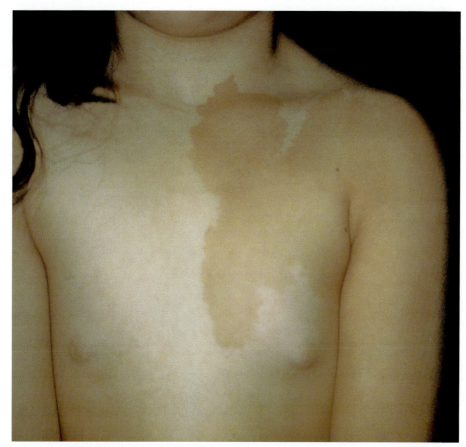

Figure 7-14 Café au lait macule (CALM)   *Large brown macule with irregular "coast of Maine" jagged borders in a girl with Albright syndrome.*

Table 7-2 CAFÉ AU LAIT MACULES AND ASSOCIATED SYNDROMES

Disorder	Synonyms	Cutaneous Findings	Associated Features
Neurofibromatosis type 1 (NF-1)	Von Recklinghausen's disease	CALM, axillary/intertriginous freckling, cutaneous neurofibromas, peripheral nerve sheath tumors, large congenital nevi, xanthogranulomas	Lisch nodules, optic gliomas, macrocephaly, CNS tumors, seizures, kyphoscoliosis, sphenoid wing dysplasia, thinning of ribs, bowing deformity of the tibia and ulna, pseudoarthroses
Watson syndrome	? Variant of NF-1	CALM, intertriginous freckling	Intellectual deficit, short stature, pulmonary valve stenosis
Neurofibromatosis type 2 (NF-2)	Central neurofibromatosis	CALM may occur, few or absent neurofibromas	Acoustic neuromas, intracranial and intraspinal tumors, lens opacities
Neurofibromatosis type 5 (NF-5)	Segmental neurofibromatosis	CALM, intertriginous freckling, neurofibromas in a segmental distribution	Deeper involvement within the involved body segment (bony or soft-tissue growths)
Neurofibromatosis type 6 (NF-6)	Familial café-au-lait macules	CALM, intertriginous freckling	Rarely skeletal or learning abnormalities, Lisch nodules
Albright syndrome	Polyostotic fibrous dysplasia, McCune–Albright syndrome	CALM with more jagged "coast of Maine" borders (Fig. 7-14)	Polyostotic fibrous dysplasia, endocrine dysfunction, sexual precocity
Jaffe–Campanacci syndrome		CALM with more jagged "coast of Maine" borders, nevi, perioral freckle-like macules	Nonossifying fibromas, mental retardation, hypogonadism, precocious puberty; ocular, skeletal, and cardiac abnormalities
Piebaldism		CALM, congenital depigmented patches	Rarely mental retardation, aganglionic megacolon, Hirschsprung disease
Westerhof syndrome		CALM, hypopigmented macules	Mild mental retardation, short stature, skeletal abnormalities
CALM, temporal dysrhythmia, and emotional instability		CALM	Headaches, depression, memory loss, syncope, temporal lobe abnormalities, cortical atrophy
Tuberous sclerosis	Epiloa, Bourneville disease	CALM, hypomelanotic macules, adenoma sebaceum, periungal fibromas, Shagreen patches	Seizures, mental retardation, rhabdomyomas, calcified brain nodules

Table 7-2   (Continued)

Disorder	Synonyms	Cutaneous Findings	Associated Features
Ataxia telangiectasia	Louis–Bar syndrome	CALM, telangiectasia of conjunctiva, neck: hyper- and hypopigmentation	Ataxia, myoclonus, choreoathetosis, impaired cell-mediated and humoral immunity
Silver–Russell syndrome	Russell–Silver syndrome	CALM, diffuse brown patches, achromic macules may be present	IUGR, macrocephaly, triangular facies, ambiguous genitalia, clinodactyly, hyperhidrosis
Bloom syndrome		CALM, photosensitivity, telangiectatic rash	Stunted growth, dolicocephaly, high-pitched voice, testicular atrophy, immune deficiencies
Multiple endocrine neoplasia type III (MEN-3)	MEN type IIb	CALM; multiple mucosal neuromas on lips, oral cavity, and eyelids; abnormal pigmentation	Marfanoid habitus, thickened corneal nerves, GI ganglioneuromatosis, pheochromocytoma, medullary throid carcinoma
Turner's syndrome	Gonadal dysgenesis, XO syndrome	CALM, epicanthal folds, hypertelorism, webbed neck, redundant neck skin, lymphedema, alopecia areata	Short stature, deafness, gonadal dysgenesis (with sexual retardation), bicuspid aortic valve, PDA, coarctation of aorta, renal abnormalities
Cowden's disease	Multiple hamartoma syndrome	CALM, multiple trichilemmomas, oral papillomatosis, acral keratoses	Breast cysts/malignancy, thyroid malignancies, GI polyps, ovarian cysts, uterus adenocarcinomas

DERMAL MELANOCYTIC DISORDERS

MONGOLIAN SPOT

Mongolian spots are benign, congenital, blue-black large macular lesions characteristically located over the lumbosacral area. Most commonly seen in Asian, black, and Hispanic populations.

EPIDEMIOLOGY

Age   Present at birth and fades during first 1 to 2 years of life.

Gender   M = F.

Race   Seen in > 80% of Asian infants, 60 to 95% of black infants, 85% of South American Indian infants, 63% of Indian infants, 46% of Hispanic infants and < 13% of white infants.

Etiology   Dermal location of melanocytes results in blue-gray appearance to the skin (Tyndall's effect).

PATHOPHYSIOLOGY

Melanocytes undergo embryonic migration from the neural crest to the epidermis. It is thought that these lesions represent migrational arrest with resultant ectopic melanocytes in the dermis.

HISTORY

Mongolian spots develop in utero and are most noticeable at birth. They are asymptomatic, benign, and darken in color until age 1 year, enlarge in size until age 2 years, and then spontaneously disappear by age 10 to 12 years. Only 3 to 4% of Mongolian spots persist for life. No melanomas have been reported to occur.

PHYSICAL EXAMINATION

Skin Findings

Type   Poorly circumscribed macule to patch.

Color   Deep brown, slate gray to blue-black.

Size   Ranges from 1 cm to extensive areas (85% of cases occupy < 5% of the body and only 5% involve > 15% of the body surface area).

Number   Typically single lesion, rarely multiple.

Distribution   Anywhere especially buttock, back, shoulders.

Sites of Predilection   Lumbosacral region (Fig. 7-15).

General Findings

Infant is otherwise well.

DIFFERENTIAL DIAGNOSIS

Mongolian spots are sometimes mistaken for ecchymoses, but the areas are nontender. Diagnosis is made on clinical presentation.

LABORATORY EXAMINATIONS

Dermatopathology on skin biopsy: Elongated spindle-shaped melanocytes are present in the mid- to deep dermis.

MANAGEMENT

Treatment is unnecessary because these lesions tend to fade by age 10 to 12 in the majority of individuals. Mongolian spots persist in only 3 to 4% of the population. Cosmetically, laser removal of the lesion is possible.

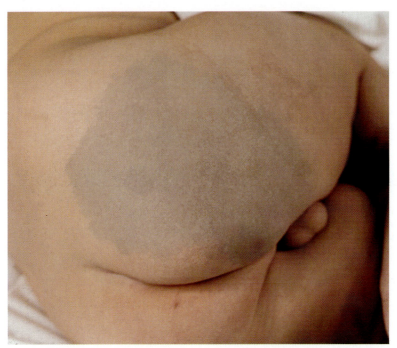

Figure 7-15 Mongolian spot *Asymptomatic macular blue-gray pigmentation on the buttock of an infant.* (Reproduced with permission from TB Fitzpatrick et al., Color Atlas and Synopsis of Clinical Dermatology, 4th edition. New York: McGraw-Hill, 2001).

NEVUS OF OTA, NEVUS OF ITO

The nevus of Ota is a unilateral bluish gray macular discoloration in the periorbital region (trigeminal nerve, first and second branches). The nevus of Ito is a similar blue-gray discoloration located on the neck and shoulder.

Synonyms Nevus fuscocaeruleus ophthalmomaxillaris and nevus fuscocaeruleus acromiodeltoideus.

EPIDEMIOLOGY

Age Bimodal age distribution: 50% are present at birth or in the first year of life, 36% appear between the ages of 11 and 20 years old.

Gender F > M, 5:1.

Race More prevalent in Asians (75% of cases); less commonly seen in East Indians and blacks; and rarely seen in whites.

Incidence Uncommon.

Prevalence Primary complaint in 0.4% of outpatient visits in Japan.

Etiology Dermal location of melanocytes results in blue-gray appearance of the skin (Tyndall effect).

PATHOPHYSIOLOGY

During embryonic development, melanocytes migrate from the neural crest to the epidermis. It is thought that the nevus of Ota and nevus of Ito represent melanocytes that have experienced migrational arrest in the dermis. Some have speculated that there is a hormonal influence as well, accounting for the lesions that appear at puberty and the female predominance. Trauma has also been reported as a triggering mechanism.

HISTORY

Nevi of Ota/Ito are sometimes present at birth, or can appear during childhood/puberty. They may increase in intensity and extent during the first year of life. They persist for life. Most nevi of Ota/Ito are benign. There are rare reports of sensorineural deafness and melanoma associated with these lesions.

PHYSICAL EXAMINATION

Skin Findings

Type Poorly demarcated macules to patches with speckled or mottled appearance.

Color Patchy blue-gray, blue-black.

Size 1-10 cm.

Distribution Ota: Typically unilateral, periorbital region, can involve sclera (Fig. 7-16). 50% of cases involve the ophthalmic and maxillary branches of the fifth cranial nerve. Rarely, pigmentation can also involve conjunctiva, cornea, retina, lips, palate, pharynx, or nasal mucosa. Ito: Typically unilateral neck/shoulder region in the distribution of the posterior supraclavicular and lateral cutaneous nerves. In < 5% of cases, these nevi can be bilateral. They may also coexist in the same patient.

General Findings

Most nevi of Ota and Ito are seen as an isolated cutaneous findings; 9% of congenital nevus of Ota is associated with open-angle glaucoma. Other rare associations include cellular blue nevi, nevus flammeus (phakomatosis pigmentavascularis), and malignant melanoma.

DIFFERENTIAL DIAGNOSIS

Nevi of Ito and Ota are sometimes mistaken for ecchymoses, but the areas are nontender. The diagnosis is made on clinical presentation.

LABORATORY EXAMINATIONS

Dermatopathology Skin biopsy demonstrates elongated dendritic melanocytes in the mid- to deep dermis.

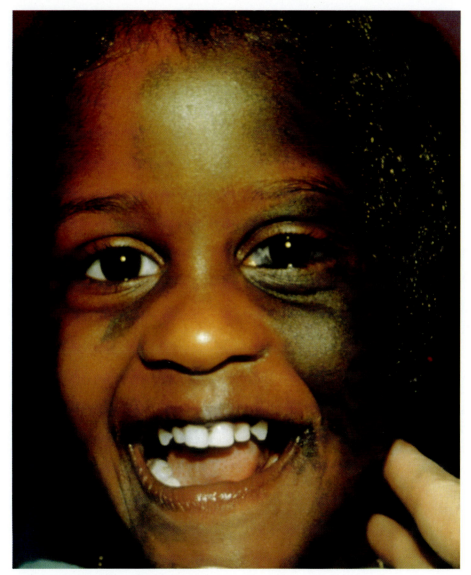

Figure 7-16 **Nevus of Ota** *Periorbital blue-gray pigmentation with scleral involvement.*

MANAGEMENT

Nevi of Ota and Ito do not require treatment. Cosmetically, they can be masked by cover-up makeup. They can also be removed by dermabrasion and laser. Because of their risk of malignancy, these nevi should be followed annually. If ocular pigmentation is present, routine ophthalmologic examination is recommended.

DISORDERS OF BLOOD AND LYMPH VESSELS

CONGENITAL VASCULAR LESIONS

SALMON PATCH

The salmon patch is the most common benign vascular lesion seen in infants, typically on the forehead, glabella, or nape of neck.

Synonyms Nevus simplex, telangiectatic nevus, "stork bite," nuchal nevus, Unna's nevus.

EPIDEMIOLOGY

Age Present at birth, fades with time.

Gender M = F.

Incidence Occurs in 30 to 40% of newborns.

Etiology Thought to be a persistence of fetal circulation.

HISTORY

Present at birth, these benign lesions fade with time. In lighter skin types, the patch may be more persistent or evident during episodes of crying or physical exertion. Fifty percent of salmon patches in the nuchal region persist for life. They are asymptomatic and benign.

PHYSICAL EXAMINATION

Skin Findings

Type Macular with telangiectasias.

Color Dull pink to red.

Distribution Head and neck.

Sites of Predilection Nape of neck (22%), glabella (20%, Fig. 8-1A), and eyelids (5%).

DIFFERENTIAL DIAGNOSIS

Salmon patch is the most common vascular birthmark. Its classic locations and self-resolving tendencies should differentiate it from other vascular birthmarks such as port-wine stains and hemangiomas.

LABORATORY EXAMINATIONS

Histopathology Skin biopsy reveals dilated dermal capillaries.

COURSE AND PROGNOSIS

Facial salmon patches fade with time (Fig. 8-1B) and only become evident in lighter skin types with crying or physical exertion. Nuchal salmon patches can persist but are asymptomatic and not usually of cosmetic concern because they are covered by the posterior hairline.

MANAGEMENT

Unlike port-wine stains, facial salmon patches fade almost completely and usually do not require treatment. Persistent lesions can occur in

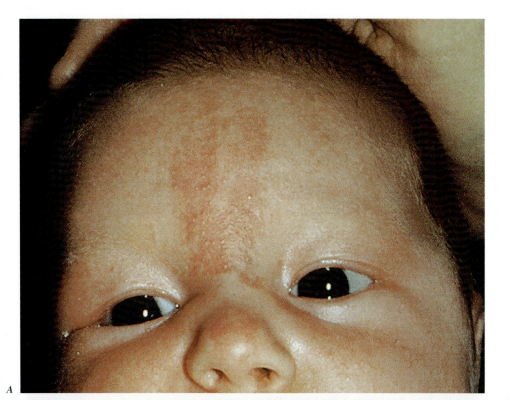

A

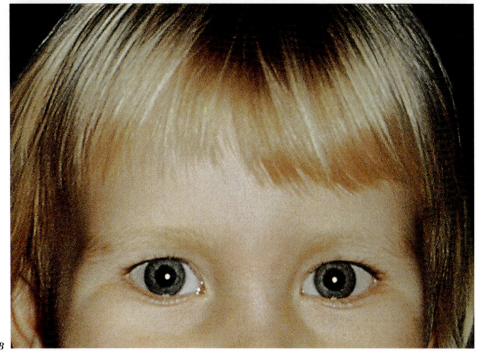

B

Figure 8-1 Salmon patch *(A) Salmon patch on the glabella of a newborn. (B) Same child at age 3 with no residual vascular lesion.*

the nuchal area, but these are typically covered with hair and not a cosmetic concern. Rare bothersome persistent lesions can be treated with laser ablation.

PORT-WINE STAIN AND ASSOCIATED SYNDROMES

A port-wine stain (PWS) is a macular vascular stain comprised of dilated blood vessels. It is present at birth, and unlike salmon patches, it persists for life. The lesions commonly involve the face and are typically benign but may be associated with other syndromes (Table 8-1).

Synonym Nevus flammeus.

EPIDEMIOLOGY

Age Present at birth, persists throughout life.

Gender M = F.

Etiology Dilated dermal capillaries.

PATHOPHYSIOLOGY

Port-wine stains are comprised of ectatic dermal capillaries thought to be due to localized neural or structural abnormalities.

HISTORY

Port-wine stains are present at birth, and grow proportionally and asymptomatically with the child. In adulthood, the blood vessels become more dilated and may form a more papular/nodular appearance.

PHYSICAL EXAMINATION

Skin Lesions

Type In infancy and childhood, PWS are macular. With increasing age of the patient, papules or nodules often develop, leading to significant disfigurement.

Color Pink to purple.

Shape Irregular. Large lesions follow a dermatomal distribution and rarely cross the midline.

Distribution Most commonly involve the face, but may occur at any cutaneous site (Fig. 8-2A).

DIFFERENTIAL DIAGNOSIS

The differential diagnosis of a port-wine stain includes a hemangioma, salmon patch, or other vascular malformation.

LABORATORY EXAMINATIONS

Histopathology Skin biopsy shows dilation of superficial capillaries. No proliferation of endothelial cells is noted.

COURSE AND PROGNOSIS

PWS do not regress spontaneously. The area of involvement tends to increase in proportion to the size of the child. In adulthood, PWS can become raised with papular and nodular areas, which leads to more severe cosmetic disfigurement. The majority of port-wine stains have no associated abnormalities. Others are associated with other abnormalities, as can be seen in Sturge–Weber syndrome (Fig. 8-2B), Klippel–Trenaunay syndrome, Parkes–Weber syndrome, and Cobb syndrome.

MANAGEMENT

PWS can be covered with waterproof cosmetics (Covermark, Dermablend). Treatment with lasers is very effective and should be considered in childhood before the lesion progresses to a more severe nodular, disfiguring form.

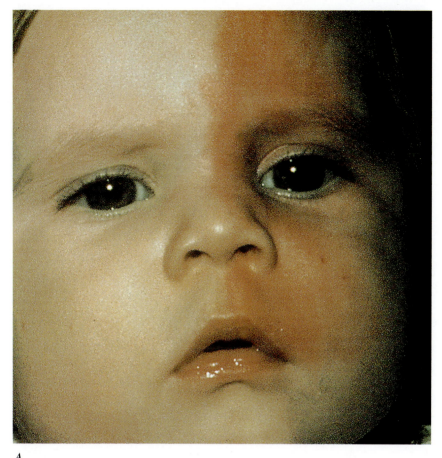

A

Figure 8-2   Port-wine stain   *(A) Macular vascular port-wine stain on the face of an infant.*

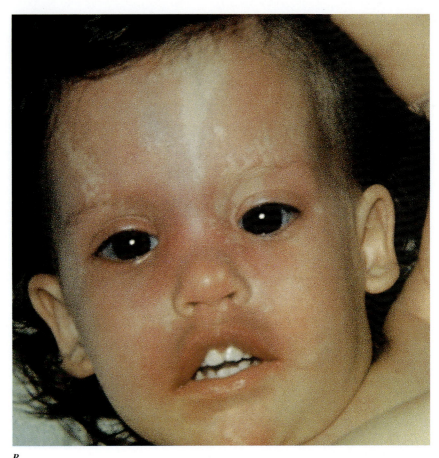

B

Figure 8-2 (continued)   Port-wine stain   *(B) Facial port-wine stain in a child with Sturge-Weber syndrome.*

Table 8-1 PORT-WINE STAINS AND ASSOCIATED SYNDROMES

Syndrome	Synonyms	Cutaneous Findings	Associated Features
Sturge–Weber syndrome	Encephalofacial angiomatosis	V1/V2 port-wine stain, can have oral telangiectatic hypertrophy	Vascular malformation of ipsilateral meninges and cerebrum, intracranial calcifications, seizures, hemiplegia, glaucoma, mental retardation
Klippel–Trenaunay syndrome	Nevus vasculosus hypertrophicus	PWS over a limb (leg much more commonly than arm), hemangiomas, varicosities	Associated limb hypertrophy
Parkes–Weber syndrome		PWS over a limb (leg more commonly than arm), hemangiomas, varicosities	Associated limb hypertrophy and AV fistulas
Cobb syndrome	Cutaneous–meningospinal angiomatosis	Cutaneous vascular nevus (PWS, hemangioma, angiolipoma, or angiokeratoma)	Angioma in the spinal cord causing pain, weakness, limb atrophy, paraplegia, and kyphoscoliosis

HEMANGIOMAS AND ASSOCIATED SYNDROMES

Hemangiomas are benign, vascular proliferations that rapidly enlarge during the first year of life and spontaneously involute by age 2 to 3 years. Superficial hemangiomas have a bright red, nodular surface and have been called strawberry hemangiomas. Deeper purple lesions are referred to as cavernous hemangiomas. Numerous hemangiomas may also be associated with more extensive malformation (Table 8-2).

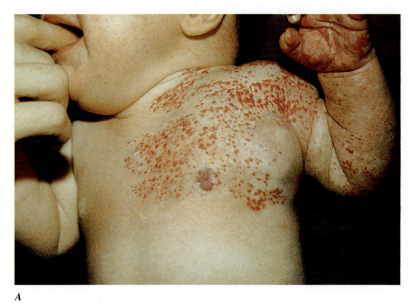

A

Figure 8-3   Hemangioma, infancy   *(A) A 10-week-old infant with a vascular lesion noted at birth.*

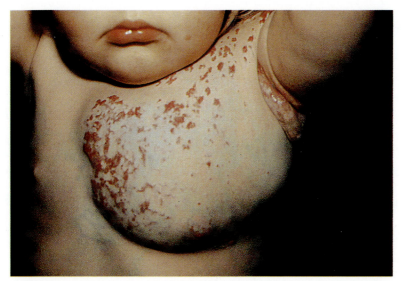

B

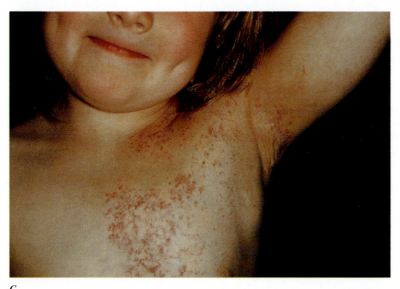

C

Figure 8-3 (continued) Hemangioma, age 1 *(B) Same child 1 year later with a fully proliferated hemangioma.* **Hemangioma, age 3** *(C) Same child 3 years later with an involuting hemangioma.*

EPIDEMIOLOGY

Age   Present at birth or onset in infancy.

Gender   F > M.

Prevalence   Seen more in premature infants (< 30 weeks gestational age or birthweight < 1500 g).

Incidence   2.6% of all newborns.

Etiology   Unclear.

PATHOPHYSIOLOGY

Hemangiomas are localized proliferations of blood vessels. Extensive study is underway to understand the signaling mechanisms that cause this benign tumor to grow, plateau, and then spontaneously involute.

HISTORY

Lesions present at or soon after birth (Fig. 8-3A), proliferate for the first year of life (Fig. 8-3B), and then spontaneously involute by age 2 to 3 years (Fig. 8-3C). Lesions are asymptomatic and benign. Complications include bleeding from trauma or ulceration; hemangiomas located near facial structures or genitourinary tract can cause obstructions. Rarely, hemangiomas can be associated with internal abnormalities. Multiple hemangiomas can be associated with hemangiomas of the CNS, GI tract, and liver.

PHYSICAL EXAMINATION

Skin Findings

Type   Nodule.

Color   Superficial lesions are pink to red; deeper lesions are blue-purple. With involution, the surface of the lesion turns white/gray and may ulcerate.

Size   Average 2 to 5 cm but can grow up to 20 cm in size.

Palpation   Superficial lesions are soft/compressible; deeper lesions are more firm.

Sites of Predilection   Face, trunk, legs, oral and genital mucous membranes.

DIFFERENTIAL DIAGNOSIS

Hemangiomas are sometimes confused with other vascular abnormalities such as port-wine stains, salmon patches, and AV malformations. Deeper lesions can mimic dermal or subcutaneous masses. The characteristic proliferative and involuting phase can clinically differentiate hemangiomas from other vascular lesions.

LABORATORY EXAMINATIONS

Histopathology   Skin biopsy of proliferating lesion would reveal numerous blood vessels. Proliferation may be capillary, subcutaneous venous, or lymphatic.

COURSE AND PROGNOSIS

Hemangiomas typically involute by age 2 to 3 years. Rarely, lesions can persist up until age 10. The residual skin changes are barely detectable but can include: skin atrophy or depigmentation. Typical spontaneous involution leaves the best cosmetic results, and thus nonintervention in uncomplicated lesions is recommended.

Numerous hemangiomas with internal involvement can lead to systemic problems. A child with numerous cutaneous hemangiomas should be evaluated for the possibility of hemangiomas of the visceral organs, GI tract, liver, CNS, or lungs.

MANAGEMENT

Treatment for the majority of lesions is unnecessary because they are asymptomatic and self-resolve with a good cosmetic result. Less than 2% of hemangiomas require intervention (for ulceration/bleeding, blocking facial structures or GI/GU tracts). These can be treated with intralesional steroids, systemic steroids, pulsed-dye laser, cryotherapy, alpha-IFN, surgery, or embolization.

Table 8-2   HEMANGIOMAS AND ASSOCIATED SYNDROMES

Disorder	Synonyms	Cutaneous Findings	Associated Features
Maffucci's syndrome	Dyschondroplasia with hemangiomas	Hemangiomas, phlebectasias, lymphangiomas	Dyschondroplasia, bony and neurologic defects
Blue-rubber-bleb syndrome		Diffuse painful hemangiomas	Angiomas of GI tract
Diffuse neonatal hemangiomatosis		Hemangiomas	Hemangiomas of GI tract, liver, CNS, lungs
Cobb syndrome	Cutaneous meningospinal angiomatosis	Hemangioma, PWS, or angiokeratoma	Angioma of spinal cord

BENIGN VASCULAR PROLIFERATIONS

SPIDER ANGIOMA

A spider angioma is a localized area of dilated capillaries, radiating from a central arteriole, occurring in healthy children.

Synonyms   Nevus araneus, spider nevus, arterial spider, spider telangiectasia, vascular spider.

EPIDEMIOLOGY

Age   Young childhood and early adulthood.

Gender   F > M.

Incidence   May occur in up to 15% of normal individuals.

Etiology   Typically idiopathic, may be associated with hyperestrogen states such as pregnancy or estrogen therapy (e.g., oral contraceptive) or hepatocellular disease (such as subacute and chronic viral hepatitis and alcoholic cirrhosis).

PHYSICAL EXAMINATION

Skin Findings

Type   Central punctum (macular or papular) at the site of the feeding arteriole with radiating telangiectatic vessels (legs); up to 1.5 cm in diameter. Usually solitary (Fig. 8-4).

Color   Red.

Shape   Round to oval.

Palpation   On diascopy, radiating telangiectasia blanches and central arteriole may pulsate.

Sites of Predilection   Face, upper trunk, arms, hands, fingers, and mucous membranes of lip or nose.

DIFFERENTIAL DIAGNOSIS

Spider angiomas can be confused with other vascular lesions such as cherry angiomas.

COURSE AND PROGNOSIS

A few spider angiomas can regress spontaneously. However, the majority of lesions will persist. They can also be associated with hereditary hemorrhagic telangiectasia, ataxia telangiectasia, progressive systemic sclerosis, and CREST syndrome.

MANAGEMENT

Spider angiomas are benign and thus do not require treatment. Lesions that are of cosmetic concern may be eradicated with electrodesiccation, electrocoagulation, or laser therapy.

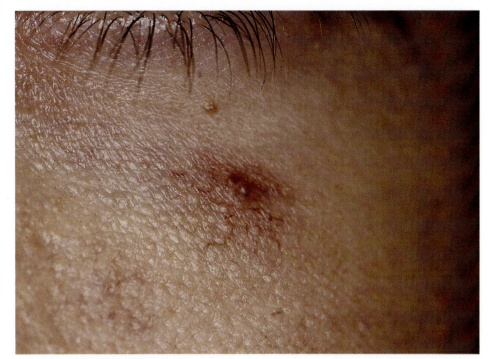

Figure 8-4   Spider angioma   *Vascular papule with radiating arterioles on the cheek of a child.* (Reproduced with permission from TB Fitzpatrick et al., Color Atlas and Synopsis of Clinical Dermatology, 4th edition. New York: McGraw-Hill, 2001).

CHERRY ANGIOMA

Cherry angiomas are benign, bright red, dome-shaped vascular lesions that usually occur on the trunk.

Synonym   Campbell de Morgan spots.

EPIDEMIOLOGY

Age   Any age, more commonly seen in adults.

Gender   M = F.

Etiology   Unknown.

HISTORY

Skin Symptoms   Usually asymptomatic. May bleed and become crusted if traumatized.

PHYSICAL EXAMINATION

Skin Findings

Type   Small macule to dome-shaped papule; surface dull to shiny (Fig. 8-5).

Color   Bright red to violaceous.

Size   1 to 8 mm in size.

Palpation   Soft, compressible. Often blanches completely with pressure.

Sites of Predilection   Trunk, proximal extremities.

DIFFERENTIAL DIAGNOSIS

The diagnosis of cherry angiomas is made clinically. They may sometimes be confused with petechiae. Larger lesions may look like a pyogenic granuloma or hemangioma.

LABORATORY EXAMINATIONS

Dermatopathology   Numerous dilated capillaries; stroma edematous with homogenization of collagen. Epidermis thinned.

COURSE AND PROGNOSIS

Begin to appear in adolescence, becoming more numerous with advancing age.

MANAGEMENT

Cherry angiomas in children are benign and hence no treatment is necessary. Lesions that are of cosmetic concern can be treated with electrocautery, electrodesiccation, or laser therapy.

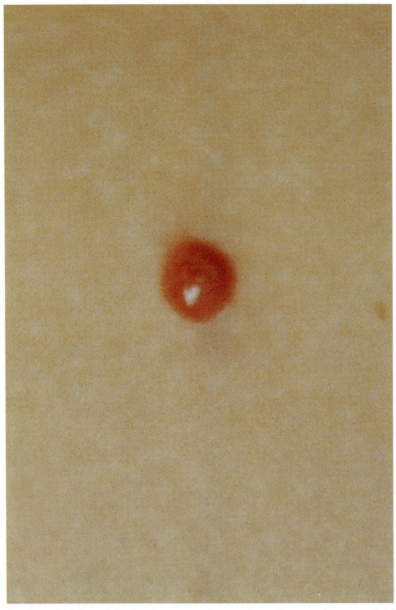

Figure 8-5 Cherry angioma *A benign 3-mm vascular papule on the arm of a young child.*

ANGIOKERATOMA

An angiokeratoma is a benign skin lesion comprised of dilated dermal capillaries with overlying epidermal hyperkeratosis. There are four major subtypes:

1. Solitary or multiple angiokeratoma.
2. Angiokeratoma circumscriptum.
3. Angiokeratoma of Mibelli.
4. Angiokeratoma of Fordyce.

Angiokeratomas can also be associated with two rare disorders: Fabry's disease and fucosidosis.

EPIDEMIOLOGY

Age Angioma circumscriptum can be seen at birth, in infancy, and in childhood. The other forms appear later in life.

Gender F > M: Angioma circumscriptum and angiokeratoma of Mibelli M > F: Angiokeratoma of Fordyce.

Prevalence Angiokeratoma of Fordyce is common. The other forms are uncommon.

Etiology Unclear. Solitary angiokeratomas are sometimes associated with trauma.

Genetics Mibelli may have an autosomal dominant inheritance with variable penetrance.

PHYSICAL EXAMINATION

Skin Findings

Type Verrucous papules coalescing into plaques (Fig. 8-6).

Color Dark red to black.

Size 1 mm to several cm.

Shape Round to stellate, can be in streaks or bands.

Palpation Soft.

Sites of Predilection

1. Solitary or multiple angiokeratoma: Lower extremities.
2. Angiokeratoma circumscriptum: Thighs, lower legs, buttocks.
3. Angiokeratoma of Mibelli: Dorsal aspect of hands/feet.
4. Angiokeratoma of Fordyce: Scrotum in males, labia in females.

General Findings

Disseminated angiokeratomas may be seen in Fabry's disease or fucosidosis. Both diseases are caused by an abnormal intracellular accumulation of glycosphingolipid in the skin and viscera with multiple systemic sequelae. Angiokeratoma of Mibelli may be associated with cold sensitivity, acrocyanosis, and chilblains.

DIFFERENTIAL DIAGNOSIS

Angiokeratomas are diagnosed and categorized by clinical presentation. Numerous angiokeratomas should alert one to check for more serious systemic disease.

LABORATORY EXAMINATIONS

Histopathology Skin biopsy reveals dilated papillary blood vessels with overlying acanthosis and hyperkeratosis of the epidermis.

COURSE AND PROGNOSIS

Angiokeratomas are typically asymptomatic but persist for life and grow proportionately with the child. Occasionally, they may bleed or warrant removal for cosmetic reasons.

MANAGEMENT

Angiokeratomas are benign and thus do not need treatment. They may, however, bleed or warrant removal for cosmetic reasons. They can be treated with surgical excision, electrodesiccation, or laser therapy.

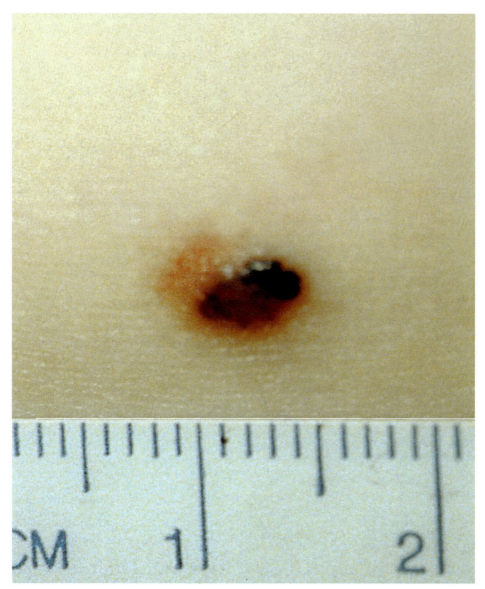

Figure 8-6 Angiokeratoma, solitary *Vascular papules coalescing into a plaque on the leg of a child.*

PYOGENIC GRANULOMA

A pyogenic granuloma is a rapidly developing, bright red papule or nodule usually occurring at a site of trauma.

Synonyms Granuloma telangiectaticum, granuloma pyogenicum.

EPIDEMIOLOGY

Age Usually children or young adults.

Gender M = F.

Etiology Unclear. May be a reactive vascular proliferation. Can be seen in patients using isotretinoin or etretinate.

HISTORY

Pyogenic granulomas are rapidly proliferating vascular nodules that typically arise at a site of minor trauma. They are benign but have a tendency to get traumatized easily and bleed copiously.

PHYSICAL EXAMINATION

Skin Lesions

Type Solitary vascular papule or nodule with smooth or warty surface (Fig. 8-7).

Color Bright red, dusky red, violaceous, brown-black.

Size 5 mm to 2 cm.

Shape Usually lesion is pedunculated, base slightly constricted, or sessile.

Sites of Predilection Area of trauma: fingers, face.

DIFFERENTIAL DIAGNOSIS

The diagnosis of a pyogenic granuloma is typically made on history and clinical examination. The differential diagnosis includes a hemangioma, nodular malignant melanoma (especially amelanotic), and metastatic carcinoma.

DERMATOPATHOLOGY

Histopathology Well-circumscribed proliferation of dermal capillaries with prominent endothelial cells.

COURSE AND PROGNOSIS

Lesions are benign but do not spontaneously disappear. They should be removed for histologic diagnosis.

MANAGEMENT

Pyogenic granuloma are benign, but have a tendency to get traumatized easily and bleed copiously. They are often precipitated by minor trauma and have a tendency to recur after (traumatic) removal. Effective treatments include surgical excision, electrodesiccation, and laser therapy. Aggressive coagulation at the base of the lesion after its removal can minimize chance of recurrence.

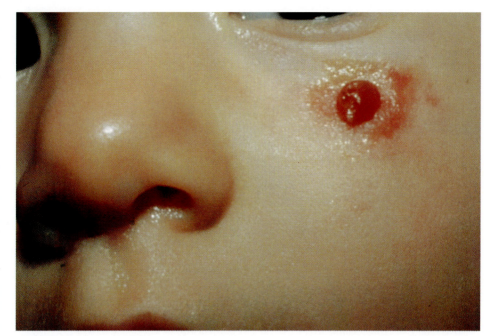

Figure 8-7   Pyogenic granuloma   *Sudden appearance of a vascular nodule on the cheek of an infant.*

VASCULAR CHANGES ASSOCIATED WITH SYSTEMIC DISEASE

LIVEDO RETICULARIS

Livedo reticularis is a mottled bluish (livid) discoloration of the skin that occurs in a net-like pattern. It is not a diagnosis in itself but a nonspecific reaction pattern.

Synonyms   Livedo racemosa, livedo annularis.

EPIDEMIOLOGY

Classification

1. *Benign idiopathic livedo reticularis.* Permanent bluish mottling for which no underlying disease is found.
2. *Secondary or symptomatic livedo reticularis.* Associated with underlying disorder such as intravascular obstruction [viscosity changes, stasis (paralysis, cardiac failure), organic disorder (atheroemboli, thrombocythemia, cryoglobulinemia, cold agglutininemia, air)]; vessel wall disease [arteriosclerosis, hyperparathyroidism, vasculitis syndromes (polyarteritis nodosa, cutaneous polyarteritis nodosa, rheumatoid vasculitis, lupus erythematosus, dermatomyositis, lymphoma, syphilis, tuberculosis, pancreatitis)]; and drugs such as amantadine (Fig. 8-8), quinine, and quinidine.
3. *Sneddon's syndrome.* Extensive livedo reticularis, hypertension, cerebrovascular accidents, and transient ischemic attacks.

Age   Adolescence to adulthood.

Gender   M = F.

Etiology   Unclear. Exposure to cold intensifies the mottling.

PATHOPHYSIOLOGY

Livedo pattern is caused by vasospasm of the arterioles in response to cold leading to hypoxia and dilation of the capillaries and venules. The slow blood flow causes a mottled cyanotic reticular pattern that persists after rewarming.

HISTORY

Appearance or worsening with cold exposure, sometimes with associated numbness and tingling.

PHYSICAL EXAMINATION

Skin Findings

Type   Netlike, blotchy, or mottled macular cyanosis. Ulceration may occur.

Color   Reddish blue.

Palpation   Skin feels cool.

Distribution

1. Benign idiopathic livedo: Symmetrical, arms/legs; less commonly, body; ulceration on lower legs.
2. Secondary livedo: Patchy, asymmetrical on extremities.

DIFFERENTIAL DIAGNOSIS

The differential diagnosis includes cutis marmorata (transient physiologic mottling of skin that resolves on warming, usually seen in infants and resolving after a few weeks of age).

LABORATORY EXAMINATIONS

Dermatopathology   On skin biopsy, there is arteriolar intimal proliferation with dilated numerous capillaries, thickening of walls of venules; and a lymphocytic perivascular infiltration.

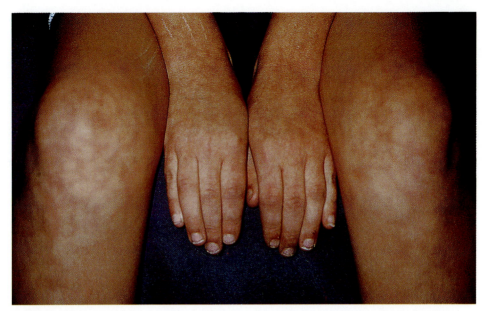

Figure 8-8 Livedo reticularis *Netlike mottled vascular pattern secondary to amantadine in a young patient.*

COURSE AND PROGNOSIS

Benign idiopathic livedo reticularis recurs with cold exposure but rarely becomes permanent. Secondary livedo reticularis is a precursor to more serious systemic sequelae.

MANAGEMENT

Benign Idiopathic Livedo Reticularis

1. Keep extremities from cold temperature exposure.

2. Low-dose aspirin (3 to 5 mg/kg per d PO divided qid).
3. Pentoxifylline (Trental) for severe refractory cases.

Secondary Livedo Reticularis
Treat associated disorder.

CUTIS MARMORATA TELANGIECTATICA CONGENITA

Cutis marmorata telangiectatica congenita (CMTC) is a reticulated mottling of the skin that is more extensive and persistent than cutis marmorata. CMTC can lead to skin ulceration and scarring.

Synonym Congenital generalized phlebectasia.

EPIDEMIOLOGY

Age Onset at birth.

Gender M = F.

Prevalence Rare.

Etiology Unknown.

Genetics Autosomal dominant with low penetrance.

PATHOPHYSIOLOGY

Ectasia of capillaries and veins may represent a mesodermal defect, which would explain CMTC's association with other mesodermal congenital abnormalities.

HISTORY

Typically mottled pattern is present at birth and improves but persists with age. Between 27 and 52% of cases can have other congenital abnormalities (vascular, skeletal, or soft-tissue defects).

PHYSICAL EXAMINATION

Skin Findings

Type Macular reticulated mottling. Ulceration may be present over the reticulated vascular pattern and may heal with depressed scars (Fig. 8-9).

Color Red to blue.

Size Dilated venous channels 3 to 4 mm in diameter.

Distribution Typically generalized. Localized forms have been seen confined to the trunk or one extremity.

DIFFERENTIAL DIAGNOSIS

Cutis marmorata telangiectatica congenita needs to be differentiated from cutis marmorata, which has a more short-lived, transient course. Both are diagnosed by clinical history and physical examination.

LABORATORY EXAMINATIONS

Histopathology Skin biopsy may show dilated capillaries and venules in all layers of the dermis and subcutaneous tissue. Histology may also be subtle and nondiagnostic.

COURSE AND PROGNOSIS

Over 50% of cases of CMTC have a good prognosis in which the skin lesions fade or persist but with no major sequelae. Other associated developmental defects that are seen in 27 to 52% of patients include vascular anomalies, cardiac defects, neurologic disorders, and soft-tissue abnormalitites.

MANAGEMENT

The skin lesions do not require therapy and the mottled vascular pigmentation usually improves. Reticulated scarring, however, is permanent. If lesions are present around the eyes, ophthalmologic evaluation may be indicated.

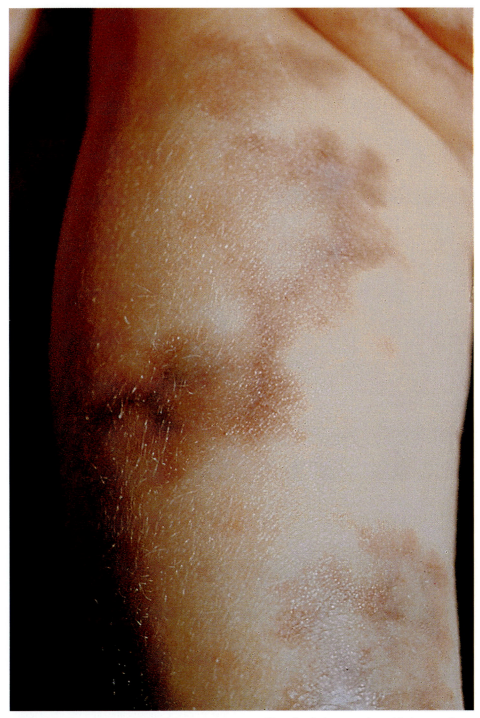

Figure 8-9 Cutis marmorata telangiectatica congenita *Vascular lesions resolve with depressed scars.*

VASCULAR CHANGES ASSOCIATED WITH SYSTEMIC DISEASE

HEREDITARY HEMORRHAGIC TELANGIECTASIA

Hereditary hemorrhagic telangiectasia (HHT) is an autosomal dominant condition that affects blood vessels, especially in the mucous membranes of the mouth and the GI tract. The disease often manifests itself by recurrent epistaxis that appears often in childhood. The telangiectasias of the skin and mucous membranes appears later in life and the clinical spectrum can range from cosmetic, asymptomatic lesions to severe pulmonary and CNS hemorrhages.

Synonyms   Osler – Weber – Rendu disease, Osler's disease.

EPIDEMIOLOGY

Age   Epistaxis may appear in childhood (average 8 to 10 years) but skin lesions begin after puberty, along with epistaxis.

Prevalence   Rare.

Genetics   Autosomal dominant.

PATHOPHYSIOLOGY

It is thought that blood vessels lack adequate perivascular support (pericytes, smooth muscle, and elastic fibers). Thus, the telangiectatic capillaries rupture easily and cause repeated nasal and GI hemorrhages.

HISTORY

The typical skin lesions (punctate red macules and papules) begin to appear after puberty but peak in the third or fourth decade. Bouts of recurrent epistaxis often begin in childhood; GI bleeding occurs in 12 to 50% of patients; pulmonary arteriovenous (AV) fistulae occur in 15% of patients; AV fistulae may occur in the liver; aneurysms of the CNS.

PHYSICAL EXAMINATION

Skin Findings

Type   Macules or papules.

Size   1 to 3 mm in diameter.

Color   Red.

Shape   Punctate (most frequent; Fig. 8-10A), stellate, or linear.

Arrangement of Multiple Lesions   Symmetrical and scattered, nonpatterned.

Distribution   Upper half of the body; begin on the mucous membranes of the nose, later develop on the lips; (Fig. 8-10B), mouth (tongue), conjunctivae (Fig. 8-10C), trunk, upper extremities, palms, soles, hands, fingers, and toes.

Nails   Nail beds of fingers and toes.

Mucous Membranes   Telangiectases appear on nasal septum, on the tip and dorsum of the tongue, nasopharynx, and throughout the GI tract.

LABORATORY EXAMINATIONS

Hematology   Anemia from chronic blood loss.

Dermatopathology   Skin biopsy reveals dilated capillaries and venules located in the dermis, lined by flattened endothelial cells.

Imaging   X-ray, CT, or MRI to rule out pulmonary AV fistulae.

DIFFERENTIAL DIAGNOSIS

Clinical diagnosis made if triad is present of (1) typical telangiectases on skin (fingers and palms) and mucous membranes (lips and tongue), (2) repeated GI hemorrhages, and (3) family history.

MANAGEMENT

In mild cases, treatment of the telangiectases is not necessary; however, iron supplementation for anemia is recommended. Troublesome or cosmetically unwanted telangiectases can be destroyed with laser therapy or cauterization. In severe cases, therapeutic approaches include estrogens and surgical resection of involved pulmonary and GI segments.

DISORDERS OF BLOOD AND LYMPH VESSELS

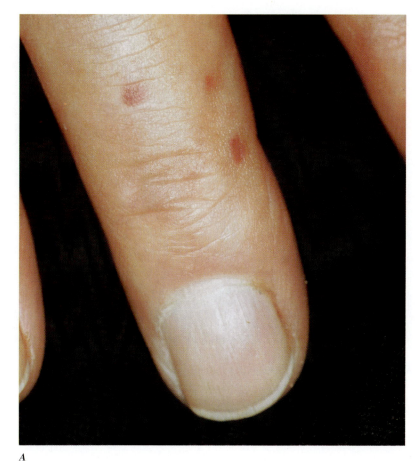

A

Figure 8-10   Hereditary hemorrhagic telangiectasia   *(A) Punctate hemorrhagic macules on the finger.*

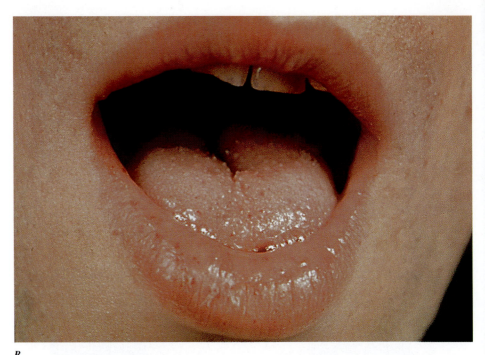

B

Figure 8-10 (continued)   Hereditary hemorrhagic telangiectasia   *(B) Punctate hemorrhagic macules on the lips.*

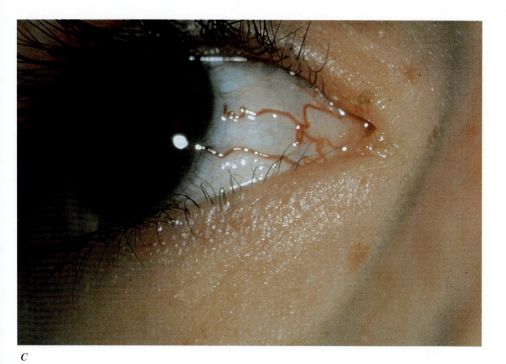

C

Figure 8-10 (continued) Hereditary hemorrhagic telangiectasia (C) *Telangiectases on the bulbar conjunctiva.*

DISORDERS OF LYMPHATIC VESSELS

LYMPHANGIOMA CIRCUMSCRIPTUM

Lymphangioma circumscriptum is a benign tumor of the lymphatic system characterized by groups of deep-seated vesicles that have been likened to "frog spawn." Often there is a hemangiomatous component.

Synonym Hemangiolymphoma.

EPIDEMIOLOGY

Age Present at birth or infancy.

Gender M = F.

Prevalence Uncommon.

Etiology Unclear.

HISTORY

Appear at birth or soon after; can remain stable or slowly grow with time.

PHYSICAL EXAMINATION

Skin Findings

Type Deep seated, thick-walled vesicles coalescing into plaques (Fig. 8-11).

Color Clear or red-purple.

Size 2- to 4-mm vesicles.

Shape Grouped vesicles.

Sites of Predilection Proximal extremities, shoulder, neck, axillae, mucous membranes.

LABORATORY EXAMINATIONS

Dermatopathology Skin biopsy reveals dilated lymph vessels with associated blood vessel dilation in the upper dermis.

DIFFERENTIAL DIAGNOSIS

The diagnosis of lymphangioma circumscriptum can be made clinically, radiologically or by biopsy. The differential diagnosis includes angiokeratoma, hemangioma, recurrent herpetic lesion, contact dermatitis, and molluscum contagiosum.

COURSE AND PROGNOSIS

Many lymphangioma circumscriptum lesions are asymptomatic and so slow-growing that no systemic effects are seen. More extensive lesions can increase in size and if bleeding (from a hemangiomatous part) occurs, they can require intervention.

MANAGEMENT

Asymptomatic, stable lesions do not need treatment. Symptomatic or cosmetically bothersome lesions can be removed by surgical excision, fulguration, coagulation, or CO_2 laser ablation. It may be more difficult to remove larger/deeper lesions, because they can be extensive and recurrent. Multiple surgical excisions may be necessary.

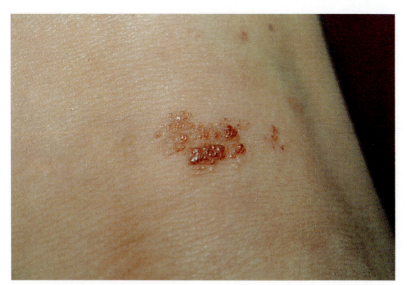

Figure 8-11 Lymphangioma circumscriptum *Hemorrhagic and clear vesicles coalescing into a well-circumscribed plaque on the back of a young child.*

CAVERNOUS LYMPHANGIOMA

Cavernous lymphangioma are large cystic dilations of the deeper lymphatics located in the dermis, subcutaneous tissue, and intramuscular septa.

EPIDEMIOLOGY

Age   Onset in childhood or adult life.

Gender   M = F.

Prevalence   Rare.

Etiology   Unclear.

PATHOPHYSIOLOGY

Dermatopathology   Histologic examination shows dilated lymph channels lined with flat or cuboidal endothelial cells.

HISTORY

Lesions appear later in life as subcutaneous swellings that involve large body surface areas. They can be quite deep and debilitating (Fig. 8-12).

PHYSICAL EXAMINATION

Skin Findings

Type   Nodular or cystic swellings.

Color   Flesh-colored.

Size   1 to several cm.

Sites of Predilection   Face, trunk, extremities.

LABORATORY EXAMINATIONS

Imaging   XRT, CT, or MRI reveal large, cystic spaces in the dermis, subcutis, or muscles.

DIFFERENTIAL DIAGNOSIS

The diagnosis of a cavernous lymphangioma is made with help from imaging studies and/or tissue sampling. The differential diagnosis includes cystic hygroma, cavernous hemangioma, and soft-tissue proliferation.

COURSE AND PROGNOSIS

Cavernous lymphangiomas can involve large parts of the face, trunk, or extremities and can be very debilitating.

MANAGEMENT

Surgical excision is the treatment of choice and it may help for well-circumscribed lesions. Recurrences are common, however, and larger lesions may require grafting to close the defect.

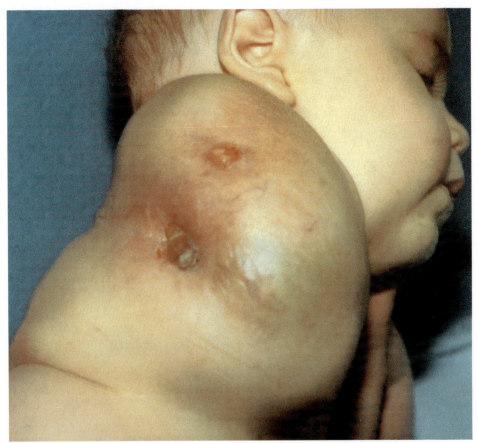

Figure 8-12 Cavernous lymphangioma *Large, cystic swelling on the neck of an infant.* (Slide courtesy of Karen Wiss.)

CYSTIC HYGROMA

Cystic hygromas are benign, loculated lymphatic proliferations.

Synonym Hygroma colli.

EPIDEMIOLOGY

Age May be present at birth or infancy.

Gender M = F.

Prevalence Rare.

Etiology Unclear.

HISTORY

Lesions present at or soon after birth. They proliferate and persist throughout life. Occasional lesions can undergo spontaneous involution.

PHYSICAL EXAMINATION

Skin Findings

Type Nodular or cystic swellings (Fig. 8-13).

Color Flesh colored to pink-red.

Size 1 to several cm in size.

Sites of Predilection Neck, axillae, groin, or popliteal fossa.

LABORATORY EXAMINATIONS

Dermatopathology Skin biopsy reveals a uniloculated or multiloculated nodule of numerous dilated lymph vessels.

DIFFERENTIAL DIAGNOSIS

The diagnosis of a cystic hygroma is made by history and clinical findings and can be confirmed by imaging studies and/or tissue diagnosis. The differential diagnosis includes cavernous lymphangioma, cavernous hemangioma, and soft-tissue proliferation.

COURSE AND PROGNOSIS

Some cystic hygromas can spontaneously involute. The majority, however, continue to grow and can affect adjacent vessels and nerves.

MANAGEMENT

Surgical excision of cystic hygromas is recommended as early as possible. Unlike lymphangiomas, recurrences of cystic hygromas are uncommon.

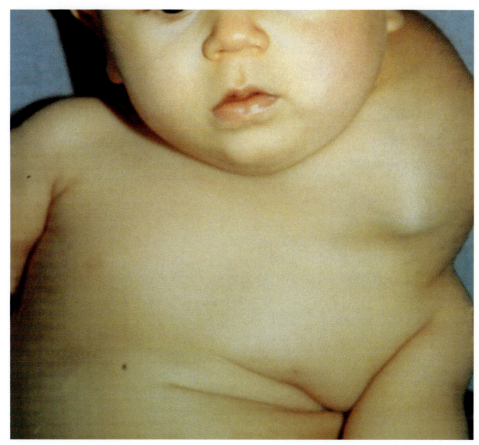

Figure 8-13 Cystic hygroma *Large, cystic swelling on the neck of an infant.*

LYMPHEDEMA

Lymphedema is diffuse soft-tissue swelling caused by poor lymphatic drainage. It may be a primary disease or secondary to pathologic obstruction of the lymph vessels.

EPIDEMIOLOGY

Age Primary lymphedema: 13% congenital, age 9 to 25 years (lymphedema praecox), > 25 years (lymphedema tarda). Secondary lymphedema: Any age.

Gender F > M, especially lymphedema praecox.

Etiology Primary: Unknown. Secondary: Postsurgery, postinfection, filariasis.

PATHOPHYSIOLOGY

The lymphatic drainage to an extremity is impaired either primarily (e.g., congenital lymphedema) or secondarily (e.g., postsurgical) and leads to swelling of the affected extremity.

HISTORY

Lymphedema of the involved area results in swelling that fluctuates in severity and gradually worsens with age. Milroy's disease is an autosomal dominant disorder with an inherited tendency for lymphedema of the legs. The etiology is unclear.

PHYSICAL EXAMINATION

Skin Findings

Type Diffuse swelling (Fig. 8-14).

Palpation Firm with pitting under pressure.

Sites of Predilection Lower extremities, upper extremities.

DIFFERENTIAL DIAGNOSIS

The diagnosis of lymphedema is made by history and clinical examination. The differential diagnosis includes cellulitis and deep tissue infection.

COURSE AND PROGNOSIS

Lymphedema slowly progresses with age, and repeated swelling of the affected area leads to worsening of the disease.

MANAGEMENT

Maintenance therapy consists of:

1. Rest and limb elevation.
2. Compression with elastic support stockings, Ace wraps, or pneumatic compression devices (Jobst or Wright pumps).
3. Reducing sodium intake.
4. Diuretics can also be helpful.
5. Subcutaneous lymphangiectomy can be attempted, but scarring is extensive and unsightly.

DISORDERS OF BLOOD AND LYMPH VESSELS

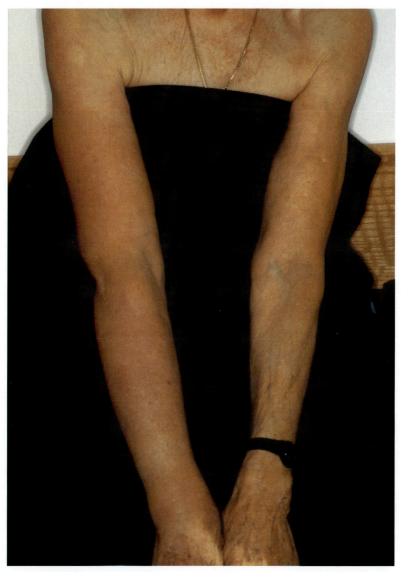

Figure 8-14   Lymphedema   *Post-surgical swelling of the right arm compared to the left arm.*

SECTION 9

BENIGN EPIDERMAL PROLIFERATIONS

EPIDERMAL NEVUS

Epidermal nevi are benign, well-circumscribed proliferations of the epidermis present at birth or infancy.

Synonyms Nevus verrucosus, nevus unius lateris, systematized epidermal nevus, ichthyosis hystrix, and linear nevus sebaceous.

EPIDEMIOLOGY

Age Usually congenital, can appear in infancy, childhood, or adult life.

Gender M = F.

Prevalence Uncommon.

Etiology Unclear.

PATHOPHYSIOLOGY

The pathophysiology of an epidermal nevus is unclear.

HISTORY

Epidermal nevi are present at or soon after birth. Solitary small lesions are common. Larger lesions can affect an entire limb or side of the body. Head and neck lesions can have associated adnexal tissue proliferations or hypertrophy.

PHYSICAL EXAMINATION

Skin Findings

Type Plaques with smooth or velvety warty/papillomatous surface (Fig. 9-1).

Number Solitary or multiple.

Color Color of the skin, light or dark brown.

Size Few mm to 2 to 5 cm.

Distribution Typically unilateral, can be bilateral.

Arrangement Linear or dermatomal large lesions follow the lines of Blaschko with whorled appearance.

Sites of Predilection Trunk or limb > head or neck.

DIFFERENTIAL DIAGNOSIS

The diagnosis of an epidermal nevus is made based upon history and physical examination. The differential diagnosis includes linear and whorled hypermelanosis, lichen striatus, incontinentia pigmenti, hypomelanosis of Ito, or an inflammatory linear verrucous epidermal nevus.

LABORATORY EXAMINATIONS

Dermatopathology Skin biopsy shows hyperkeratosis, acanthosis, and papillomatosis. There may be increased melanin in the basal layer in places. There may be ballooning of the cells (epidermolytic hyperkeratosis) in places.

COURSE AND PROGNOSIS

Epidermal nevi are typically asymptomatic and grow proportionately with the child. Malignant degeneration of epidermal nevi is rare. Adults with epidermal nevi can have a keratin mutation in their germ line resulting in offspring with epidermolytic hyperkeratosis.

MANAGEMENT

Treatment of the skin lesions is not necessary. Symptomatic or cosmetically unwanted lesions can be treated with:

1. Shave excision.
2. Dermabrasion.
3. Laser ablation.
4. Electrodesiccation.
5. Cryotherapy.
6. Surgical removal is curative but not realistic for extensive lesions.

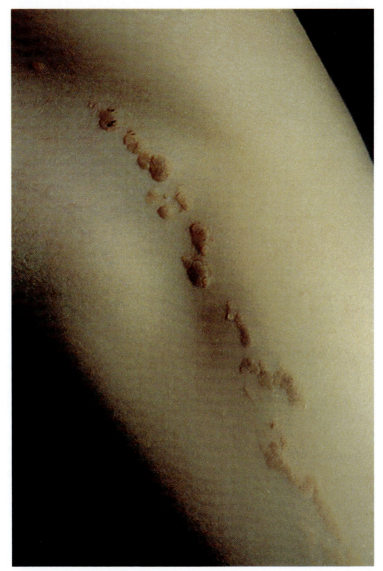

Figure 9-1　Epidermal nevus　*Brown verrucous papules in a linear arrangement on the arm of a child.*

INFLAMMATORY LINEAR VERRUCOUS EPIDERMAL NEVUS

Inflammatory linear verrucous epidermal nevus (ILVEN) is a subtype of epidermal nevus comprised of pruritic, erythematous, linearly arranged papules and plaques.

EPIDEMIOLOGY

Age   Usually present at birth; 95% present by age 7 years.

Prevalence   Uncommon.

Etiology   Unclear. ILVEN is thought to be a developmental defect.

PATHOPHYSIOLOGY

Developmental abnormality with unclear etiology.

HISTORY

Initial presentation of ILVEN is of a barely palpable lesion or a confluence of smooth-topped papules. This progresses to a more wart-like and scaly lesion. During the newborn period, there are episodes of redness and inflammation. Other skin findings include: an increased number of cutaneous lesions including café au lait spots, congenital hypopigmented macules, and congenital nevocellular nevi. There may also be associated skeletal defects, seizure disorders, mental retardation, and ocular abnormalities.

PHYSICAL EXAMINATION

Skin Findings

Type   Scaling papules coalescing into plaques (Fig. 9-2).

Color   Erythematous.

Size   2 to 5 cm in length.

Shape   Linear or oval.

Distribution   Anywhere on the body. The long axis of the lesion parallels the long axis of the dermatome.

DIFFERENTIAL DIAGNOSIS

The diagnosis of ILVEN is made on morphologic appearance of lesions, intense pruritus, and resistance to therapy. ILVEN can be confused with warts, psoriasis, lichen simplex chronicus, lichen striatus, incontinentia pigmenti, linear and whorled hypermelanosis, or hypomelanosis of Ito.

LABORATORY EXAMINATIONS

Dermatopathology   Skin biopsy reveals hyperkeratosis, focal parakeratosis, acanthosis with elongation of the rete ridges, spongiosis, and a perivascular lymphocytic and histiocytic infiltrate.

COURSE AND PROGNOSIS

ILVEN runs a chronic course and is generally resistant to therapy with episodes of intense pruritus.

MANAGEMENT

Pruritus and inflammatory episodes may benefit from:

1. Topical steroids.
   a. Low potency steroids (Desowen, 1% hydrocortisone, 2.5% hydrocortisone) should be used on face or groin area, no more than bid × 2 weeks.
   b. Medium potency steroids (Elocon, Dermatop, Cutivate) should be used on the body or extremities no more than bid × 2 weeks.
   c. Strong steroids (Ultravate, Psorcon, Diprolene) are reserved for older children/adults on severely affected areas bid for no more than 2 weeks.
   Patients need to be cautioned about steroid side effects. See page 48 for more details.
2. Intralesional steroids.

The verrucous appearance can be improved with:

1. Mild keratolytics:
   a. Hydroxy acid creams (Lac-Hydrin, Aquaglycolic).

b. Retinoic acid creams (Retin A, Renova, or Differin).
2. Emollients such as hydrated petrolatum, Vaseline, mineral oil, Aquaphor, Lubriderm, Moisturel, and Eucerin.

With noncompliance or discontinuation of therapy, lesions revert to their hyperkeratotic form.

Curative approaches include dermabrasion, laser ablation, and surgical removal.

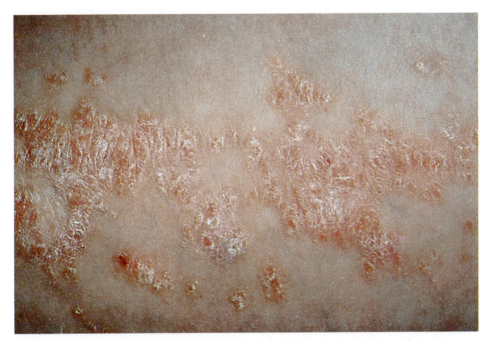

Figure 9-2 Inflammatory linear verrucous epidermal nevus *Inflammatory, scaly erythematous papules coalescing into plaques.*

EPIDERMAL NEVUS SYNDROMES

A congenitally acquired syndrome characterized by the presence of epidermal nevi in association with various developmental abnormalities of the skin, eyes, and nervous, skeletal, cardiovascular, and urogenital systems.

Synonyms Schimmelpenning syndrome, linear nevus sebaceous syndrome, Feuerstein and Mims syndrome.

EPIDEMIOLOGY

Age Birth to 40 years of age.

Gender M = F.

Incidence Unknown; may be as high as 16% in cases of epidermal nevi.

Etiology Believed to occur sporadically.

Genetics Isolated instances of autosomal dominant inheritance pattern have been documented.

PATHOPHYSIOLOGY

Developmental abnormality of unclear etiology affecting skin, skeletal, and cardiovascular and CNS systems. Proposed mechanisms for the phenotypes seen include loss of heterozygosity, nonallelic twin spotting, paradominant inheritance, and mosaicism.

HISTORY

A spectrum of epidermal nevi may be represented in this syndrome. Epidermal nevi seen, from most to least common, include: nevus unius lateris, icthyosis hystrix, acanthotic form of epidermal nevus, inflammatory linear verrucous epidermal nevus, nevus sebaceus, Becker nevus, and nevus comedonicus. Other mucocutaneous lesions include: hemangiomas, pigmentary changes, hair and dental abnormalities, and dermatomegaly (increase in skin thickness, warmth, and hairiness).

Review of Symptoms Skeletal abnormalities (15 to 70%): bone deformities, cysts, atrophies, and hypertrophies; neurologic abnormalities (15 to 50%): mental retardation and seizures; ocular abnormalities (9 to 30%).

PHYSICAL EXAMINATION

Skin Findings

Type Hypertrophic warty papules coalescing into plaques.

Color Orange, brown, or dark brown.

Size and Shape 2- to 4-mm papules coalescing to larger plaques.

Distribution May be single linear lesion or more extensive spiraling lesion, unilateral (Fig. 9-3) or bilateral.

Sites of Predilection Trunk, extremities, head, neck.

LABORATORY EXAMINATIONS

Dermatopathology Skin biopsy shows findings consistent with an epidermal nevus. Biopsy of a lesion on the face, scalp, or ears, may show sebaceous gland hyperplasia.

DIFFERENTIAL DIAGNOSIS

Diagnosis should be suspected on presentation with extensive epidermal nevi or epidermal nevi associated with systemic abnormalities. Pertinent medical history includes developmental history, specifically attainment of developmental milestones, history of seizures, and abnormalities of bones, eyes, and urinary tract. Mucocutaneous, neurologic, ophthalmologic, and orthopedic examinations must be performed.

COURSE AND PROGNOSIS

Rarely, malignant transformation of epidermal nevi may occur. Transformation most common with nevus sebaceus. Syndrome may also be associated with various visceral malignancies:

Wilms' tumor, astrocytoma, adenocarcinoma, ameloblastoma, ganglioneuroblastoma, esophageal and stomach carcinoma, and squamous cell carcinoma.

MANAGEMENT

The treatment of skin lesions in the epidermal nevus syndrome is difficult given their extensive distribution. To smooth the verrucous surface, therapies include:

1. Keratolytics:
   a. Hydroxy acid creams (Lac-Hydrin, Aquaglycolic).
   b. Retinoic acid creams (Retin A, Renova, or Differin).
2. Emollients such as hydrated petrolatum, Vaseline, mineral oil, Aquaphor, Lubriderm, Moisturel, and Eucerin.

Curative approaches to the skin manifestations include dermabrasion, laser ablation, and surgical removal. More importantly for systemic disease, regular follow-up should be instated. Periodic electroencephalograms and skeletal radiologic analysis may be important to the long-term care of the patient.

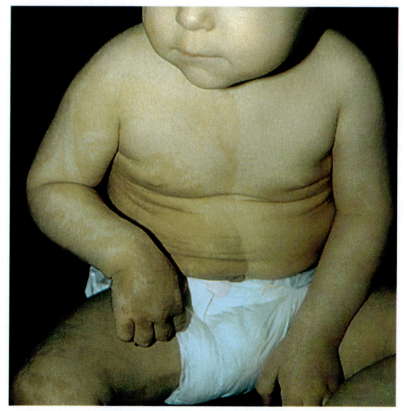

Figure 9-3 Epidermal nevus syndrome *Large, unilateral brush-like strokes in a young infant.*

BENIGN APPENDAGEAL PROLIFERATIONS

NEVUS SEBACEUS

A nevus sebaceus is a solitary, well-circumscribed, yellow-orange hairless plaque located on the face or scalp, which later in life can give rise to neoplastic changes.

Synonyms   Nevus sebaceus of Jadassohn, organoid nevus.

EPIDEMIOLOGY

Age   Usually present near birth. May appear in childhood or adulthood.

Gender   M = F.

Prevalence   Uncommon.

Genetics   Usually sporadic, rare familial forms reported.

HISTORY

A nevus sebaceus is typically present near birth and has 2 stages: prepubertal (infantile phase) and pubertal (adolescent phase).

PHYSICAL EXAMINATION

Skin Findings

Type   Hairless plaque surface may be velvet-like, verrucous, or papillomatous (Fig. 10-1).

Color   Yellow, yellow-brown, orange, pink.

Size   Few millimeters to several centimeters.

Shape   Round, oval, or linear.

Distribution   Head and neck.

Arrangement   Solitary, rarely, multiple lesions have been reported.

General Findings

Typically there are no systemic symptoms. Rarely, extensive lesions can be associated with ocular, CNS, or skeletal abnormalities.

DIFFERENTIAL DIAGNOSIS

The differential diagnosis includes other appendageal tumors; smaller lesions can resemble warts.

LABORATORY EXAMINATION

Dermatopathology   Early skin lesions reveal numerous immature sebaceus glands and cords or buds of undifferentiated hair follicles. Later lesions show papillomatous hyperplasia of the epidermis with hyperkeratosis and hypergranulosis. There are also typically ectopic apocrine glands located deep in the dermis.

COURSE AND PROGNOSIS

Nevus sebaceus tend to grow slowly and become thicker and more papillomatous with age. About 10 to 15% may have neoplastic changes: 8 to 19% syringocystadenoma papilliferum (Fig. 10-2), 5 to 7% basal cell carcinoma, 2% squamous cell carcinoma.

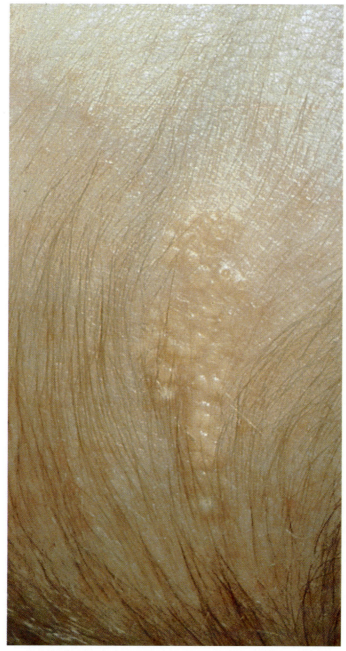

Figure 10-1   Nevus sebaceus, infant   *(A) Verrucous yellow-orange plaque on the scalp of an infant.*

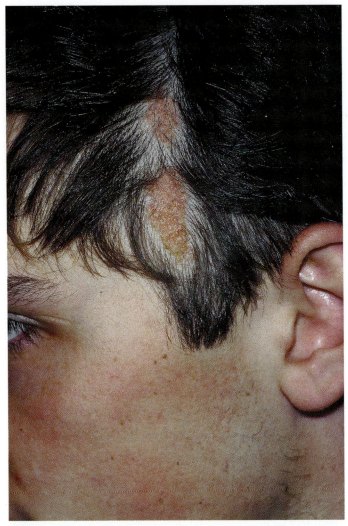

Figure 10-1 Nevus sebaceus, 14-year-old *(B) Same nevus 14 years later with a more orange-brown appearance.*

MANAGEMENT

Small facial lesions can be observed regularly for any signs or symptoms of neoplastic change.

Scalp or larger lesions that are difficult to monitor or have a higher risk of neoplastic change should be removed before puberty with surgical excision.

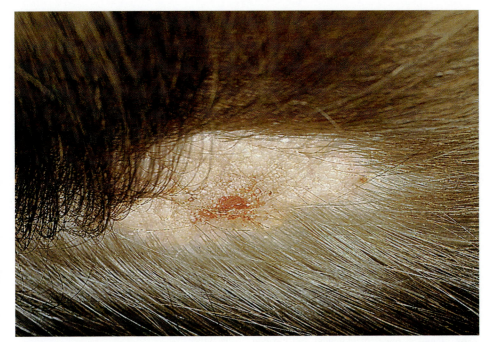

Figure 10-2　Nevus sebaceus, adult　*Central ulceration and crusting in a post-pubertal nevus sebaceus. Skin biopsy revealed neoplastic changes suggestive of syringocystadenoma papilliferum.*

NEVUS COMEDONICUS

A nevus comedonicus is a congenital, well-circumscribed area of comedones.

Synonym Comedo nevus.

EPIDEMIOLOGY

Age Present at birth in 50% others appear before age 10 to 15 years.

Gender M = F.

Prevalence Rare.

Etiology Suspected to be either a mesodermal developmental defect or a variant of an epidermal nevus.

PHYSICAL EXAMINATION

Skin Findings

Type Papules, open (blackheads) and closed (whiteheads) comedones (Fig. 10-3).

Arrangement Linear or band-like configuration.

Distribution Unilateral solitary lesion on any part of the body.

Sites of Predilection Face, neck, upper arm, chest, abdomen.

DIFFERENTIAL DIAGNOSIS

Nevus comedonicus can be confused clinically with comedonal acne or hidradenitis suppurativa, but the congenital onset and localized nature is diagnostic.

LABORATORY EXAMINATIONS

Dermatopathology Skin biopsy shows multiple dilated follicles filled with keratin plugs.

COURSE AND PROGNOSIS

Nevi comedonicus are typically asymptomatic but can occasionally become inflamed and painful. Pustules, abscesses, and scarring may occur. The lesions persist throughout life but are benign. Rarely, they may be associated with systemic abnormalities (ipsilateral cataract and skeletal defects). This is termed the nevus comedonicus syndrome.

MANAGEMENT

Nevus comedonicus with active acneiform outbreaks may be treated like localized acne with the following.

1. Topical antibiotics such as clindamycin (Cleocin) or erythromycin (Emgel, Erycette, or Akne-mycin) help decrease bacterial load and inflammation.
2. Topical benzoyl peroxide (Benzac, Brevoxyl, or Desquam-E) also suppresses *Propionibacterium acnes.*
3. Topical salicylic acid (SalAc, Stridex) or hydroxy acid preparations (Aqua Glycolic) help slough the outer layer of skin preventing follicular blockage.
4. Topical retinoids (Retin A, Differin) are effective, but require detailed instructions and gradual increases in concentration. Retinoids help the skin turnover more rapidly to decrease possible follicular blockage and rupture.
5 Topical sulfur (Sulfacet) is antimicrobial and keratolytic.

More extensive or refractory cases may benefit from systemic acne treatment. More troublesome lesions can also be resurfaced with surgical excisions, dermabrasion, or laser ablation.

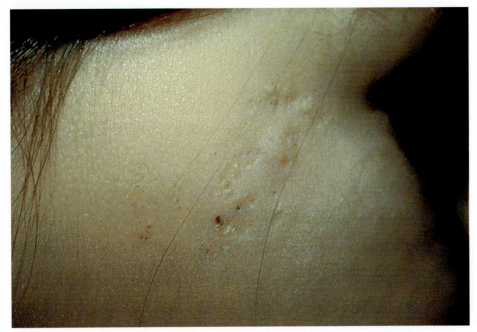

Figure 10-3 Nevus comedonicus *Localized area of open comedones on the cheek of a child present since birth.*

TRICHOEPITHELIOMA

Trichoepitheliomas are benign appendageal tumors that appear in childhood and occur on the face and, less often, on the scalp, neck, or trunk.

Synonyms Brooke's tumor, epithelioma adenoides cysticum, multiple benign cystic epithelioma.

EPIDEMIOLOGY

Age Early childhood or puberty.

Gender M = F.

Prevalence Uncommon.

Genetics Autosomal dominant inheritance.

HISTORY

Multiple trichoepitheliomas appear during early childhood or at puberty and are asymptomatic but permanent.

PHYSICAL EXAMINATION

Skin Findings

Type Firm papules and nodules.

Color Color of the skin or slightly pink and translucent with fine telangiectasia present on larger lesions.

Size and Shape 2 to 5 mm in diameter, round. Lesions may enlarge to 5 mm on face and ears and up to 2 to 3 cm in other sites.

Number Few at onset to multiple after puberty (Fig. 10-4).

Distribution Face, ears, and trunk.

Sites of Predilection Nasolabial folds, nose, forehead, upper lip, and eyelids.

DIFFERENTIAL DIAGNOSIS

The diagnosis of trichoepitheliomas is based on clinical findings and confirmed by skin biopsy.

Trichoepitheliomas are most commonly confused with basal cell carcinomas or other appendageal tumors.

LABORATORY EXAMINATIONS

Dermatopathology Microscopic investigation of dominantly inherited multiple trichoepitheliomas reveals horn cysts (fully keratinized inner shell) surrounded by solid nests and lace-like strands of flattened basophilic epithelial cells. Solitary trichoepitheliomas histologically show numerous horn cysts and abortive attempts to form hair papillae and hair shafts.

COURSE AND PROGNOSIS

Trichoepitheliomas are benign lesions that persist for life. Clinically, more lesions may appear on the face, but the patient is otherwise asymptomatic.

MANAGEMENT

Trichoepitheliomas must be histologically differentiated from basal cell carcinomas. They are benign and cosmetically may be treated with:

1. Surgical excision.
2. Electrodesiccation and curettage.

Other destructive methods such as cryosurgery, dermabrasion, or laser often result in recurrences.

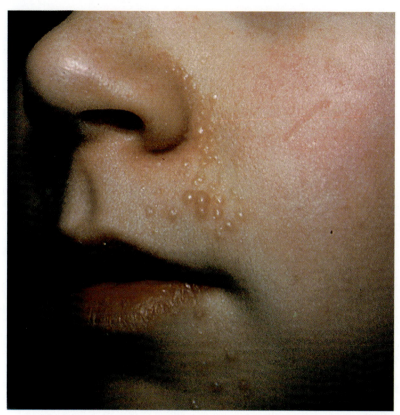

Figure 10-4 **Multiple trichoepitheliomas** *Numerous 2- to 5-mm skin-colored papules on the face of a child.*

SYRINGOMA

Syringomas are benign tumors of the eccrine duct that appear as tiny papules on the lower eyelids.

EPIDEMIOLOGY

Age Typically appear at puberty or adolescence.

Gender F = M.

Incidence One percent of population.

Etiology Unclear.

Other Factors Higher incidence (19 to 37%) in patients with Down's syndrome.

HISTORY

Syringomas are asymptomatic benign skin lesions that appear and proliferate at puberty. They may be influenced by hormones (increases in estrogen).

PHYSICAL EXAMINATION

Skin Findings

Type Tiny papules or nodules.

Color Yellow.

Size 1 to 5 mm.

Number Few to numerous.

Distribution Eyelids, neck, thorax, abdomen, back, upper arms, thighs, and genitalia.

Sites of Predilection Lower eyelids (Fig. 10-5).

DIFFERENTIAL DIAGNOSIS

The diagnosis of syringomas can usually be made clinically. The differential diagnosis includes other appendageal tumors, milia, or acne.

LABORATORY EXAMINATIONS

Dermatopathology Skin biopsy reveals many small ducts in the dermis with comma-like tails commonly referred to as "tadpoles."

COURSE AND PROGNOSIS

Syringomas enlarge and proliferate during puberty and then typically persist asymptomatically for life. Rare cases of spontaneous regression are reported.

MANAGEMENT

Syringomas are benign and treatment is not necessary. Therapeutic methods for cosmetic purposes include surgical removal, electrodesiccation, cryotherapy, and laser ablation.

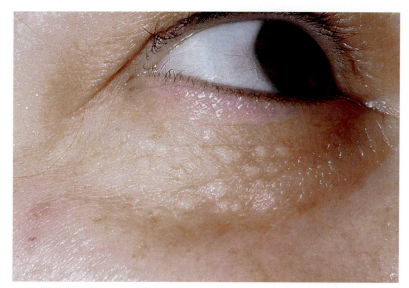

Figure 10-5 Syringomas *Small 3- to 5-mm yellowish papules on the lower eyelid of a young adult.*

PILOMATRIXOMA

A pilomatrixoma is a benign hair follicle tumor that clinically presents as a solitary calcified nodule on the face, neck, or arms of children or young adults.

Synonyms Calcifying epithelioma of Malherbe, pilomatricoma.

EPIDEMIOLOGY

Age Develops before age 21 years.

Gender F > M.

Prevalence Uncommon.

Genetics Usually not inherited although there are some rare familial forms reported.

HISTORY

Pilomatrixomas are not present at birth, appear suddenly, and persist throughout life.

PHYSICAL EXAMINATION

Skin Findings

Type Solitary papule or nodule (Fig. 10-6).

Color Color of the skin or reddish-blue.

Size 0.5 to 3 cm.

Palpation Firm and lobular. When skin is stretched lesion has a "tent" appearance with multiple angles.

Distribution Face, neck, arms or genital area.

Sites of Predilection More than 50% on head or neck.

General Findings

Rare familial forms associated with myotonic dystrophy (Steinert's disease).

DIFFERENTIAL DIAGNOSIS

The differential diagnosis includes other dermal tumors and cysts. The firmness to palpation and distinct color of a pilomatrixoma can help differentiate it from other entities.

LABORATORY EXAMINATIONS

Dermatopathology Skin biopsy reveals sheets of compact basal cells alternating with "ghost" or "shadow" cells. Calcification may also be present.

COURSE AND PROGNOSIS

Pilomatrixomas are typically asymptomatic. Occasionally, lesions may become inflamed or swollen. Uncommonly, calcified material may perforate through the skin. Rarely, lesions may grow rapidly and behave in a malignant form.

MANAGEMENT

The treatment of choice for pilomatrixomas is surgical excision and is usually done for both cosmetic and therapeutic purposes.

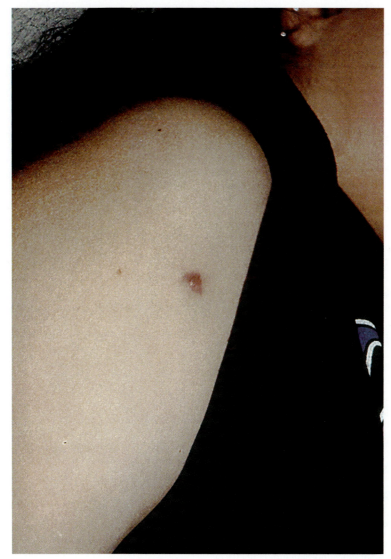

Figure 10-6 Pilomatrixoma *Reddish-blue nodule on the arm of a young girl.* (Slide courtesy of Lisa M. Cohen.)

STEATOCYSTOMA MULTIPLEX

Steatocystoma multiplex is a benign disorder characterized by multiple cutaneous cystic nodules located mainly on the chest of affected individuals.

Synonym Sebocystomatosis.

EPIDEMIOLOGY

Age Adolescence.

Gender M = F.

Prevalence Uncommon.

Etiology Unclear.

Genetics Autosomal dominant inheritance resulting from a mutation of keratin 17 on chromosome 17.

Other Features May occur concomitantly with pachyonychia congenita.

PATHOPHYSIOLOGY

Steatocystoma multiplex are hamartomas; histologic variants of dermoid or vellus hair cysts.

HISTORY

Steatocystoma multiplex arise at puberty or thereafter and persist. They may become larger at puberty but are usually asymptomatic.

PHYSICAL EXAMINATION

Skin Findings

Type Numerous firm, slow-growing, cutaneous cystic nodules, no punctum (Fig. 10-7).

Color Yellow.

Size and Shape 2 to 4 mm in diameter.

Shape Round.

Palpation Firm.

Distribution Chest, face, arms, scrotum, thighs.

Sites of Predilection Sternal areas, axillae, neck, and scrotum.

DIFFERENTIAL DIAGNOSIS

Steatocystomas are diagnosed by history and clinical findings. Steatocystomas can be confused with sebaceous, keratin-inclusion cysts or pilar cysts. Unlike the other cysts, steatocystomas have odorless, syrup-like fluid when expressed.

LABORATORY EXAMINATIONS

Dermatopathology Steatocystomas have cystic spaces lined by a corrugated thin epidermal lining. Abortive hair follicles and groups of sebaceous, eccrine, or apocrine structures are often incorporated into the cyst wall. Glycogen and amylophosphorylase are present in the invaginations and cyst wall.

COURSE AND PROGNOSIS

Steatocystomas appear at puberty and persist for life. They are asymptomatic but can become quite numerous and troublesome cosmetically.

MANAGEMENT

Steatocystomas are benign, thus no treatment is necessary. They can be removed for cosmetic reasons by:

1. Surgical excision.
2. Incision and drainage.
3. Electrodesiccation.
4. Dermabrasion.
5. Laser resurfacing.

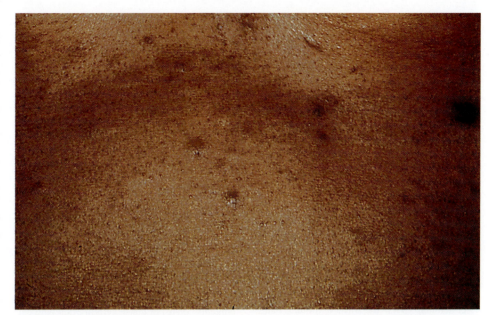

Figure 10-7   Steatocystoma multiplex   *Multiple asymptomatic flesh-colored cysts on the chest of a young woman. The lesion on the righthand side of the photograph is a supernummary nipple.* (Slide courtesy of Lisa M. Cohen.)

TRICHILEMMAL CYST

A trichilemmal cyst is the second most common type of cutaneous cyst occurring most often on the scalp. It is often an inherited trait and can be single or multiple in number.

Synonyms Pilar cyst, isthmus catagen cyst, wen.

EPIDEMIOLOGY

Age Adolescence to adulthood.

Gender F > M.

Prevalence Common.

Genetics May be inherited as an autosomal dominant trait.

PATHOPHYSIOLOGY

Trichilemmal cysts are formed around hairs with trapping of the keratin intradermally leading to cyst formation and enlargement.

HISTORY

Cysts appear in the scalp and are usually asymptomatic. They grow then plateau in size and persist for life. Ruptured cysts may become inflamed and painful.

PHYSICAL EXAMINATION

Skin Findings

Type Smooth, firm, dome-shaped nodules to tumors (Fig. 10-8). Lacks the central punctum seen in epidermal inclusion cysts. Overlying scalp hair usually normal; may be thinned if cyst is large.

Color Color of the skin.

Size 0.5 to 5 cm.

Distribution Occur on scalp in 90%.

DIFFERENTIAL DIAGNOSIS

Other cysts can mimic pilar cysts, but the scalp location is usually diagnostic.

LABORATORY EXAMINATIONS

Dermatopathology Cyst excisions reveal a cyst with a stratified squamous epithelial lining and a palisaded outer layer resembling the outer root sheath of a hair follicle. The inner layer is corrugated with no granular layer and the cyst contents consist of dense keratin often with calcified cholesterol.

COURSE AND PROGNOSIS

Trichilemmal cysts begin on the scalp during adolescence and persist for life. They can become inflamed or painful. They may also become quite large in size.

MANAGEMENT

Asymptomatic lesions can be left untreated. Symptomatic lesions can be:

1. Incised and the cyst contents can be expressed, however they often recur.
2. Surgically excised with removal of the cyst capsule for permanent cure. These surgical removals are often very bloody given the well-vascularized scalp location of these lesions.

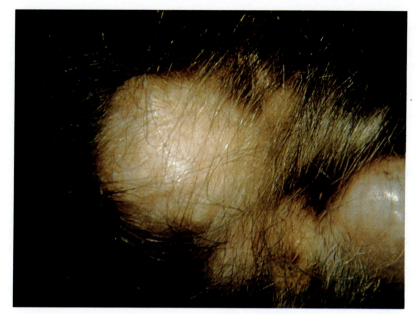

Figure 10-8 **Trichilemmal cyst** *Smooth cystic growth on the scalp.*

EPIDERMAL INCLUSION CYST

Epidermal inclusion cyst (EIC), the most common cutaneous cyst, is caused by epidermal implantation of the epidermis within the dermis. This causes a cyst filled with keratin debris to form. Cyst contents are cream-colored with a pasty consistency, and smell like rancid cheese.

Synonyms Epidermoid cyst, sebaceous cyst, infundibular cyst, epidermal cyst.

EPIDEMIOLOGY

Age Adolescence to adulthood.

Gender: M > F.

Prevalence Common.

PATHOPHYSIOLOGY

Epidermal cysts are formed when skin desquamation is blocked and keratin gathers in a little ball under the skin, instead of normally shedding to the skin surface.

HISTORY

Cysts appear, occasionally drain from a central punctum but often recur. They are benign but can persist for life.

PHYSICAL EXAMINATION

Skin Findings

Type Nodule, usually with central punctum (Fig. 10-9).

Color Color of the skin.

Size 0.5 to 5 cm.

Arrangement Usually solitary, may be multiple.

Distribution Face, neck, upper trunk, scrotum.

DIFFERENTIAL DIAGNOSIS

Epidermal cysts can be confused with other cysts, however the rancid white yellow cyst contents is diagnostic.

LABORATORY EXAMINATIONS

Dermatopathology Skin excisions reveal a cyst lined by structural squamous epithelium and the cyst space filled with keratin.

COURSE AND PROGNOSIS

EICs are benign; however, they may grow to disfiguring sizes or become recurrently inflamed. If the cyst ruptures, the irritating cyst contents initiate an inflammatory reaction, and the lesion becomes painful.

MANAGEMENT

Asymptomatic lesions can be left untreated. Symptomatic lesions can be:

1. Incised and cyst contents can be expressed, however they often recur.
2. Surgically excised with removal of the cyst capsule for permanent cure.

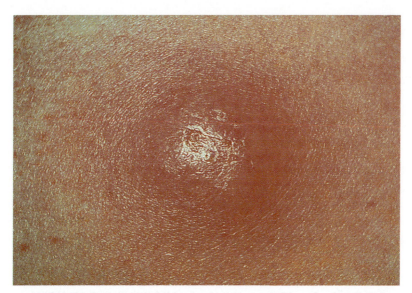

Figure 10-9   Epidermal inclusion cyst   *A 1-cm erythematous painful ruptured cyst on the arm.*

BENIGN DERMAL PROLIFERATIONS

CONNECTIVE TISSUE NEVUS

Connective tissue nevi are benign, slightly elevated, well-circumscribed plaques that are often seen as an isolated skin finding, but can also be associated with other systemic disease (Table 11-1).

Synonyms   Nevus elasticus, juvenile elastoma, collagenoma, collagen hamartomas.

EPIDEMIOLOGY

Age   Young children, adolescence.

Gender   M = F.

Prevalence   Uncommon.

Genetics   May have an autosomal dominant inherited form.

PATHOPHYSIOLOGY

Connective tissue nevi are localized malformations of dermal collagen and/or elastic fibers.

HISTORY

Connective tissue nevi appear in childhood or adolescence and are asymptomatic but can be disfiguring.

PHYSICAL EXAMINATION

Skin Findings

Type   Slightly raised plaque (Fig. 11-1).

Color   Skin-colored to yellow.

Size   Few mm to several cm.

Distribution   Symmetrically over abdomen, back, buttocks, arms, thighs.

General Findings

Can be associated with systemic disease (see Table 11-1).

DIFFERENTIAL DIAGNOSIS

Connective tissue nevi can be diagnosed clinically and confirmed by skin biopsy. They can be confused with other dermal or subcutaneous processes such as lipomas, scars, or keloids. The presence of connective tissue nevi should alert the clinician to check carefully for other signs of tuberous sclerosis. Connective tissue nevi can also be confused with pseudoxanthoma elasticum or the mucopolysaccharidoses.

LABORATORY EXAMINATIONS

Dermatopathology   Skin biopsy reveals disorganized collagen and/or elastin fibers. Typically, there is an increase in collagen and a decrease or normal amount of elastin. Biopsies of the lesion can be easily mistaken for normal skin.

COURSE AND PROGNOSIS

Connective tissue nevi are benign. They persist for life and can increase in number during pregnancy. They are typically asymptomatic but can be cosmetically troublesome. They may also rarely be associated with systemic syndromes (Table 11-1).

MANAGEMENT

Treatment for connective tissue nevi is not necessary. Early recognition and evaluation for pos-

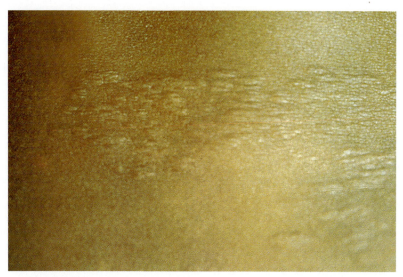

Figure 11-1 **Connective tissue nevus** *Skin-colored, slightly raised plaque on the torso of an infant.*

sible associated syndromes (see Table 11-1), such as tuberous sclerosis, is recommended. Cosmetically, the lesions tend to be too large yet subtle to warrant treatment. Cosmetic im-

provement can be attempted by surgical excision, dermabrasion, electrodesiccation, curettage, and laser ablation.

Table 11-1 CONNECTIVE TISSUE NEVI AND ASSOCIATED SYNDROMES

Syndrome	Synonyms	Cutaneous Findings	Associated Features
Familial cutaneous collagenomas	—	Multiple collagenomas	May have associated cardiomyopathy
Tuberous sclerosis	Epiloa, Bourneville disease	Shagreen patch, adenoma sebaceum, ashleaf macules, café au lait spots, periungual fibromas	Epilepsy, mental retardation, rhabdomyomas, calcified brain nodules
Buschke-Ollendorf syndrome	Albers-Schonberg disease	Dermatofibrosis lenticularis disseminata	Osteopoikilosis, dysplasia of bone (leg bones, pelvis, hands, feet)

BECKER'S NEVUS

A Becker's nevus is a common acquired benign hamartoma that occurs as a unilateral brown pigmented plaque, typically on the shoulder of adolescent boys. Over time, the lesion becomes hairy and may become slightly raised.

EPIDEMIOLOGY

Age   Onset before age 10 (50%), between ages 10 and 15 (25%), and after 15 years of age (25%).

Gender   M > F.

Prevalence   Common.

Incidence   In males ages 17 to 26 years old, 0.5%. Incidence much less in females.

Etiology   Unclear.

Genetics   May be familial in some cases.

HISTORY

Pigmentation appears at puberty, and terminal hairs (in males) begin within a year. Lesions persist for life but are otherwise asymptomatic.

PHYSICAL EXAMINATION

Skin Findings

Type   Isolated macule or plaque, smooth or verrucous surface, increased hair growth (in 56%, Fig. 11-2).

Color   Light tan to brown, blotchy.

Size   One to several cm (average size ~125 cm^2).

Shape   Large irregular shape.

Distribution   Shoulder (32%), lower back (23%), upper back (19%), arms (3%), legs (3%).

Side-lighting   Oblique lighting of the lesion will help to detect subtle elevation.

General Findings

Associated findings are uncommon. In rare instances, underlying hypoplasia of the tissue may be present (i.e., shortened extremity).

DIFFERENTIAL DIAGNOSIS

The diagnosis of a Becker's nevus is often made by history and clinical examination. The increased hair growth (seen in 56% and predominantly in males) is distinctive for Becker's nevi. Becker's nevi can be confused with café au lait macules. They may also be confused with giant congenital nevi, which can be differentiated based on age of onset.

LABORATORY EXAMINATIONS

Dermatopathology   Epidermal acanthosis, hyperkeratosis, and occasional horn cysts. No nevomelanocytes are present. Melanocyte numbers are not increased. Basal cell keratinocytes are packed with melanin.

COURSE AND PROGNOSIS

Pigmentation occurs in adolescence usually followed by increased coarse hair growth (56%) in males that are affected. Females with Becker's nevi have less of a tendency to have hair growth in the lesion. After 2 years, the lesion stabilizes and may fade slightly but persists for life. They may be associated with a smooth muscle hamartoma. Very rarely, Becker's nevi can have an associated underlying hypoplastic limb or bony defect (Becker's nevus syndrome).

MANAGEMENT

Becker's nevi are benign and thus no treatment is necessary. Lesions tend to be quite large and treatment becomes impractical. Cosmetically, lesions can be lightened or the hair can be removed with laser therapy.

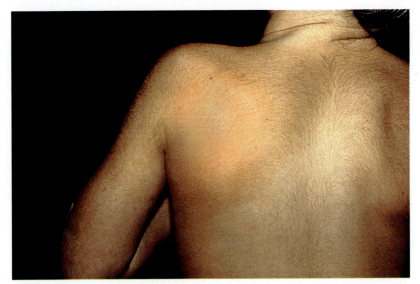

Figure 11-2 Becker's nevus *Large brown plaque that becomes noticeable at puberty with increased pigment followed by hair growth.*

RECURRENT INFANTILE DIGITAL FIBROMA

Recurrent infantile digital fibromas are single or multiple fibrous nodules occurring on the fingers and toes, during infancy or early childhood.

Synonyms Infantile digital fibromatosis, Reye's tumor.

EPIDEMIOLOGY

Age At birth or during the first years of life.

Gender M = F.

Etiology Unknown.

PATHOPHYSIOLOGY

Immunohistochemical and ultrastructural studies have shown that the fibroblasts contain myofilaments. Eosinophilic inclusions are suggestive of a possible viral etiology.

PHYSICAL EXAMINATION

Skin Findings

Type Solitary or multiple well-circumscribed nodules (Fig. 11-3).

Size 1 to 2 cm.

Color Skin-colored to pink.

Palpation Firm.

Distribution Extensor surfaces of the digits, especially on the knuckle area. Thumbs and great toes usually spared.

DIFFERENTIAL DIAGNOSIS

History, physical examination, and skin biopsy can differentiate recurrent digital fibromas from verruca, other fibromas, fibroepithelial polyps, or other dermal nodules.

LABORATORY EXAMINATIONS

Dermatopathology Skin biopsy reveals many spindle cells and collagen bundles arranged in interlacing fascicles in the dermis. The cells contain characteristic perinuclear eosinophilic inclusions measuring 3 to 10 μm in diameter (collection of actin microfilaments by ultrastructural studies).

COURSE AND PROGNOSIS

The lesions of recurrent infantile digital fibromas appear in infancy and spontaneous involution may occur after several years.

MANAGEMENT

For smaller asymptomatic lesions, no treatment is necessary. Larger lesions can lead to functional impairment or deformity. Removal of these lesions by surgical excision is recommended for cosmetic and functional purposes. In 75% of cases, recurrences are observed in late childhood, at which time wide surgical excision may be required.

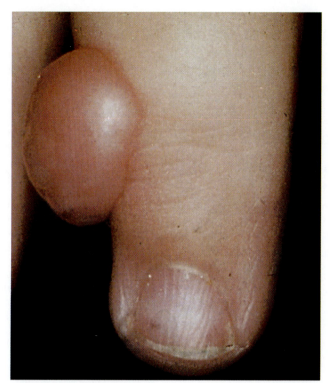

Figure 11-3 Recurrent infantile digital fibroma *Two-year-old with a recurrent nodule on the index finger.* (Reproduced with permission from IM Freedberg et al., Dermatology in General Medicine, 5th edition. New York: McGraw-Hill, 1999).

HYPERTROPHIC SCARS AND KELOIDS

Hypertrophic scars and keloids are formed when there is an exaggerated fibrous tissue response to cutaneous injury. A hypertrophic scar remains confined to the site of original injury; a keloid, however, extends beyond this site with clawlike extensions.

EPIDEMIOLOGY

Age   Puberty to 30 years old.

Gender   M = F.

Race   Much more common in darker skin types.

Etiology   Unknown. Usually follow injury to skin (i.e., surgical scar, laceration, abrasion, cryosurgery, electrocoagulation, as well as vaccination, acne, etc.). May also arise spontaneously without history of injury.

HISTORY

Scars or keloids appear and are usually asymptomatic. May be pruritic or painful at onset. Symptoms fade with time.

PHYSICAL EXAMINATION

Skin Findings

Type   Papules to nodules to tumors to large nodular lesions (Fig. 11-4).

Color   Skin-colored to pink.

Shape   May be linear following traumatic or surgical injury. Hypertrophic scars tend to be dome shaped and are confined to the site of the original injury. Keloids, however, may extend in a clawlike fashion far beyond the site of original injury.

Palpation   Firm to hard; surface smooth.

Sites of Predilection   Ear lobes, shoulders, upper back, chest.

DIFFERENTIAL DIAGNOSIS

The diagnosis of a hypertrophic scar or keloid is made clinically. A biopsy is usually not warranted unless there is clinical doubt, because it may induce new hypertrophic scarring or keloid formation. The differential diagnosis includes a scar, dermatofibroma, dermatofibrosarcoma protuberans, desmoid tumor, sarcoidosis, foreign body granuloma, or lobomycosis.

LABORATORY EXAMINATIONS

Dermatopathology   A hypertrophic scar appears as whorls of young fibrous tissue and fibroblasts in haphazard arrangement. A keloid has an added feature of thick, eosinophilic, acellular bands of collagen.

COURSE AND PROGNOSIS

Hypertrophic scars tend to regress in time becoming flatter and softer. Keloids, however, may continue to slowly expand in size for years.

MANAGEMENT

A person with a history of hypertrophic scars and/or keloids should avoid skin trauma and elective procedures (e.g., ear-piercing) to reduce the risk of scar formation.

Once formed, the treatment for hypertrophic scars and keloids include:

1. Topical steroids with or without occlusion. Flurandrenolide-impregnated tape (Cordran) can be used as a steroid under occlusion. Patients need to be cautioned about steroid side effects. See page 48 for more details.

2. Intralesional steroids.
   a. Triamcinolone (3 to 10 mg/mL, intralesional 0.1 to 1 mL) every month often reduces pruritus or sensitivity of lesion, as well as reducing its volume and flattening it.
   b. Combined treatment of intralesional triamcinolone and cryotherapy may be a little more effective.

Lesions that are excised surgically often recur larger than the original lesion. Thus, careful plastic surgery and occlusive wound care is recommended if excision is to be attempted.

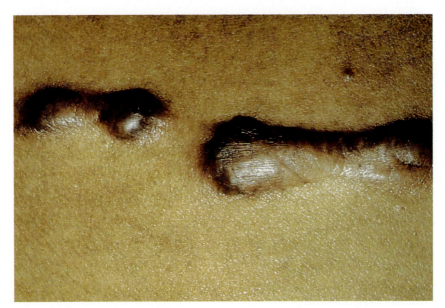

Figure 11-4   Keloid   *Spontaneous keloids on the chest of an adolescent.*

DERMATOFIBROMA

Dermatofibromas are very common, benign, button-like skin lesions, usually occurring on the extremities, important only because of their cosmetic appearance or their being mistaken for other lesions.

Synonyms Solitary histiocytoma, sclerosing hemangioma, histiocytoma cutis.

EPIDEMIOLOGY

Age Occasionally seen in children, more common in adolescence and adulthood.

Gender F > M.

Etiology Unknown, may be chronic histiocytic-fibrous reaction to insect bite, skin injury, or ingrown hair.

PHYSICAL EXAMINATION

Skin Findings

Type Papule or nodule. Surface domed (Fig. 11-5), but may be depressed below plane of surrounding skin. Texture of surface may be dull, shiny, or scaling. Top may be crusted or scarred secondary to excoriation or shaving. Borders ill-defined, fading to normal skin.

Size 3 to 10 mm in diameter.

Color Variable; color of the skin and/or pink, brown, tan, dark brown. Usually darker at center, fading to the normal skin color at margin. Often, center shows postinflammatory hypo- or hyperpigmentation secondary to repeated trauma.

Palpation Firm dermal button- or pea-like papule or nodule. *Dimple sign:* lateral compression with thumb and index finger produces a depression or dimple.

Distribution Legs > arms > trunk. Uncommonly occur on head, palms, soles. Usually solitary, may be multiple, and are randomly scattered.

DIFFERENTIAL DIAGNOSIS

Dermatofibromas are diagnosed clinically and the dimpling sign is a useful clinical diagnostic tool. Dermatofibromas may be confused with nevi, scars, cysts, lipomas, or histiocytomas.

LABORATORY EXAMINATIONS

Dermatopathology Skin biopsy can have several different appearances. Some show a proliferation of spindle shaped fibroblasts/collagen fibers and/or histiocytes.

COURSE AND PROGNOSIS

Lesions appear gradually over several months, and persist for years to decades; few lesions regress spontaneously.

MANAGEMENT

Dermatofibromas are benign and typically best left untreated. Surgical removal is not usually indicated because the resulting scar is often worse cosmetically. Indications for excision include repeated trauma, unacceptable cosmetic appearance, or uncertainty of clinical diagnosis. Cryotherapy may be used to flatten raised lesions.

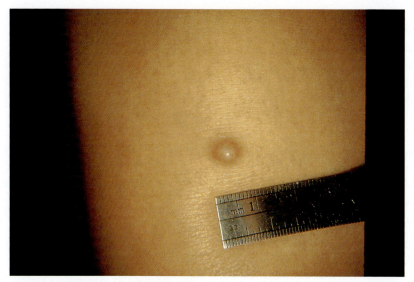

Figure 11-5   **Dermatofibroma**   *Raised dome-shaped 5-mm papule on the leg of a child.*

SKIN TAG

A skin tag is a benign, pedunculated lesion the color of the skin or darker, occurring at intertriginous sites. In some locations (i.e., in the preauricular or perianal region), they can be a sign of systemic disease.

Synonyms Acrochordon, cutaneous papilloma, soft fibroma.

EPIDEMIOLOGY

Age Adolescence and adulthood.

Gender F > M.

Incidence Very common.

Etiology Unknown. Often familial. More common in overweight individuals.

HISTORY

Skin Symptoms Usually asymptomatic but skin tags may become inflamed or irritated. Occasionally, they may become tender or bleed following trauma or torsion.

PHYSICAL EXAMINATION

Skin Findings

Type Pedunculated papilloma (Fig. 11-6), usually constricted at base. At times, crusted or hemorrhagic following trauma.

Size 1 to 10 mm.

Color Range of skin colors; may be the same color or darker than the racial pigmentation of the patient.

Shape Usually round to oval.

Number One to several.

Palpation Soft, pliable.

Distribution Intertriginous areas.

Sites of Predilection Eyelids (upper > lower), neck, axillae, inframammary, groin.

General Findings Preauricular skin tags can be associated with first arch embryonic developmental abnormalities. Perianal skin tags may be an indicator of associated GI polyps.

DIFFERENTIAL DIAGNOSIS

The diagnosis of skin tags is typically made clinically. The differential diagnosis includes a pedunculated dermal or compound melanocytic nevus, neurofibroma, or wart.

LABORATORY EXAMINATIONS

Dermatopathology Skin biopsy shows a pedunculated lesion of fibrous tissue stroma.

COURSE AND PROGNOSIS

Skin tags tend to become larger and more numerous over time. Following torsion, autoamputation can occur.

MANAGEMENT

Skin tags are benign thus no treatment is necessary. Symptomatic skin tags can be removed by snipping them off with scissors, electrodesiccation, or cryosurgery.

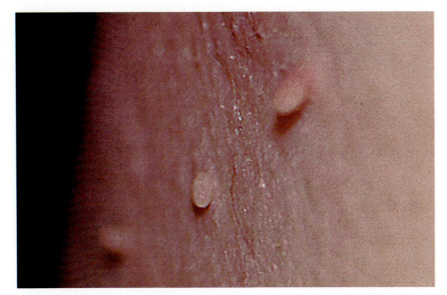

Figure 11-6 Skin tag *2- to 3-mm pedunculated skin-colored growths on the neck.*

LEIOMYOMA

Leiomyomas are benign smooth muscle growths clinically characterized by solitary or multiple red dermal nodules subject to episodes of paroxysmal pain.

EPIDEMIOLOGY

Classification (1) Angioleiomyomas, arising from vascular smooth muscle; (2) solitary pilar leiomyomas arising from the arrector pili muscles (majority); (3) multiple pilar leiomyomas: inherited with autosomal dominant trait; and (4) genital leiomyomas originating in the dartoic, vulvar, or mamillary muscles of the scrotum, labia, or nipple.

Age Can be seen in childhood. More common in adults.

Gender M = F.

Prevalence Uncommon.

Etiology Usually acquired, except multiple piloleiomyomas.

Genetics Multiple piloleiomyomas are inherited in an autosomal dominant trait.

HISTORY

Skin Symptoms Chronic lesions can be sensitive to touch or cold; spontaneously painful.

PHYSICAL EXAMINATION

Skin Findings

Type Solitary or multiple nodules with a waxy appearance, measuring from a few mm to 1 cm (Fig. 11-7).

Size 1 to 10 mm.

Color Reddish brown to blue.

Palpation Firm, fixed to skin but freely movable over the underlying structures.

Shape Round.

Arrangement Grouped when multiple; tend to coalesce into plaques with arciform or linear configuration.

Distribution Back, sides of face and neck, extensor surfaces of extremities.

General Findings

Leiomyomas typically have no associated systemic findings. Rarely, women with multiple inherited piloleiomyomas may have associated painful smooth muscle tumors of the uterus (familial leiomyomatosis cutis et uteri).

DIFFERENTIAL DIAGNOSIS

History, physical examination, and skin biopsy can help differentiate leiomyomas from angiolipomas, glomus tumors, osteoma cutis, eccrine spiradenomas, neuromas, and neurilemmomas. Rarely, there can be leiomyosarcomas, which are typically larger than their benign counterparts.

LABORATORY EXAMINATIONS

Dermatopathology Pilar leiomyomas reveal a proliferation of haphazardly arranged smooth muscle fibers in the dermis, separated from the epidermis with a Grenz zone. Angioleiomyomas reveal a well-demarcated dermal nodule composed of concentrically arranged smooth muscle fibers around numerous slit-like vascular spaces.

COURSE AND PROGNOSIS

Leiomyomas are benign and are typically asymptomatic. Some lesions are painful. They have a high incidence of recurrence (50%) following removal.

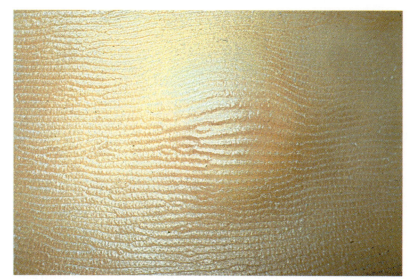

Figure 11-7 **Angioleiomyoma** *Ill-defined 1-cm painful nodule on the plantar surface.*

MANAGEMENT

Leiomyomas are benign and thus no treatment is necessary. For symptomatic lesions, possible treatments include:

1. Wide surgical excision but the recurrence rate is high (50%).
2. Alpha-adrenergic blockers (phenoxybenzamine).
3. Calcium channel antagonists (nifedipine).
4. Acetaminophen.
5. Lidocaine.
6. Scopolamine.
7. Glycerol.
8. Topical nitroglycerin.

LIPOMA

A lipoma is a common benign tumor characterized by an asymptomatic, well-demarcated, soft nodule of mature fat cells. They are typically solitary lesions and benign, but can be associated with more diffuse disease (Table 11-2).

EPIDEMIOLOGY

Age   Any age, but most have an onset at or after puberty.

Gender   M = F.

Incidence   Very common.

Genetics   Familial multiple lipomatosis is inherited as an autosomal dominant trait.

HISTORY

Lipomas are asymptomatic nodules that are stable or slowly growing in size for years. They may become tender to palpation.

PHYSICAL EXAMINATION

Skin Findings

Type   Single or multiple nodules.

Size   1 to 10 cm.

Color   Skin-colored.

Shape   Round, disc-shaped, or lobulated.

Distribution   Anywhere.

Sites of Predilection   Neck, shoulders, back (Fig. 11-8), and abdominal wall.

DIFFERENTIAL DIAGNOSIS

The diagnosis of a lipoma is made by history and clinical examination. It can be confirmed by skin biopsy or fine needle aspiration.

Variants

1. Nevus lipomatosus superficialis of Hoffman-Zurhelle: Soft, color of the skin or yellowish papules, nodules, and plaques on the sacrococcygeal areas or thighs.
2. Angiolipomas: Multiple and tender nodules resembling lipomas. The differential diagnosis includes a cavernous hemangioma, cavernous lymphangioma, or liposarcoma.

LABORATORY EXAMINATIONS

Dermatopathology   Encapsulated tumors composed of mature fat cells (large polygonal or spherical cells with lipid vacuole and peripherally displaced nucleus) intersected by thin strands of fibrous tissue.

COURSE AND PROGNOSIS

Most lipomas remain stable and asymptomatic. They may enlarge or become tender. Malignant transformation (liposarcoma) is extremely rare and typically occurs in lesions of 10 cm or more in diameter.

MANAGEMENT

Lipomas are usually benign and asymptomatic and thus no treatment is required. For symptomatic or enlarging lesions, surgical excision or liposuction can be performed.

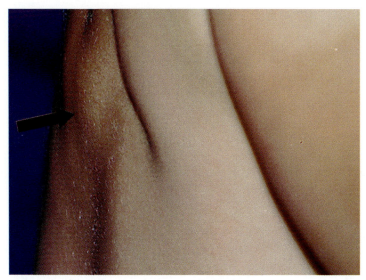

Figure 11-8 Lipoma *Soft asymptomatic nodule on the midback of an infant. Imaging studies were normal.*

Table 11-2 LIPOMAS AND ASSOCIATED SYNDROMES

Syndrome	Synonym	Cutaneous Findings	Associated Findings
Multiple familial lipomatosis		Multiple asymptomatic diffuse lipomas	Inherited in an autosomal dominant fashion
Nevus lipomatosis superficialis	Hoffman-Zurhelle disease	Buttocks, sacrococcygeal, and thigh lipomas	—
Adiposis dolorosa	Dercum's disease	Tender lipomas on arms and legs	Usually in post-menopausal women; paresthesias, weakness, arthralgias, obesity, mental disturbances, amenorrhea, alcoholism
Benign symmetric lipomatosis	Madelung's disease	Symmetric neck and upper trunk lipomas	Usually in alcoholic men
Michelin-tire baby	—	Embryonic overgrowth of fatty tissue causing deep conspicuous cutaneous folds	Mental retardation, microcephaly, rocker-bottom feet, metatarsus abductus, hemiplegia, hemihypertrophy, abnormal chromosomes and neurologic defects
Proteus syndrome	—	Congenital lipomas, nevi	Gigantism, hemihypertrophy, mesenchymal neoplasms

DISORDERS OF PIGMENTATION

Skin color is genetically determined and is due to the total amount of melanin pigment in the skin. Normal constitutive melanin pigmentation determines skin type, which is currently classified by the Fitzpatrick phototypes as follows:

Skin Phototypes	Ability to Tan	Susceptibility to Burns
SPT I	Never tans	Sunburns easily
SPT II	Tans with difficulty	Sunburns easily
SPT III	Can tan with time	Occasionally burns
SPT IV	Tans easily	Rarely burns
SPT V	Tans easily, brown skin	Rarely burns
SPT VI	Tans easily, black skin	Rarely burns

Disorders of hypopigmentation are caused by decreased melanin content in the skin due to decreased or absent melanin production or melanocytes. Disorders of hyperpigmentation are caused by increased melanin content in the skin due to an increase in melanin production or melanocytes.

DISORDERS OF HYPOPIGMENTATION

Decreased or absent melanin in the skin can lead to hypomelanosis and can occur by two main mechanisms.

1. Absent or decreased melanocytes in the epidermis producing _melanocytic hypomelanosis_ (e.g., vitiligo).

2. Normal melanocyte numbers in the epidermis, but decreased or absent melanin production producing _melanotic hypomelanosis_ (e.g., postinflammatory hypopigmentation).

PITYRIASIS ALBA

Pityriasis alba is a common asymptomatic, sometimes scaly, hypopigmentation of the face, neck, and body.

EPIDEMIOLOGY

Age Young children, often ages 3 to 16 years.

Gender M = F.

Race All races, more common in darker skin types. Cases reported from North America, South America, Europe, and Africa.

Prevalence Common

Etiology Likely a form of atopic dermatitis.

PATHOPHYSIOLOGY

Thought to be an eczematous dermatosis, with hypomelanosis resulting from postinflammatory changes and ultraviolet screening effects of the hyperkeratotic and parakeratotic epidermis.

HISTORY

Hypopigmented areas are usually stable then gradually disappear with age. Some lesions may persist into adulthood. The areas are typically asymptomatic, but can sometimes burn or itch.

PHYSICAL EXAMINATION

Skin Findings

Type Two or 3 macules with indistinct margins, may have slight scale.

Number One to 20 lesions may be present.

Color Subtle erythema fades, leaving an off-white to tan-white color.

Size and Shape 5 to 30 mm or larger.

Distribution Face, neck, trunk, back, limbs, and scrotum.

Sites of Predilection Face, especially the cheeks (Fig. 12-1), mid-forehead, and around the eyes and mouth.

General Findings

May be associated with atopy (eczema, allergies, hayfever, asthma).

DIFFERENTIAL DIAGNOSIS

Pityriasis alba can be confused with other hypopigmented skin disorders such as vitiligo, tinea versicolor, tinea corporis, and the ash leaf or confetti macules of tuberous sclerosis.

Pityriasis alba is differentiated from tinea infections by the absence of a positive scraping. A Wood's lamp examination can differentiate pityriasis alba from the depigmented skin lesions of vitiligo (the latter will light up brightly compared to the former).

LABORATORY EXAMINATIONS

Dermatopathology Histology reveals hyperkeratosis, parakeratosis, moderately dilated vessels of the superficial dermis, slight perivascular infiltrate, and edema of the papillary dermis. The number of melanocytes is reduced and those present contain fewer and smaller melanosomes.

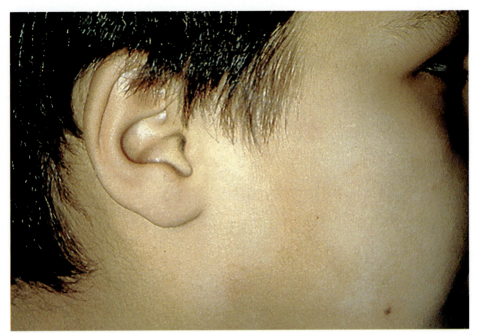

Figure 12-1   Pityriasis alba   *Faint hypopigmented slight scaly macules located on the cheeks and periauricular area of a child.*

COURSE AND PROGNOSIS

Pityriasis alba is a benign condition and often is self-limited.

MANAGEMENT

Treatment is unnecessary. The condition improves with age. For cosmetic reasons, lubrication with moisturizers followed by sun exposure may be useful to diminish the dry scales and repigment the area. Phototherapy alone is often ineffective. Moisturizers should be applied to normal and abnormal (affected) skin after prescription ointments have been applied. The most useful time to apply these is immediately after bathing or showering. Some moisturizers contain perfumes, alcohol, and preservatives—these should be avoided if possible. Generally, for dry skin, the more greasy creams and lotions are best. Some moisturizers are: hydrated petrolatum, Vaseline, mineral oil, Aquaphor, Lubriderm, Moisturel, and Eucerin creams.

In severe cases of pityriasis alba, a topical steroid can be used sparingly in appropriate strengths. (See page 48 for more details.)

POSTINFLAMMATORY HYPOPIGMENTATION

A common cause of benign hypopigmentation characterized by decreased melanin formation following cutaneous inflammation.

Synonym   Postinflammatory hypomelanosis.

EPIDEMIOLOGY

Age   Any age.

Gender   M = F.

Etiology   Usually follows involution of any inflammatory skin disorders (e.g., eczematous or psoriatic lesions, pityriasis rosea, burns, bullous disorders, infections, etc.).

PATHOPHYSIOLOGY

Inflammatory conditions of the epidermis may result in transient keratinocyte injury and may render them temporarily unable to accept melanin from melanocytic dendrites.

HISTORY

Skin Symptoms   None.

PHYSICAL EXAMINATION

Skin Findings

Type   Macules and patches usually with ill-defined borders.

Color   Off-white to tan.

Shape   Linear, oval, round, punctate depending on primary process (Fig. 12-2).

Distribution   Localized or diffuse depending on primary process.

DIFFERENTIAL DIAGNOSIS

A clinical history of an antecedent inflammatory dermatosis is helpful to differentiate postinflammatory hypopigmentation from tinea versicolor, tuberous sclerosis, vitiligo, albinism, or infectious disease (leprosy, pinta, etc.).

LABORATORY EXAMINATIONS

Dermatopathology   Skin biopsy may show decreased melanin in keratinocytes, inflammatory infiltrate may or may not be present depending on the etiologic primary process.

COURSE AND PROGNOSIS

Hypopigmentation gradually self-resolves over a period of months provided that the affected areas are kept disease-free.

MANAGEMENT

No treatment is necessary. Prevention would focus on eliminating the primary inflammatory process.

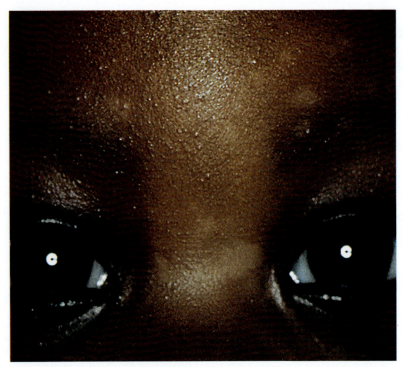

Figure 12-2 Post-inflammatory hypopigmentation *Residual hypopigmented macules after resolution of tinea versicolor in a young child.*

DISORDERS OF PIGMENTATION

VITILIGO

Vitiligo is a pigmentary disorder characterized clinically by the development of completely white macules, microscopically by the absence of melanocytes, and medically by the increased risk of autoimmune mediated disease (i.e., thyroid disorders).

EPIDEMIOLOGY

Age   Any age, 50% begin between ages 10 to 30 years. In rare instances, it is present at birth.

Gender   M = F.

Race   All races. Apparent prevalence in darker-skinned persons is because the disease is more noticeable.

Incidence   Common. Affects up to 1% of the population.

Genetics   Up to 30% of patients have a first-degree relative with vitiligo. As many as 4 genetic loci have been implicated in vitiligo. Families with thyroid disease, diabetes, and other autoimmune processes are at increased risk of developing vitiligo.

Etiology   Likely autoimmune mediated.

PATHOPHYSIOLOGY

Three pathophysioloic mechanisms for vitiligo have been proposed.

1. Autoimmune (activated lymphocytes attack melanocytes).
2. Neurogenic (melanocytes interacting with nerve cells).
3. Self-destructive (melanin production makes a toxin that destroys melanocytes).

HISTORY

Both genetics and environment play a role in vitiligo. Many patients attribute the onset of their vitiligo to trauma, as with cuts, suture sites, etc. (Koebner or isomorphic phenomenon). Emotional stress (e.g., grief over lost partner) is also mentioned by patients as a cause. The white areas gradually appear and 30% or more can undergo spontaneous repigmentation.

PHYSICAL EXAMINATION

Skin Findings

Type of Lesion   Typically pure white macules. Occasionally, hypomelanotic macules may also be observed.

Size   Can vary from a few confetti-sized macules to larger extensive regional areas (Fig. 12-3A).

Color   Chalk-white depigmentation is classic but newly developing lesions may be "off-white" in color; follicular areas of repigmentation may be noted (Fig. 12-3B).

Palpation   Rarely, there is a raised erythematous border. This is called "inflammatory" vitiligo but it has no special significance.

Shape of Individual Lesion   Oval, geographic patterns; the borders may often be scalloped. There may be linear patterns or artifactual type areas (as under a neck pendant); these represent the isomorphic or Koebner phenomenon.

Distribution of Lesions   Isolated macules, unilateral, quasidermatomal, or generalized lesions at sites of repeated trauma, such as the bony prominences (malleoli, tip of the elbow, necklace area in females).

Wood's Lamp Examination   It is essential to examine patients with a light skin color with the Wood's lamp to detect all the areas of vitiligo. The depigmented areas will light up brightly with the Wood's lamp examination.

Associated Cutaneous Findings

Hair   White hair and premature gray hair, alopecia areata, and halo nevi.

Mucous Membranes   Rarely present in the mouth (gums).

Eye   Iritis in 10%, but may not be symptomatic; retinal changes consistent with healed chorioretinitis in up to 30% of patients.

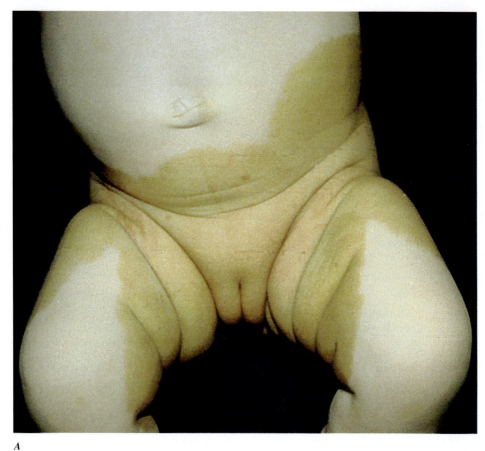

A

Figure 12-3 Vitiligo *(A) Extensive areas of depigmentation on the legs and the abdomen of an infant with vitiligo. Normal skin color of the child is the darker area in the diaper region.*

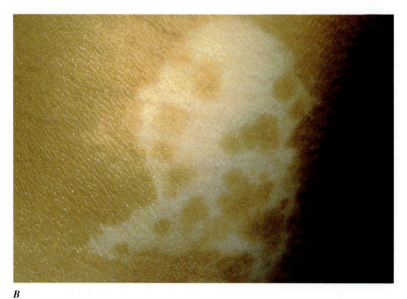

B

Figure 12-3 (continued)   Vitiligo   (B) *Area of vitiligo with characteristic "islands of repigmentation" indicative of follicular-based repigmentation.*

General Examination

Thyroid disease present in up to 30% of patients with vitiligo, diabetes mellitus (more than 5%), pernicious anemia (uncommon), Addison's disease (uncommon), syndrome of polyendocrinopathy with mucocutaneous candidiasis (rare).

DIFFERENTIAL DIAGNOSIS

Physical examination is diagnostic, but in certain cases a skin biopsy can differentiate vitiligo from lupus erythematosus, pityriasis alba, tinea versicolor, piebaldism, chemical leukoderma, leprosy, nevus depigmentosus, tuberous sclerosis, leukoderma with metastatic melanoma, and postinflammatory hypomelanosis.

LABORATORY EXAMINATIONS

Dermatopathology On skin biopsy, melanocytes are completely absent in fully developed vitiligo macules, but at the margin of the white macules, there may be melanocytes present and a mild lymphocytic response.

Laboratory Examination of Blood Blood tests for T4, TSH, glucose, CBC, and cortisol (in high-risk patients) may be indicated to rule out autoimmune diseases.

COURSE AND PROGNOSIS

The course of vitiligo is unpredictable; lesions may remain stable for years or progress rapidly. About 30% of patients have some degree of spontaneous repigmentation. In rare instances, the total melanin pigmentation of the skin is lost except for the eyes.

MANAGEMENT

Sunscreen: Protect involved skin from burns and to limit uninvolved skin from tanning:

Cosmetic cover-up: Vitadye and DyoDerm stains can be used. Covermark and Dermablend are cosmetics mixed to match skin hues to mask white areas.

Topical steroids may be used with careful physician monitoring.
1. Low potency steroids (Desowen, 1% hydrocortisone, 2.5% hydrocortisone) can be used on the youngest patients (younger than 10) or on the face and groin area of older children bid.
2. Medium potency steroids (Elocon, Dermatop, Cutivate) can be used on older children (ages 10 to 20) on the body or extremities bid.
3. Strong steroids (Ultravate, Psorcon, Diprolene) are reserved for older children and adults (older than age 10) on severely affected or refractory areas bid.

Patients need to be cautioned about steroid side effects. (See page 48 for more details.)

Topical photochemotherapy (PUVA) topical psoralens such as 8-methoxypsoralen (8-MOP) and artificial UVA (in a doctor's office) may be tried but require regular, biweekly light treatments and is not a permanent cure.

Systemic photochemotherapy may be attempted in older children (typically older than 10 years).
1. Oral trimethylpsoralen (TMP) and sunlight under the guidance of a physician.
   OR
2. Oral TMP or 8-MOP (8-MOP Ultra 0.3 mg/kg) and artificial UVA (in a doctor's office) biweekly.

Ophthalmologic examination and an ANA are required before starting light treatment. Side effects include nausea and GI upset acutely. Long-term phototherapy can lead to photoaging, lentigenes, and an increased risk of cutaneous carcinomas.

Minigrafting: Grafts of pigmented skin are transplanted to non-pigment areas.

Bleaching: Widespread cases may benefit more from bleaching residual pigmented areas. Bleaching can be accomplished with 20% monobenzoether cream to the skin qd to bid or 20% hydroquinone cream to the skin qd to bid.

Depigmentation of the normal skin color takes 2 to 3 months to see initial lightening and may take 1 to 3 years to complete. It is important to warn the patient that the bleaching of the skin color is permanent.

ALBINISM

Albinism is an uncommon inherited disorder that presents as a congenital absence of pigment in the skin, eyes, and hair. Albinism can principally affect the eyes, *ocular albinism* (OA, X-linked recessive or autosomal recessive) or the eyes and skin, *oculocutaneous albinism* (OCA, autosomal recessive or dominant). There are many types of albinism with involvement of several different genes (Table 12-1).

EPIDEMIOLOGY

Age   Present at birth.

Race   There is no racial predilection except for Hermansky-Pudlak syndrome (OCA and a platelet disorder), which is seen in Hispanics from Puerto Rico, in persons of Dutch origin, and in East Indians from Madras.

Incidence   OCA 1:20,000.

Genetics   OA: X-linked recessive or autosomal recessive. OCA: autosomal recessive autosomal dominant.

PATHOPHYSIOLOGY

The defect in melanin synthesis has been shown to result from absence of the activity of the enzyme, tyrosinase in OCA 1A. Tyrosinase is a copper-containing enzyme that catalyzes the oxidation of tyrosine to dopa and the subsequent dehydrogenation of dopa to dopaquinone. Recent cloning of complementary DNAs (cDNAs) encoding tyrosinase has made it possible to directly characterize the mutations in the tyrosinase gene responsible for deficient tyrosinase activity in type 1A albinism. Two different missense mutations, one from each parent, result in amino acid substitutions within one of the two copper-binding sites.

OCA 1B individuals have mutations in the tyrosinase gene which lead to yellow, minimal-pigment and temperature-sensitive OCA.

OCA 2 individuals have mutations in the P gene.

HPS individuals have OCA and a bleeding diathesis secondary to ceroid storage defects and defective platelets.

CHS individuals have hematologic abnormalities (thrombocytopenia) and repeated bacterial infections from a defective degranulation response to infection.

HISTORY

Patients with albinism learn early in life to avoid the sun because of repeated sunburns, especially as toddlers. They have a normal life span but can have problems with vision, to the point of blindness, and skin cancers later in life.

PHYSICAL EXAMINATION

Skin Findings

Type   White to light tan coloring of the skin (Fig. 12-4).

Color   Chalk white, yellow, cream, or light tan (tyrosinase-negative).

Hair   White, yellow cream, or light brown (tyrosinase-positive), red, platinum.

Eyes: Iris translucency, nystagmus.

General Findings

Reduction of visual acuity and squinting in sunlight. In Hermansky-Pudlak syndrome (HPS): epistaxis, gingival bleeding, excessive bleeding after childbirth or dental procedures, fibrotic restrictive lung disease.

LABORATORY EXAMINATIONS

Dermatopathology

Light Microscopy   Melanocytes are present in the skin and hair bulb in all types of albinism. The dopa reaction of the skin and hair is markedly reduced or absent in melanocytes of the skin and hair depending on the type of albinism (tyrosinase-negative or tyrosinase-positive).

Electron Microscopy   Melanosomes are present in melanocytes in all types of albinism but, depending on the type of albinism, there is a reduction of the melanization of melanosomes, with many being completely unmelanized (stage I) in tyrosinase-negative albinism. Melanosomes in the albino melanocytes are transferred in a normal manner to the keratinocytes.

Tyrosine Hair Bulb Test (tyrosinase-negative and tyrosinase-positive) Hair bulbs are incubated in tyrosine solutions for 12 to 24 h and develop new pigment formation from normal and tyrosinase-positive patients, but no new pigment formation is present in tyrosinase-negative albinism.

Hematology In instances of Hermansky-Pudlak syndrome (albinism with platelet disorder), defects in platelets are detected. In instances of Chédiak-Higashi syndrome (albinism with depressed degranulation and bactericidal functions), defects in platelets and leukocytes are detected.

DIFFERENTIAL DIAGNOSIS

Iris translucency and the presence of other eye findings in the fundus are reliable signs of albinism. The hair and skin color may vary from normal to absent melanin and the types are listed in Table 12-1.

COURSE AND PROGNOSIS

Patients with tyrosinase-positive OCA form some melanin pigment in the hair, skin, and eyes during early life, the hair becoming cream, yellow, or light brown, and the eye color changing from light gray to blue, hazel, or even brown.

Patients with albinism who are unprotected in sunny climates can develop squamous cell carcinomas and they are particularly at risk for metastases. Dermatoheliosis and basal cell carcinomas are frequent in patients with albinism living in temperate climates. Melanomas are less frequently seen in albinos and are typically of the amelanotic variety.

MANAGEMENT

Recognition of albinism early in life is important to begin early patient education about prophylactic daily skin care.

1. Daily application of topical, potent, broad-spectrum sunblocks, including lip protection (SPF higher than 30).
2. Wide brim hats and long-sleeved clothing to reduce exposed areas.
3. Avoidance of direct sun exposure between the hours of 10 AM and 2 PM, especially in high-intensity seasons.
4. Regular periodic skin examinations to detect and treat skin cancers as early as possible.
5. Regular opthalmologic care.

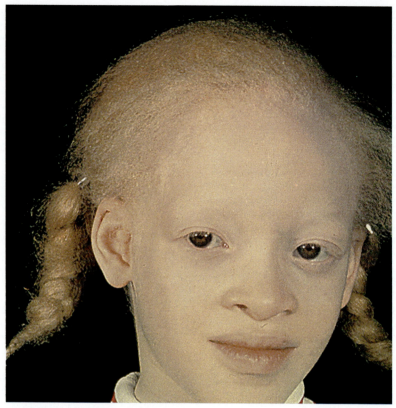

Figure 12-4 Albinism *A black child with albinism. Note the light colored hair, skin, and eyes in a child whose familial constitutional skin color is much darker.*

DISORDERS OF PIGMENTATION

Table 12-1 CLASSIFICATION OF ALBINISM

Type	Subtypes	Gene Locus	Includes	Clinical Findings
OCA1	OCA1A	Tyrosinase	Tyrosinase-negative OCA	White hair and skin, eyes (pink at birth → blue)
	OCA1B	Tyrosinase	Minimal pigment OCA	White to near-normal skin and hair pigmentation
			Yellow OCA	Yellow (pheomelanin) hair, light red or brown hair
			Temperature-sensitive OCA	May have near-normal pigment but not in axillas
			Autosomal recessive OA (some)	
OCA2	P		Tyrosinase-positive	Yellow hair, "creamy" white (Africa)
			Brown OCA	Light brown/tan skin (Africa)
OCA3	TRP1		Autosomal recessive OCA (some)	
			Rufous OCA	Red and red-brown skin and brown eyes (Africa)
HPS	HPS		Hermansky-Pudlak syndrome	Skin/hair as in OCA1A or OCA1B or OCA2, bleeding diathesis (Puerto Rico)
CHS	CHS		Chédiak-Higashi syndrome	Silver hair/hypopigmentation/ serious medical problems
OA1	OA1		X-linked OA	Normal pigmentation of skin, any hair

ABBREVIATIONS: OA, ocular albinism; OCA, oculocutaneous albinism; TRPI, tyrosine-related protein 1.

SOURCE: Reproduced with permission from TB Fitzpatrick et al., *Color Atlas and Synopsis of Clinical Dermatology*, 4th edition. New York; McGraw-Hill, 2001.

NEVUS DEPIGMENTOSUS

Nevus depigmentosus is a congenital hypomelanotic lesion characterized by a singular spot or streak of hypopigmentation with a chronic persistent course.

Synonym Nevus achromicus.

EPIDEMIOLOGY

Age Present at birth.

Gender M = F.

Prevalence Uncommon.

Etiology Unclear.

PATHOPHYSIOLOGY

Proposed mechanism for nevus depigmentosus is melanosome aggregation in melanocytes and a block of transfer to keratinocytes.

HISTORY

Patients are born with the depigmented area of skin and the area is asymptomatic but persists for life.

PHYSICAL EXAMINATION

Skin Findings

Type Depigmented macules or patches with irregular, serrated, or geographic margins.

Color Depigmented white or light tan (Fig. 12-5).

Size Few mm to several cm.

Number Typically solitary, may have several quasidermatomal lesions.

Distribution Usually on the trunk, lower abdomen, and proximal extremities. Face and neck may be involved.

General Findings

May rarely be associated with hemihypertrophy and/or mental retardation.

DIFFERENTIAL DIAGNOSIS

Nevus depigmentosus must be differentiated from vitiligo, nevus anemicus, and lesions of tuberous sclerosis. The diagnosis is usually made clinically.

LABORATORY EXAMINATIONS

Wood's Lamp Examination Accentuation of depigmented areas.

Dermatopathology The number of melanocytes is normal but a dopa reaction would be diminished.

Electron Microscopy Reveals melanocytes with poorly developed dendrites. Melanosomes tend to aggregate in melanocytes and are reduced in keratinocytes. Melanization is decreased or normal.

COURSE AND PROGNOSIS

Lesions persist for life, but remain asymptomatic.

MANAGEMENT

No treatment is necessary. Cosmetically, the lesion is less noticeable if the patient is not tan. Good sunscreen use and sun avoidance is recommended.

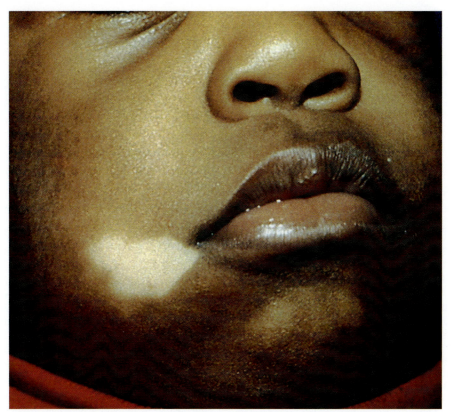

Figure 12-5 Nevus depigmentosus *Depigmented area on the cheek of an infant present since birth.*

NEVUS ANEMICUS

Nevus anemicus is a rare congenital vascular disorder that presents with a benign patch of pale or mottled skin.

Synonym   Pharmacologic nevus.

EPIDEMIOLOGY

Age   Newborn.

Gender   F > M.

Prevalence   Rare.

Etiology   Unclear.

PATHOPHYSIOLOGY

It has been suggested that nevus anemicus arises from a focal decreased blood vessel sensitivity to endogenous vasodilatory mediators (acetylcholine, histamine, serotonin) or an increased sensitivity to endogenous constricting catecholamines. There also could be a defect at the smooth muscle effector cells of the blood vessels. Intralesional injection of histamine or serotonin, acetylcholine failed to produce vasodilatation in the affected areas.

HISTORY

Lesions are present at birth and persist asymptomatically for life.

PHYSICAL EXAMINATION

Skin Findings

Type   Well-demarcated macule or patch with irregular margins and satellite macules (Fig. 12-6).

Size   Few mm to several cm.

Color   Hypopigmented, avascular.

Distribution   Most commonly on the chest although can occur on face and extremities.

Wood's Lamp   Does not enhance the lesion(s).

DIFFERENTIAL DIAGNOSIS

Three factors may be helpful for differentiating a nevus anemicus from a pigmentary problem: (1) a nevus anemicus does not accentuate by Wood's lamp; (2) pressure on the lesion by a glass slide makes the lesion unapparent from surrounding normal skin; and (3) friction or heat application fails to induce erythema to the hypomelanotic areas.

The differential diagnosis includes nevus depigmentosum, tuberous sclerosis, vitiligo, hypomelanosis of Ito, and incontinenti pigmenti.

LABORATORY EXAMINATIONS

Dermatopathology   A skin biopsy would be interpreted as normal skin.

COURSE AND PROGNOSIS

Nevus anemicus persists for life and is usually asymptomatic.

MANAGEMENT

No treatment is necessary.

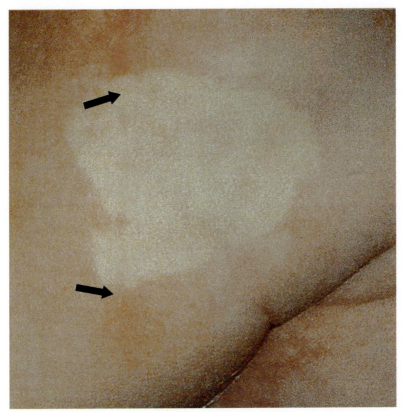

Figure 12-6 Nevus anemicus *Hypopigmented macule present since birth. Stroking of the lesion produces a normal erythematous response at the periphery (see arrow), but not within the lesion, indicative of its avascularity.*

DISORDERS OF HYPERPIGMENTATION

Increased melanin in the skin can lead to hypermelanosis and can occur by two main mechanisms.

1. Increased melanocytes in the epidermis producing *melanocytic* hypermelanosis.

2. Normal melanocyte numbers in the epidermis, but increased amounts of melanin producing *melanotic* hypermelanosis (e.g., postinflammatory hyperpigmentation).

POSTINFLAMMATORY HYPERPIGMENTATION

Postinflammatory hyperpigmentation is a common entity characterized by increased melanin formation and deposition following cutaneous inflammation.

Synonym Postinflammatory melanosis.

EPIDEMIOLOGY

Age Any age.

Gender M = F.

Race More severe and longer lasting in darker skin types.

Etiology Pigment incontinence leading to hyperpigmentation can result from inflammation (following physical trauma, friction, irritant dermatitis, eczematous dermatitis, lichen simplex chronicus, psoriasis, pityriasis rosea, fixed drug eruptions, pyoderma, photodermatitis, dermatitis herpetiformis, lupus erythematosus, etc.).

PATHOPHYSIOLOGY

Inflammatory conditions of the epidermis may result in disruption of the dermal-epidermal junction and basal layer with resultant pigment incontinence. Melanin drops from the normal epidermal counterpart and passes into the dermal melanophages.

PHYSICAL EXAMINATION

Skin Findings

Type Macules and patches usually with ill-defined borders (Fig. 12-7).

Size Few mm to several cm.

Color Dark or light brown.

Shape Linear, oval, round, punctate depending on primary process.

Distribution Localized or diffuse depending on primary process.

Wood's Lamp Examination Accentuation of dermal pigmentation.

DIFFERENTIAL DIAGNOSIS

A clinical history of a previous inflammatory process is helpful to distinguish postinflammatory hyperpigmentation from melanocytic proliferations (ephelides, lentigines, nevi), endocrine abnormalities (Addison's disease, estrogen therapy, ACTH and MSH producing tumors, hyperthyroidism), metabolic disorders (hemochromatosis, porphyria cutanea tarda, ochronosis), melasma, melanoma, scleroderma, pregnancy, drug-induced hyperpigmentation, ashy dermatosis, and macular amyloidosis.

LABORATORY EXAMINATIONS

Dermatopathology Epidermis normal to slightly atrophic depending on etiologic agent, prominent vacuolization on the dermoepidermal junction, and scattered perivascular and intervascular melanophages in papillary dermis.

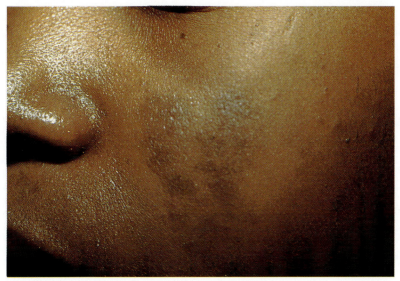

Figure 12-7   Postinflammatory hyperpigmentation   *Hyperpigmentation on the cheek following a contact dermatitis.*

COURSE AND PROGNOSIS

Hyperpigmentation gradually fades over a period of months provided that the affected areas are protected from ultraviolet exposure. Darker skin types have a more persistent and refractory course.

MANAGEMENT

Treatment is not necessary because the hyperpigmentation will resolve slowly.
For mild cases a low potency corticosteroid (Desowen, 1% hydrocortisone, 2.5% hydrocortisone) can be helpful.

For patients who desire more active therapy, hydroquinone formulations are available (Solaquin, Eldoquin, Melanex, Lustra) and can be applied qhs. Patients should be warned about cautious use of hydroquinone preparations for a limited period of time as excessive pigmentary loss may occur. Further worsening of the hyperpigmentation is also possible. They should also be informed about sun protection when using these products as well as about their slow therapeutic action (3 to 4 months are required before a therapeutic effect is achieved).

LINEAR AND WHORLED NEVOID HYPERMELANOSIS

Linear and whorled nevoid hypermelanosis is a benign, congenital, streaky hyperpigmentation along Blaschko's lines.

EPIDEMIOLOGY

Age At or soon after birth.

Gender M = F.

Race No racial predilection.

Prevalence Rare.

Etiology Unclear.

PATHOPHYSIOLOGY

Nevoid hyperpigmentation along Blaschko's lines is thought to be due to mosaicism likely due to a heterogenous group of genetic abnormalities rather than just one specific entity.

HISTORY

Whorled "marble cake-like" streaks of hyperpigmentation appear soon after birth with no antecedent rash, persists asymptomatically for life and may become less prominent with time.

PHYSICAL EXAMINATION

Skin Findings

Type Macular whorled hyperpigmentation (see Fig. 12-8).

Color Light to dark brown.

Size Few mm to several cm.

Distribution Asymmetric or symmetric. Can affect a localized area or an entire limb, quadrant, or the whole body may be involved.

General Findings

Most reported cases of linear and whorled nevoid hypermelanosis have no associated abnormalities. Other cases may have been reported as incontinentia pigmenti lacking an inflammatory or verrucous phase or hypomelanosis of Ito. Associated congenital malformations and immune deficits have been reported.

DIFFERENTIAL DIAGNOSIS

History and physical examination with no antecedent rash and no associated anomalies differentiates linear and whorled nevoid hypermelanosis from incontinentia pigmenti (third stage), hypomelanosis of Ito, epidermal nevi, or other reticulated pigmentary syndrome.

LABORATORY EXAMINATIONS

Dermatopathology Skin biopsy shows basilar hyperpigmentation with a slight increase in basal melanocytes without incontinence of pigment.

COURSE AND PROGNOSIS

Skin findings are congenital, asymptomatic, and persist for life without complications. A few cases fade in pigmentation with time.

MANAGEMENT

No treatment is needed.

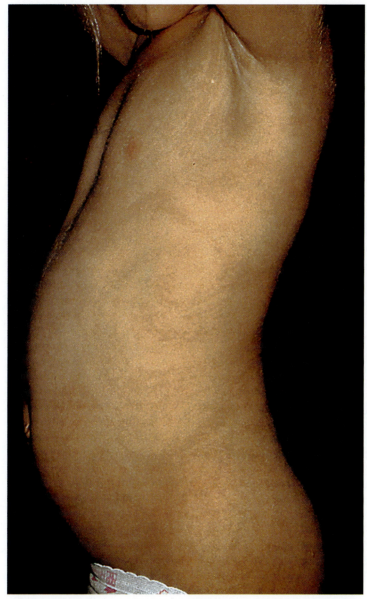

Figure 12-8 Linear and whorled hypermelanosis *Congenital whorled pigmentation present since birth in an otherwise well child.*

NEUROCUTANEOUS DISORDERS

The neurocutaneous disorders are a group of inherited conditions with skin, central nervous system, and other systemic abnormalities. Embryologically, the skin and nervous system are derived from the same neural crest origin and thus it is not surprising that many neurologic disorders have associated skin abnormalities.

NEUROFIBROMATOSIS

Neurofibromatosis (NF) is an autosomal dominant disorder characterized by café au lait spots and tumors of the nervous system. Two main forms of NF are now recognized: (1) classical von Recklinghausen disease, termed NF-1 and first described in 1882; and (2) central or acoustic NF, termed NF-2. Both types have café au lait macules and neurofibromas, but only NF-2 has *bilateral* acoustic neuromas (unilateral acoustic neuromas are a variable feature of NF-1). An important diagnostic sign present only in NF-1 is pigmented hamartomas of the iris (Lisch nodules).

Synonym   Von Recklinghausen disease.

EPIDEMIOLOGY

Age   Café au lait macules appear in the first 3 years of life. Neurofibromas appear in adolescence.

Gender   Males slightly more than females.

Race   All races.

Incidence   NF-1, 1:4,000; NF-2, 1:50,000.

Heredity   Autosomal dominant, the gene for NF-1 is on chromosome 17, and for NF-2 on chromosome 22; 50% of cases are new mutations

PATHOPHYSIOLOGY

Neurofibromatosis-1 is an autosomal dominantly inherited disorder caused by a mutation in chromosome 17q11.2. The gene product, "neurofibromin," negatively regulates the *ras*-family of signal molecules through GTP activating protein (GAP) function. Neurofibromatosis-2 is an autosomal dominantly inherited disorder caused by a mutation in chromosome 22q12.2. The gene product, "merlin," is thought to be involved in actin cytoskeletal signaling.

HISTORY

Café au lait macules (CALMs) are not usually present at birth but appear during the first 3 years; neurofibromas appear during late adolescence and may be tender to palpation. Clinical manifestations can vary depending on which organ is affected: hypertensive headache (pheochromocytomas), pathologic fractures (bone cysts), mental retardation, brain tumor (astrocytoma), short stature, precocious puberty (early menses, clitoral hypertrophy).

PHYSICAL EXAMINATION

Skin Findings

Café au lait Macules (CALMs)   Light or dark brown *uniform* melanin pigmentation. Lesions vary in size from multiple "frecklelike" tiny macules to larger patches (Fig. 13-1). Less than

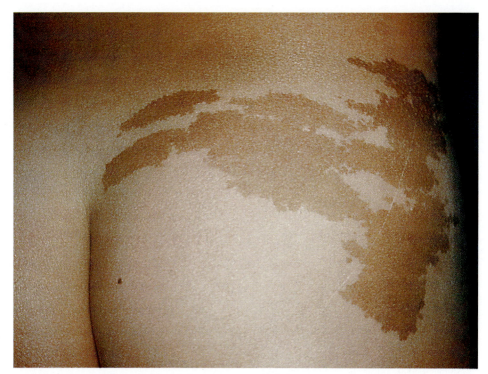

Figure 13-1   Neurofibromatosis, café au lait macule   *Well-demarcated uniform brown macule on the buttock of a patient with neurofibromatosis.*

2.0 mm to very large; larger than 20 cm, brown macules. The common size, however, is 2 to 5 cm. Tiny frecklelike lesions in the axillae are highly characteristic (Crowe's sign, Fig. 13-2).

Neurofibromas Color of the skin, pink, or brown; pedunculated; soft or firm nodules with "button hole sign"—invagination with the tip of the index finger is diagnostic (Fig. 13-3).

Plexiform Neuromas Drooping, soft, doughy loose lesions the color of the skin, described as a "bag of worms."

Distribution of Lesions Randomly distributed but may be localized to one region (segmental NF-1).

Wood's Lamp Examination Café au lait macules are more easily visualized with Wood's lamp examination.

Other Physical Findings

Eye Pigmented hamartomas of the iris (Lisch nodules) present after the age of 16 years and in 92% of patients with NF-1, but not present in NF-2. These are visible only with slit lamp examination and appear as "glassy," transparent, dome-shaped, yellow-to-brown papules up to 2.0 mm. They do not correlate with the severity of the disease.

Musculoskeletal Cervicothoracic kyphoscoliosis, segmental hypertrophy.

Adrenal Pheochromocytoma Elevated blood pressure and episodic flushing.

Peripheral Nervous System Elephantiasis neuromatosa (gross disfigurement from neurofibromatosis of the nerve trunks).

Central Nervous System Optic glioma, acoustic neuroma (rare in NF-1 and unilateral, bilateral in NF-2), astrocytoma, meningioma, neurofibroma.

LABORATORY EXAMINATIONS

Dermatopathology Café au lait macules demonstrate more than 10 *melanin macroglobules* per 5 high-power fields in "split" dopa preparations. Neurofibromas demonstrate proliferation of irregular nerve fascicles.

DIFFERENTIAL DIAGNOSIS

Neurofibromatosis-1 The diagnosis of NF-1 can be made if two of the following criteria are met:

1. Multiple café au lait macules, > 6.
   a. Age less than 5: six CALMs, > 5 mm.
   b. Age greater than 5: six CALMs > 1.5 cm.
2. Multiple freckles in the axillary and inguinal regions (Crowe's sign).
3. Based on clinical and histologic grounds, two or more neurofibromas of any type, or one plexiform neurofibroma.
4. Sphenoid wing dysplasia or congenital bowing or thining of long bone cortex, with or without pseudoarthrosis.
5. Optic nerve glioma.
6. Two or more iris hamartomas (Lisch nodules) on slit lamp examination.
7. First-degree relative (parent, sibling, or child) with NF-1 by the above criteria.

Neurofibromatosis-2 The diagnosis of NF-2 can be made by:

1. CT or MRI demonstrating bilateral acoustic neuromas or
2. A first-degree relative (parent, sibling, child) with NF-2 and either:

   a. Unilateral nerve VIII mass or
   b. Two of the following: Neurofibroma, meningioma, glioma, schwannoma, juvenile posterior subcapsular lenticular opacity.

Differential Diagnosis
Café au lait macules can also be present in Albright's syndrome (polyostotic fibrous dysplasia). The CALMs in Albright's frequently have a jagged "coast of Maine" border as compared to the CALMs in NF-1, which have smooth "coast of California" borders. Other criteria listed above are required to establish a diagnosis of neurofibromatosis.

COURSE AND PROGNOSIS

There is a variable involvement of the organs affected over time, with neurofibromatosis-1 patients being more severely affected than neu-

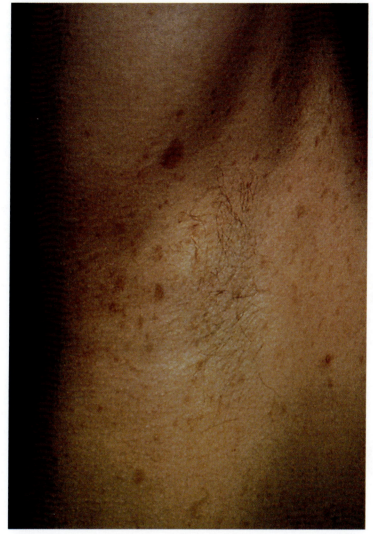

Figure 13-2 **Neurofibromatosis, Crowe's sign** *Axillary freckling in a child with neurofibromatosis.*

rofibromatosis-2 patients. Skin problems can range from just a few pigmented macules to marked disfigurement with thousands of nodules, segmental hypertrophy, and plexiform neurofibromas. The mortality rate is higher than in the normal population, principally because of the development of neurofibrosarcoma during adult life.

MANAGEMENT

It is important to establish the diagnosis to follow patients with a multidisciplinary approach. Support groups help with social adjustment in severely affected persons. An orthopedic physician should manage the two major bone problems: kyphoscoliosis and tibial bowing. The plastic surgeon can do reconstructive surgery on the facial asymmetry. The language disorders and learning disabilites should be evaluated by psychological assessment. Close follow-up annually should be mandatory to detect sarcomas and leukemias.

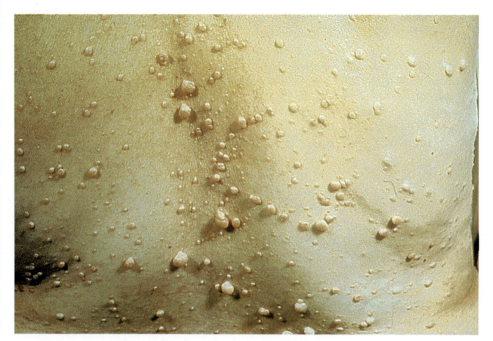

Figure 13-3 **Neurofibromatosis, neurofibromas** *Skin-colored soft papules and nodules on the back are neurofibromata appearing in late adolescence in a patient with neurofibromatosis.*

TUBEROUS SCLEROSIS

Tuberous sclerosis is an autosomal dominant disease arising from a genetically programmed hyperplasia of ectodermal and mesodermal cells and manifested by a variety of lesions in the skin, CNS, heart, kidney, lungs, and bones. The principal early manifestations are the triad of seizures, mental retardation, and congenital white spots (macules). Facial angiomata are pathognomonic but do not appear until the third or fourth year of life.

Synonyms Epiloia, Bourneville disease.

EPIDEMIOLOGY

Age Infancy.

Gender M = F.

Race All races.

Incidence 1:9400.

Genetics Can be autosomal dominantly inherited; greater than 50% of cases are new mutations.

Etiology Unclear.

PATHOPHYSIOLOGY

Gene defects in chromosome 16p13 (termed TSC2, 50 to 64% of patients) and chromosome 9p34 (termed TSC1, 33 to 50% of patients) have been identified. Chromosome 16p13 affects the gene product "tuberin," a protein that may regulate *ras* proteins through GAP domain. Chromosome 9q34 affects the gene product "hamartin," a protein that interacts with tuberin in some fashion. Both chromosome mutations lead to genetic alterations of ectodermal and mesodermal cells with hyperplasia, with a disturbance in embryonic cellular differentiation.

HISTORY

White macules appear at birth or in infancy (80% occur by 1 year of age, 100% appear by the age of 2 years) followed by a shagreen patch (seen in) 21 to 83% of patients between ages 2 to 5 years) and angiofibromata (more than 20% are present at 1 year of age, 50% occur by the age of 3 years, the rest become evident at puberty). The skin changes often precede the systemic symptoms. Seizures (infantile spasms) occur in 86% of patients; earlier onset of seizures leads to more marked mental retardation.

PHYSICAL EXAMINATION

Skin Findings (96% incidence of skin lesions)

Types of Lesions

1. Hypomelanotic macules (ashleaf spot, confetti macules, and thumbprint macules) are present in more than 80% of patients—"off-white"; one or many, usually more than three; 80% appear by 1 year of age (Fig. 13-4).
2. Papules/nodules (adenoma sebaceum, angiofibromas) on the face are present in 70% of patients (Fig. 13-5)—red and the skin color, but these appear more in adolescence (fewer than 20% at 1 year of age).
3. Plaques (shagreen patch) are present in 40% of patients—yellow-brown plaques favor buttock area (Fig. 13-6).
4. Peri/subungual papules fibromas—present in 22% of patients, arise late in childhood and have the same pathology (angiofibroma) as the facial papules (Fig. 13-7).
5. Fibrous plaques (hamartomas)—plaque the color of the skin usually on forehead (Fig. 13-8).

Wood's Lamp Examination Accentuates depigmented lesions.

Distribution of Lesions
White macules occur on the trunk (56%), lower extremities (32%), upper extremities (7.0%), head and neck (5.0%). Angiofibromatous papules and nodules occur on the face. Shagreen patches occur on the back or buttocks.

Hair

Depigmented tufts of hair may present at birth.

Associated Systems

CNS (tumors producing seizures), eye (gray or yellow retinal plaques, 50%), heart (benign

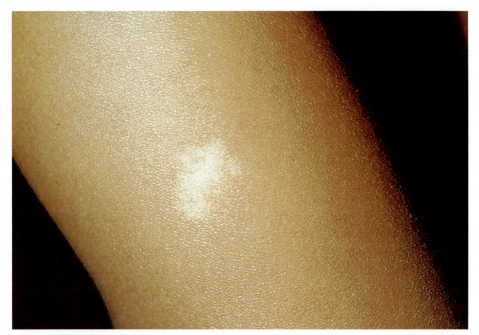

Figure 13-4   Tuberous sclerosis, ashleaf macule   *Ashleaf (oval-shaped) hypomelanotic macule on the lower leg of a child.*

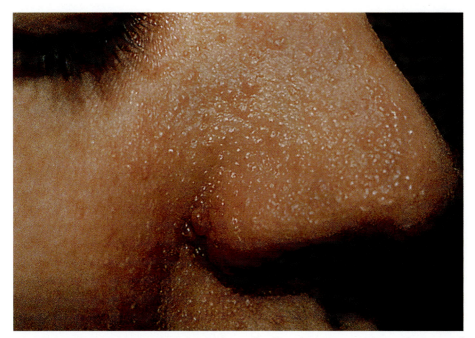

Figure 13-5   Tuberous sclerosis, adenoma sebaceum   *Small erythematous papules on the nose and cheeks of a child representing angiofibromata.*

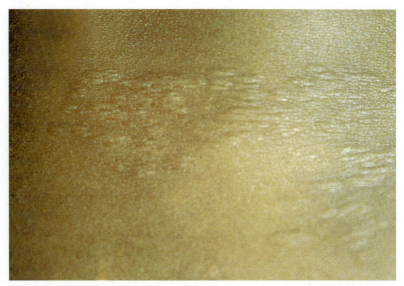

Figure 13-6   Tuberous sclerosis, Shagreen patch   *Raised skin-colored plaque on the torso of a child representing a connective tissue nevus.*

NEUROCUTANEOUS DISORDERS

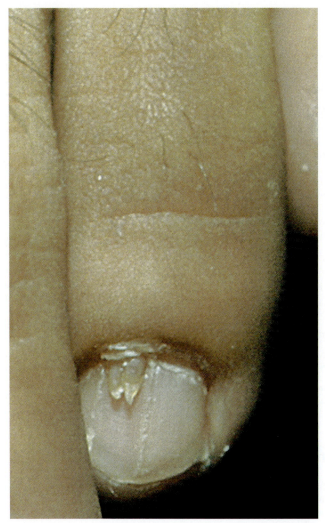

Figure 13-7   Tuberous sclerosis, periungual fibroma   *Flesh-colored periungual papule appearing in adolescence in an individual with tuberous sclerosis.*

rhabdomyomas), hamartomas of mixed-cell type (kidney, liver, thyroid, testes, and GI system).

LABORATORY EXAMINATIONS

Dermatopathology

Light Microscopy

1. White macules: (ashleaf spot, confetti macules, and thumbprint macules). Decreased number of melanocytes, decreased melanosome size, decreased melanin in melanocytes and keratinocytes.
2. Angiofibromata: (adenoma sebaceum, peri/subungual fibromas). Dermal fibrosis, capillary dilation, absence of elastic tissue.
3. Brain: "Tubers" are gliomas.

Dopa Reaction Demonstrates decreased melanin formation.

Transmission Electron Microscopy Shows decreased size and decreased melanin in the melanosomes.

Electroencephalography Abnormal.

Skull X-ray Multiple calcific densities are seen in 50 to 75% of individuals.

MRI or CT scan In smaller children when skull radiographs are not diagnostic, small calcifications and ventricular dilation are helpful in diagnosis.

DIFFERENTIAL DIAGNOSIS

The diagnosis may be difficult or impossible in an infant or child if white macules are the only cutaneous finding. Nevus depigmentosus may,

however, be a confounding lesion, as the white macules in tuberous sclerosis and nevus depigmentosus contain a normal number of melanocytes. Other white macules (vitiligo and piebaldism) contain few or no melanocytes. The angiofibromata (adenoma sebaceum) of the face are almost pathognomonic but do not appear until late infancy or older.

Even when typical white ash leaf or thumbprint macules are present, it is necessary to confirm the diagnosis. A pediatric neurologist can then evaluate the patient with a study of the family members, and by obtaining various types of imaging as well as electroencephalography. It should be noted that mental retardation and seizures may be absent.

COURSE AND PROGNOSIS

In severe cases, 30% die before the fifth year of life, and 50 to 75% before reaching adult age. Most die from CNS tumors of status epilecticus.

MANAGEMENT

Treatment is targeted at affected organs. Seizures can be controlled with anticonvulsant therapy. Genetic counseling is helpful, but because more than 50% are new mutations, the disorder is difficult to prevent. Skin lesions do not need treatment but can be surgically excised or electrodesiccated for cosmetic or symptomatic improvements.

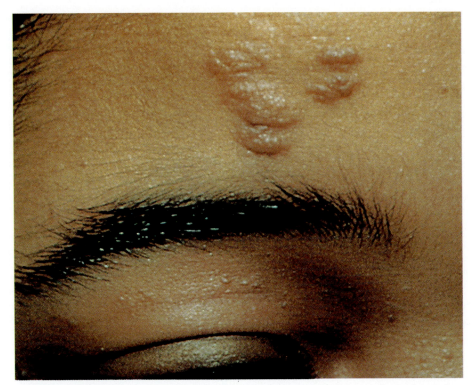

Figure 13-8 **Tuberous sclerosis, fibrous plaque** *Raised skin-colored plaque on the forehead of a child representing a connective tissue nevus.*

INCONTINENTIA PIGMENTI

Incontinentia pigmenti (IP) is a rare congenital disease affecting the skin, central nervous system, eyes, and skeletal system. The skin has a "marble cake" appearance and goes through four stages: inflammatory, verrucous, hyperpigmented, and finally, hypopigmented stages. About 79% of IP patients have internal manifestations.

Synonym Bloch-Sulzberger syndrome.

EPIDEMIOLOGY

Age Appears at birth or shortly after (90% of patients have cutaneous lesions within first 2 weeks of life).

Gender Females, 97%. Disease is prenatally lethal to hemizygous males. The disease in living male patients is usually the result of spontaneous mutation.

Prevalence Rare.

Mode of Transmission X-linked dominant, some cases are new mutations.

PATHOPHYSIOLOGY

Two gene loci for IP have been identified: (1) a locus at Xp11.21 (IP1) and (2) a locus at Xq28 (IP2). These mutations are suspected to produce a failure of immune tolerance in ectodermal tissues resulting in an autoimmune-like reaction in heterozygote girls and a fatal graft-versus-host-like disease in homozygous boys.

PHYSICAL EXAMINATION

Clinical Appearance Four distinct cutaneous stages have been designated, which may frequently overlap: (1) *inflammatory stage* (newborn to few months): vesicles or bullae developing in a linear distribution over trunk and extremities at birth or immediately after (Fig. 13-9); (2) *verrucous stage* (few months of age to 1 year old): follows the vesicular lesions and is characterized by irregular linear warty or verrucous lesions on one or more extremities that resolve spontaneously after a period of several months (Fig. 13-10); (3) *hyperpigmentary change* (age 1 to 2 up to adolescence): band of slate-brown to blue-gray patches in whorled patterns on trunk and extremities (seen in 100% of patients, Fig. 13-11); (4) *hypopigmentary changes* (adulthood): hypopigmented atrophic linear streaks on arms, trunk, thighs, and calves, devoid of hair and sweat pores.

General Findings CNS manifestations in 30% of patients including seizures (3.3%), mental retardation (16%), spastic abnormalities (13%). Ophthalmic changes in 35% (strabismus, cataracts, optic atrophy, retinal damage), alopecia (38%), nail dystrophy (7%), dental anomalies (64% with delayed dentition, partial anodontia, pegged or conical teeth), cardiac anomalies, skeletal malformations (microcephaly, syndactyly, hemiatrophy, shortening of arms and legs). Prominent peripheral eosinophilia in 74% of patients during the inflammatory stage.

DIFFERENTIAL DIAGNOSIS

Diagnosis is made based on history, physical examination, and histologic confirmation. Peripheral eosinophilia and radiographic changes of distal phalanges are suggestive signs in early stages. The differential can vary from stage to stage: (1) inflammatory-> epidermolysis bullosa, linear IgA, childhood bullous pemphigus; (2) verrucous-> epidermal nevus; (3) hyperpigmented-> lichen planus, lichen nitidis; and (4) hypopigmented-> hypomelanosis of Ito.

LABORATORY EXAMINATIONS

Dermatopathology: (1) Inflammatory-> intraepidermal vesicles with a dermal infiltrate composed of PMNs, lymphocytes, mononuclear cells, and eosinophils; (2) verrucous stage-> acanthosis, irregular papillomatosis, hyperkeratosis, basal cell vacuolization with decrease in melanin content, and a mild chronic inflammatory infiltrate; (3) hyperpigmented stage-> and extensive deposits of melanin with melanophages in the upper dermis; and (4) hypopigmented stage -> decrease melanin as well as appendages in affected skin.

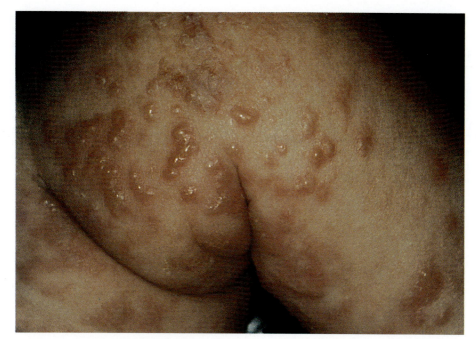

Figure 13-9 Incontinentia pigmenti, inflammatory stage *Inflammatory papules and vesicles on the leg of a newborn.*

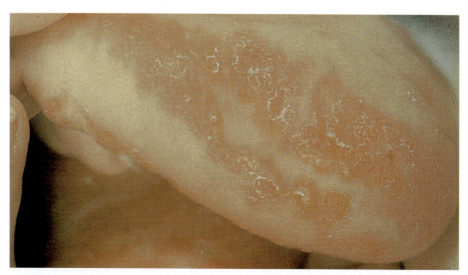

Figure 13-10 Incontinentia pigmenti, verrucous stage *Verrucous linear streaks on the arms of an infant.*

Hematology Peripheral eosinophilia in early stages.

Radiography Lytic effects on distal phalanges.

COURSE AND PROGNOSIS

Up to 80% of patients have systemic disease. There is a poor prognosis and developmental delay in patients who develop seizures during the first week of life. Absence of seizures and normal developmental milestones appears to predict a good prognosis. The pigmentary changes may persist for many years and gradually fade, completely disappearing in adolescence or early adulthood.

MANAGEMENT

No special treatment is required for the cutaneous lesions of IP. Genetic counseling for carrier females is advisable because up to 80% of affected children have associated congenital defects.

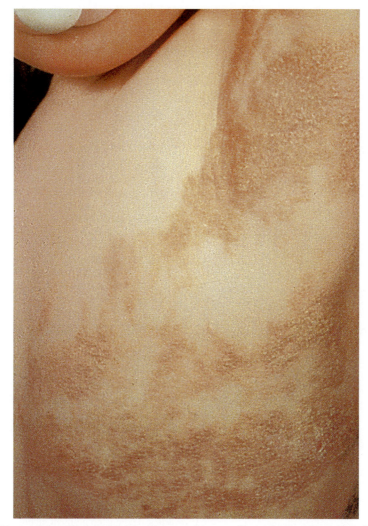

Figure 13-11   Incontinentia pigmenti, hyperpigmented stage   *Hyperpigmentation along the lines of Blaschko in a child with incontinentia pigmenti.*

HYPOMELANOSIS OF ITO

A familial disorder of hypopigmentation characterized by linear swirled hypopigmented streaks. Resembles the negative image of hyperpigmentation in incontinentia pigmenti (IP). More than 50% of patients with hypomelanosis of Ito have internal manifestations.

Synonym   Incontinentia pigmenti achromians.

EPIDEMIOLOGY

Age   Onset at birth or early infancy or childhood.

Gender   F > M, 2:1.

Prevalence   Estimated prevalence in pediatric hospital: 1:8000.

Incidence   Rare.

Genetics   Usually sporadic, familial cases with autosomal dominant pattern have been reported.

PATHOPHYSIOLOGY

Possibly a result of chromosomal mosaicism or random distribution of two cellular clones with different pigment potential. Chromosomal abnormalities (translocation of Xp11, microdeletion of 15q1) have been reported.

HISTORY

Skin hypopigmentation is whorled pattern; present at birth or early childhood. It is asymptomatic but persists for life. Internal symptoms may include seizures, mental retardation, skeletal abnormalities, and strabismus.

PHYSICAL EXAMINATION

Skin Findings

Type   Macular hypopigmentation.

Color   Tan to off-white.

Shape   Linear, streaked, whorled.

Pattern   "Marble cake" following lines of Blaschko (Fig. 13-12).

Distribution   More pronounced on the ventral surface of the trunk or flexor surfaces of limbs. Scalp, palms, soles are not involved.

General Findings

Internal manifestations occur in 75 to 94% of patients. CNS disorders (seizures, mental retardation), ocular disturbances (strabismus, heterochromia iridis, microphthalmia, nystagmus), musculoskeletal anomalies (macrocephaly, scoliosis, asymmetry of limbs, dwarfism, small stature, polydactyly, syndactyly, spina bifida occulta), hair anomalies (diffuse alopecia, hirsutism, facial hypertrichosis), dental anomalies (anodontia, dental dysplasia), hepatomegaly, diaphragmatic hernia.

DIFFERENTIAL DIAGNOSIS

Diagnosis is made on history and physical examination. The differential diagnosis includes IP, Goltz syndrome, nevus depigmentosus, depigmented lichen striatus, or vitiligo.

LABORATORY EXAMINATIONS

Dermatopathology   Skin biopsy reveals a decrease in number of melanin granules in the basal layer and complete absence of melanin in other areas. The hypopigmented areas contain smaller melanocytes with sparse, short dendrites. There is no pigment incontinence in contrast to incontinentia pigmenti.

MANAGEMENT

No treatment for the skin lesions is needed. The skin lesions may slowly repigment in late childhood. Most therapeutics are directed towards controlling neurologic symptoms and correcting skeletal malformations.

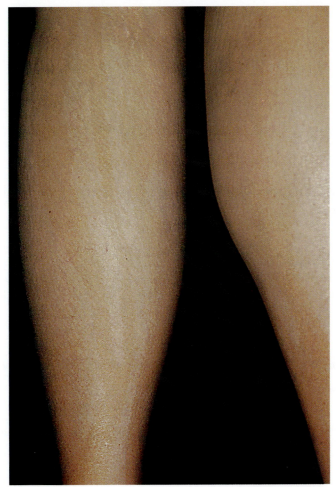

Figure 13-12 Hypomelanosis of Ito *Whorled hypopigmented streaks along the lines of Blaschko, a negative image of the hyperpigmented stage of IP.*

MISCELLANEOUS INFLAMMATORY DISORDERS

PAPULOSQUAMOUS ERUPTIONS

PITYRIASIS ROSEA

Pityriasis rosea (PR) is a common, benign, self-limited whole body rash with a seasonal prevalence that is clinically characterized by a solitary "herald patch" lesion followed by a whole body exanthem.

EPIDEMIOLOGY

Age   10 to 35 years. Rare in children under 5 years old.

Incidence   Represents 2% of all dermatology visits.

Prevalence   Common especially in fall, winter, and spring.

Etiology   Unclear. The season prevalence suggests a viral etiology but no virus has yet been isolated as the causative agent.

HISTORY

A "herald" patch precedes the exanthematous phase by 1 to 2 weeks. The exanthematous phase develops over a period of a week and self-resolves in 6 to 14 weeks without intervention. The rash may be pruritic or completely asymptomatic. There may be a mild prodrome of headache, malaise, pharyngitis, or lymphadenitis but often this is absent.

PHYSICAL EXAMINATION

Skin Lesions

Herald Plaque   In 80% of patients there is a preceding 2- to 5-cm, erythematous plaque with a marginal collarette of fine scale.

Exanthem   Fine scaling macules and papules with a marginal collarette of scale (Fig. 14-1).

Color   Dull pink or red.

Size   5 mm to 3 cm.

Shape   Round to oval.

Arrangement   Scattered discrete lesions.

Distribution   Characteristic pattern of lesions—the long axes of the lesions follow the lines of cleavage in a "Christmas tree" distribution. Lesions usually confined to trunk and proximal aspects of the arms and legs. Head and face involvement not seen in adults but can be seen in children (Fig. 14-2).

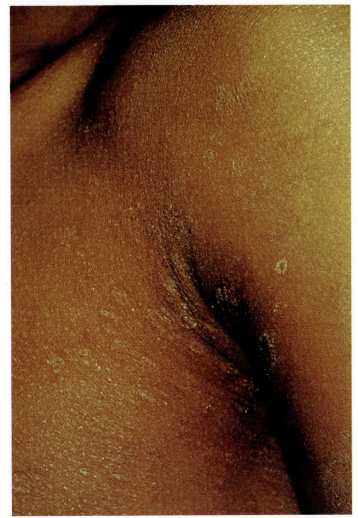

Figure 14-1 Pityriasis rosea *Scattered erythematous plaques with a collarette of scale concentrated in the axillary area.*

Sites of Predilection Bilateral axillary area and back.

DIFFERENTIAL DIAGNOSIS

The diagnosis of pityriasis rosea is made on history, especially of a preceding herald patch and on clinical findings. PR can be confused with tinea, secondary syphilis (obtain serology), guttate psoriasis (no marginal collarette), tinea, parapsoriasis seborrheic dermatitis, drug eruption, and nummular eczema.

LABORATORY EXAMINATIONS

Dermatopathology Skin biopsy reveals a superficial lymphohistiocytic infiltrate, acanthosis, spongiosis, mild exocytosis, and patchy parakeratosis with vascular dilatation and eczema.

Bloodwork An RPR should be checked in atypical presentations or at-risk individuals because secondary syphilis can be indistinguishable from the rash of PR.

COURSE AND PROGNOSIS

Lesions of pityriasis rosea self-resolve in 6 to 14 weeks. Lesions that persist longer than 14 weeks may need a biopsy to rule out parapsoriasis.

MANAGEMENT

No treatment is needed. Pruritus may be improved with:

1. Topical steroids
   a. Low potency steroids (Desowen, 1% hydrocortisone, 2.5% hydrocortisone) should be used on face or groin area, no more than bid × 2 weeks.
   b. Medium potency steroids (Elocon, Dermatop, Cutivate) should be used on the body or extremities no more than bid × 2 weeks.
   c. Strong steroids (Ultravate, Psorcon, Diprolene) are reserved for older children and adults on severely affected areas bid for no more than 2 weeks. (See page 48 for more details.)
2. Sunlight exposure can also help clear the rash.
3. With severe pruritus in older children (>10 years old), UVB light treatment is a possibility.

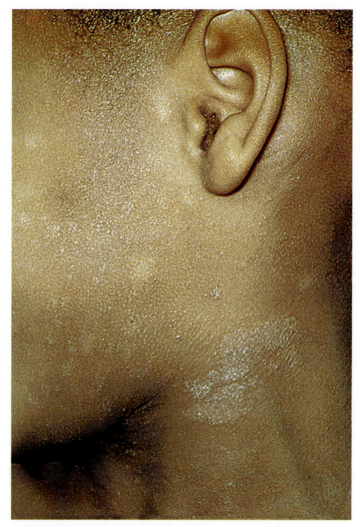

Figure 14-2 Pityriasis rosea *Lesions spreading to the face, which is uncommon, but can be seen in childhood PR.*

PITYRIASIS LICHENOIDES

Pityriasis lichenoides (PL) is a self-limited eruption of unknown etiology, characterized clinically by successive crops of a wide range of morphologic lesions, (i.e., macules, papules, vesicles, pustules, and crusts in the acute form, and by reddish brown papules with adherent central scale in the chronic form). The acute form is called pityriasis lichenoides et varioliformis acuta (PLEVA). The chronic form is called pityriasis lichenoides chronica (PLC).

Synonyms Acute guttate parapsoriasis, parapsoriasis varioliformis, Mucha-Habermann disease, guttate parapsoriasis of Juliusberg.

EPIDEMIOLOGY

Age

1. PLEVA: Any age.
2. PLC: Adolescents and adults.

Gender M > F.

Etiology Unknown.

PATHOPHYSIOLOGY

The etiology of PLEVA and PLC is unclear. Theories include an infectious course, an autoimmune mechanism, or a hypersensitivity reaction. No etiologic agent has yet been identified.

HISTORY

Skin lesions tend to appear in crops over a period of weeks or months. Uncommonly, patients with an acute onset of the disorder may have symptoms of an acute viral infection with fever, malaise, and headache. Cutaneous lesions are usually asymptomatic, but may be pruritic or sensitive to touch. PLEVA has a self-limited course of a few weeks to months. PLC may last up to years. Both disorders need careful follow-up because there are a few rare instances in which they evolve into cutaneous T-cell lymphoma (CTCL).

PHYSICAL EXAMINATION

Skin Lesions

Type Initial edematous papules (i.e., lichenoides, Fig. 14-3). Less commonly, vesicles-to-bullae, which undergo necrosis with central vesiculation and hemorrhagic crusting (i.e., varioliformis). In the chronic form, scaling papules are seen. Postinflammatory macular hypo- or hyperpigmentation is often present after lesions resolve and the sites may heal with depressed or elevated scars.

Color Acute: pink-to-erythematous. Chronic: reddish brown. Scars may be hypopigmented or depigmented.

Arrangement Random.

Distribution Most commonly, trunk, proximal extremities (Fig. 14-4). Lesions may occur in a generalized distribution, including palms and soles.

Oral and Genital Mucosa Inflammatory papules and necrotic lesions may occur.

DIFFERENTIAL DIAGNOSIS

The diagnosis of PLEVA and PLC are made based on history and physical examination, which may be confirmed by lesional skin biopsy. PLEVA and PLC are often confused with varicella, lichen planus, guttate psoriasis, prurigo nodularis, lymphomatoid papulosis, bites, impetigo, folliculitis, scabies, secondary syphilis or allergic reaction.

LABORATORY EXAMINATIONS

Dermatopathology Skin biopsy shows epidermal spongiosis, keratinocyte necrosis, vesiculation, ulceration, and exocytosis. There is also dermal edema, a wedge-shaped chronic inflammatory cell infiltrate extending to deep reticular dermis; hemorrhage; vessels congested with blood, and swollen endothelial cells.

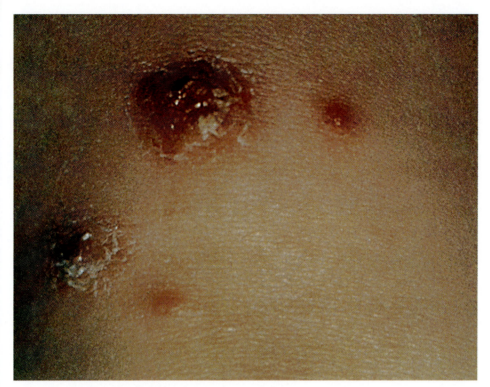

Figure 14-3 Pityriasis lichenoides, crusted keratotic *Inflammatory edematous papules on the fore-arm of a child.*

COURSE AND PROGNOSIS

Skin lesions continue to appear in crops . PLEVA tends to self-resolve after weeks to months. PLC can last years. Both disorders tend to have a relapsing but benign course. They should always have continued follow-up because rare cases have been reported to progress to cutaneous T-cell lymphoma (CTCL).

MANAGEMENT

Most patients do not require any therapeutic intervention. For symptomatic relief:

1. Topical corticosteroid preparations can be useful.
   a. Low potency steroids (Desowen, 1% hydrocortisone, 2.5% hydrocortisone) should be used on face or groin area, no more than bid × 2 weeks.
   b. Medium potency steroids (Elocon, Dermatop, Cutivate) should be used on the body or extremities no more than bid × 2 weeks.
   c. Strong steroids (Ultravate, Psorcon, Diprolene) are reserved for older children and adults on severely affected areas bid for no more than 2 weeks. (See page 48 for more details.)
2. Oral antibiotics (e.g., erythromycin, 30 to 50 mg/kg per d divided qid, not to exceed 2 g/d or tetracycline, 25 to 50 mg/kg per d divided bid not to exceed 3 g/d) have been used with mixed results.
3. Ultraviolet radiation, whether natural sunlight or artificial UVB and PUVA in older children (>10 years old), seem to clear skin lesions well.
4. Follow-up of these children (acutely: every few months, then chronically: an annual skin examination) is needed to ensure that they do not go on to develop the rare disease CTCL.

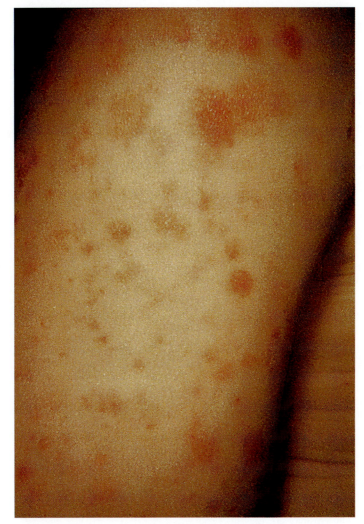

Figure 14-4 Pityriasis lichenoides *Scattered inflammatory papules on the right arm of a child. The lesions are in different stages of evolution characteristic of PLEVA.*

LICHENOID ERUPTIONS

LICHEN SCLEROSIS

Lichen sclerosis (LS) is a benign mucocutaneous disorder, characterized by white angular, well-defined, indurated papules and plaques. In males, it is called balanitis xerotica obliterans (BXO).

Synonyms   Guttate morphea, guttate scleroderma, white-spot disease, lichen sclerosis et atrophicus.

EPIDEMIOLOGY

Age   Occurs in children, 1 to 13 years. Also occurs in adults. Up to 70% of patients had the onset of the disorder before age 7 years.

Gender   F >> M (10:1).

Etiology   Unknown.

HISTORY

Asymptomatic genital lesions may be present for years prior to detection. Often the skin findings are mistaken for sexual abuse in young children and are thus brought to medical attention. Older patients are diagnosed when atrophic changes are noted by a gynecologist or internist during pelvic examination. Spontaneous involution occurs in children more than adults. Persistent lesions can be sensitive especially while walking; pruritus and pain can occur especially if erosions are present. Other complications include dysuria; dyspareunia and stricture of the introitus. In males, chronic BXO can lead to phimosis and recurrent balanitis.

PHYSICAL EXAMINATION

Skin Lesions

Type   Flat-topped papules coalescing to plaques. Older lesions show atrophy and delling (fine follicular plugs).

Color   Papules: pink. Plaques: ivory white semitransparent resembling mother-of-pearl.

Arrangement   In females, the lesion is perianal and perivulvar forming an "hourglass" or "figure-of-eight" pattern (Fig. 14-5).

Nongenital Distribution   Trunk especially upper back, periumbilical, neck, axillae; flexor surface of wrists; rarely palms and soles.

Genital Distribution   In females the vulva and perianal regions as well as the perineum; inguinal line. In males the under surface of prepuce and glans (Fig. 14-6).

Oral Mucosa Distribution   Bluish-white plaques on buccal or palatal mucosa; tongue. Superficial erosions. Hyperkeratotic, macerated lesions may have reticulate pattern resembling lichen planus.

DIFFERENTIAL DIAGNOSIS

Diagnosis is made on history and clinical presentation, and may be confirmed by skin biopsy. LS can be confused with morphea, lichen simplex chronicus, discoid lupus erythematosus, leukoplakia, lichen planus, condyloma acuminatum, intertrigo candidiasis, pinworm infestation, or bacterial vulvovaginitis.

LABORATORY EXAMINATIONS

Dermatopathology   On skin biopsy, early lesions will show hyperkeratotic, follicular plugging and edema with a lymphocytic bandlike infiltrate subepidermally. Later lesions show epidermis atrophic with band of homogenized dermal collagen below epidermis.

COURSE AND PROGNOSIS

The prognosis is good for patients with childhood onset. Most clear in 1 to 10 years and 60% to 70% improve substantially by puberty. A small number persist into adulthood.

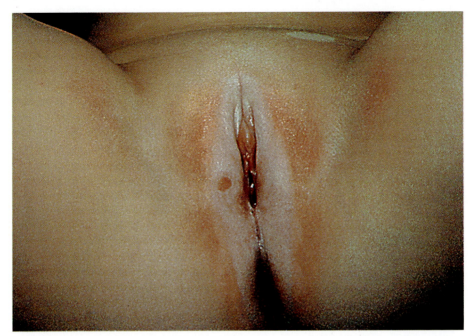

Figure 14-5 Lichen sclerosis *Hypopigmented "hourglass" or "figure-of-eight" configuration around the vulva and the perianal area of a young girl. Lichen sclerosis is often mistaken for child abuse.*

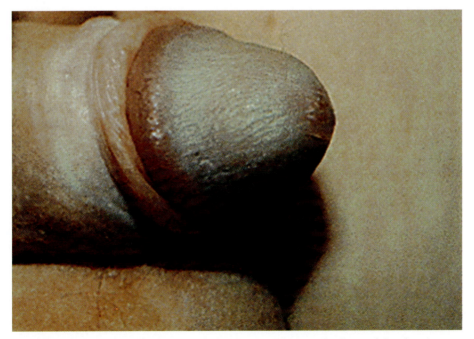

Figure 14-6 Balanitis xerotica obliterans *Hypopigmented area on the dorsa of the glans in a young man.*

MANAGEMENT

Topical treatments include:

1. Topical corticosteroids
   a. Low potency steroids (Desowen, 1% hydrocortisone, 2.5% hydrocortisone) qd–bid can be used.
   b. Short courses of medium potency steroids (Elocon, Dermatop, Cutivate) or strong steroids (Ultravate, Psorcon, Diprolene) can be used qd–bid for short periods of time (< 4 weeks).
2. Emollients and antipruritic agents (Pramasone) bid can also be tried for symptomatic relief.

3. Use of 2% testosterone propionate in petrolatum is effective but the side effects of clitoral hypertrophy and increased libido are usually not acceptable in children. A weaker 1% progesterone (100 mg/30 g of petrolatum) can be tried.

Close follow-up is warranted especially in chronic cases because adulthood LS is more problematic. Involution in adults is uncommon and LS needs to be chronically monitored for progression towards leukoplakia and squamous cell carcinoma (seen in 4.4% of adult cases). In adults, new nodules or ulcers that persist for weeks warrant a skin biopsy to rule out leukoplakia or carcinoma.

LICHEN PLANUS

This acute or chronic inflammation of the skin and mucous membranes has characteristic flat-topped (Latin planus, "flat"), violaceous, shiny, pruritic papules, and milky-white papules in the mouth.

EPIDEMIOLOGY

Age   30 to 60 years.

Gender   F > M.

Other Factors   The etiology is unknown. Severe emotional stress can precipitate an attack.

HISTORY

Duration of Lesions   Acute (days) or insidious onset in weeks.

Symptoms

Skin   Pruritus, which may be severe or absent.

Mucous Membrane   Painful, especially when ulcers present.

PHYSICAL EXAMINATION

Skin Lesions

Type   Papules, 1 to 10 mm, shiny (Fig. 14-7).

Color   Violaceous, with white lines (Wickham's striae) seen best with hand lens after application of mineral oil.

Shape   Polygonal or oval.

Arrangement   Grouped, linear (isomorphic phenomenon), annular, or disseminated scattered discrete lesions.

Distribution   Wrists (flexor, Fig. 14-8), lumbar region, eyelids, shins (thicker, hyperkeratotic lesions), and scalp.

Mucous Membranes   In 40 to 60% of patients, the buccal mucosa, tongue and lips show milky-white papules, with white lacework on the buccal mucosa. Carcinoma may develop in mouth lesions.

Scalp   Atrophic scalp skin with alopecia.

Nails   In 10% of patients, destruction of the nail fold and nail matrix, especially the large toe, can be seen.

DIFFERENTIAL DIAGNOSIS

Drug-induced lichen planus (See Table 14-1).

LABORATORY EXAMINATIONS

Dermatopathology   In the epidermis and dermis there is inflammation with hyperkeratosis, an increased granular layer, irregular acanthosis, liquefaction degeneration of the basal cell layer, and bandlike mononuclear infiltrate that hugs the epidermis.

COURSE AND PROGNOSIS

Spontaneous resolution in weeks is possible; lesions may also persist for years, especially on the shins and in the mouth.

MANAGEMENT

Symptomatic treatment includes:

1. Topical corticosteroids with or without occlusion. Patients should be forewarned that occlusion increases the steroid strength.
    a. Low potency steroids (Desowen, 1% hydrocortisone, 2.5% hydrocortisone) should be used on face or groin area, no more than bid × 2 weeks.
    b. Medium potency steroids (Elocon, Dermatop, Cutivate) should be used on the body or extremities no more than bid × 2 weeks.
    c. Strong steroids (Ultravate, Psorcon, Diprolene) are reserved for older children and adults on severely affected areas bid for no more than 2 weeks.
    Patients need to be cautioned about steroid side effects. (See page 48 for more details).
2. Oral prednisone (1 to 2 mg/kg per d divided qd–bid for 5 to 14 d can be used in severe cases, and only in short courses.
3. PUVA (psoralen plus artificial UVA exposure) photochemotherapy may be used in

older children (older than age 10) in generalized or resistant cases.

4. Topical steroids, and topical or oral retinoids are helpful for erosive lichen planus of the mouth.

    a. Oral 13-*cis*-retinoic acid (Accutane, 0.5 to 1 mg/kg per d) can be used. As retinoids are teratogenic in females, it is necessary that female patients have a pretreatment pregnancy test and they must be on two forms of birth control at least 1 month prior to beginning treatment, throughout treatment, and for 1 month after treatment is discontinued. Furthermore, a patient must have a negative serum pregnancy test within the 2 weeks prior to beginning treatment. Careful monitoring of the blood is necessary during therapy, especially in patients with elevated blood triglycerides before therapy is begun.

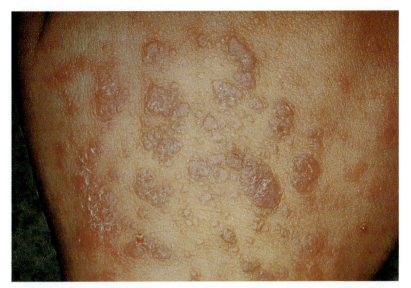

Figure 14-7 Lichen planus *Flat-topped erythematous papules on the elbow of a child.*

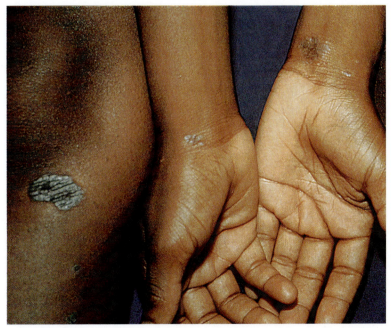

Figure 14-8 Lichen planus *Flat-topped, violaceous plaques on the wrist and leg of a young child.*

Table 14-1 AGENTS REPORTED TO INDUCE CUTANEOUS DISORDERS THAT VERY CLOSELY RESEMBLE TYPICAL LICHEN PLANUS

Types of Agents	Special Agents
Angiotensin-converting enzyme inhibitors	Captopril
	Enalapril
Antiarthritic	Gold
Antibiotic	Streptomycin
	Tetracycline
Antimalarial	Quinacrine
	Chloroquine
	Quinine isomer, quinidine
Antitubercular	*p*-Amino salicylic acid
Ataractic	Phenothiazine derivatives
	Metopromazine
	Levomepromazine
Chelator	Penicillamine
Color film developer	*p*-Phenylenediamine salts
	2-Amino-5-diethylaminotoluene monochloride (CD2)
	4-Amino-*N*-diethyl-aniline sulfate (TTS)
	Antimony trioxide
Diuretic	Chlorothiazide
	Hydrochlorothiazide
Hypoglycemic agents	Chloropropamide
	Tolazamide

SOURCE: Reproduced with permission from IM Freedberg et al., *Dermatology in General Medicine*, 5th edition. New York: McGraw-Hill, 1999.

LICHEN NITIDUS

Lichen nitidus is a benign dermatosis commonly seen in childhood, characterized by asymptomatic, small, pinpoint, papules the color of the skin located on the penis, lower abdomen and groin, flexor surface of the arms and wrists, and submammary region.

EPIDEMIOLOGY

Age All ages but commonly in preschool and school age children.

Gender M = F.

Prevalence Uncommon.

Etiology Unknown, possibly a form of lichen planus.

PATHOPHYSIOLOGY

Due to ultrastructural and immunophenotypic studies, lichen nitidus is thought to share a similar pathogenesis to lichen planus. Antigen presentation by Langerhans cells to helper T cells with subsequent lymphokine production recruits more T cells and induces cytokine production of keratinocytes.

HISTORY

The skin lesions appear suddenly and are typically asymptomatic (some cases have pruritus). Lesions may regress spontaneously after weeks to months but other cases persist for years.

PHYSICAL EXAMINATION

Skin Findings

Type Multiple, sharply demarcated, slightly elevated, flat-topped, glistening papules. In the generalized form, lesions appear plaque-like with a fine scale.

Color Papules are the color of the skin, occasionally pink. Plaques are red-yellow, brown, or red-violet.

Size and Shape Pinpoint to pinhead in size (Fig. 14-9A) and round or polygonal in shape *or* plaque formation with grouping and confluence.

Sites of Predilection Shaft and glans of the penis, lower abdomen and groin (Fig. 14-9B), flexor surface of the arms, anterior wrist surface, and breasts.

Other Findings

Linear lesions in lines of trauma (Koebner reaction) is common. Mild rubbing of papules may raise a tiny scale; diascopy reveals papules darker than surrounding skin.

DIFFERENTIAL DIAGNOSIS

The finding of numerous asymptomatic, discrete, pinpoint, shiny papules the color of the skin in typical locations is pathognomonic of lichen nitidus. Histopathology may be confirmatory. It can be confused with lichen planus, psoriasis, flat warts, keratosis pilaris, lichen spinulosa, or an id reaction.

LABORATORY EXAMINATIONS

Dermatopathology Skin biopsy reveals sharply circumscribed nests of lymphocytes and histiocytes in the uppermost dermis (often confined to two to three dermal papillae) with overlying thin, scaling epidermis. Dermis and epidermis are often detached at central portion of lesion. Rete ridges extend down around the infiltrate in a claw-like manner.

Electron Microscopy Prominent staining for T-helper lymphocytes with several Langerhans cells in the dermal infiltrate.

COURSE AND PROGNOSIS

Typical lichen nitidus lesions self-resolve in less than 1 year. In other instances, lesions may persist for several years despite treatment. After papules clear, skin is without atrophy or pigmentary changes.

MANAGEMENT

For symptomatic relief, topical regimens include:

1. Topical steroids
   a. Low potency steroids (Desowen, 1% hydrocortisone, 2.5% hydrocortisone) should be used on face or groin area, no more than bid × 2 weeks.

b. Medium potency steroids (Elocon, Dermatop, Cutivate) should be used on the body or extremities no more than bid $\times$ 2 weeks.

c. Strong steroids (Ultravate, Psorcon, Diprolene) are reserved for older children and adults on severely affected areas bid for no more than 2 weeks.

Patients need to be cautioned about steroid side effects. (See page 48 for more details.)

2. Antihistamines may be somewhat helpful in controlling itching. They are particularly useful at bedtime when itching is usually the worst. They often have the side effect of producing drowsiness and, in rare instances, hyperactivity. The most commonly prescribed antihistamines are Atarax (hydroxyzine, 2 to 4 mg/kg per d divided tid or qid) and Benadryl (diphenhydramine, 5 mg/kg per d divided tid or qid, not to exceed 300 mg per d). With continued use, antihistamines may lose their effectiveness, and higher doses may be required. Therefore, use of these should be limited to times of greatest discomfort.

3. Antipruritic agents (Pramasone) may also be helpful.

More severe cases may be treated with:

1. PUVA (psoralen plus artificial UVA light) photochemotherapy.

2. Systemic steroids (prednisone 1 to 2 mg/kg per d divided qd to bid for 5 to 14 days).

3. Oral retinoids (e.g., 13-*cis*-retinoic acid, Accutane, 0.5 to 1 mg/kg per d) can be used. As retinoids are teratogenic in females, it is necessary that female patients have a pretreatment pregnancy test and they must be on two forms of birth control at least 1 month prior to beginning treatment, throughout treatment, and for 1 month after treatment is discontinued. Furthermore, a patient must have a negative serum pregnancy test within the 2 weeks prior to beginning treatment. Careful monitoring of the blood is necessary during therapy, especially in patients with elevated blood triglycerides, before therapy is begun.

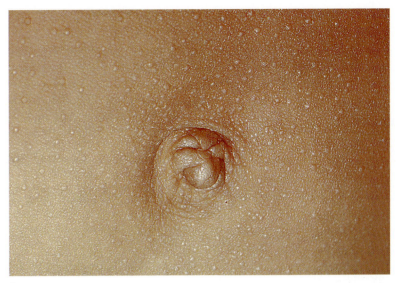

A

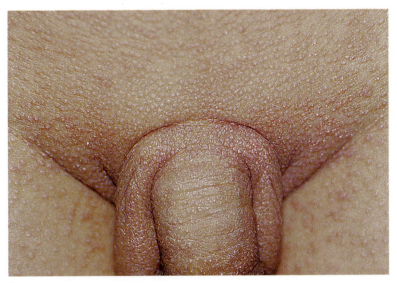

B

Figure 14-9   Lichen nitidus   *(A) Scattered small pinpoint papules on the abdomen of a child. (B) Same child with extensive groin involvement.*

LICHEN STRIATUS

A benign, self-limiting dermatitis characterized by a unilateral, linear papular eruption on the extremities of children.

EPIDEMIOLOGY

Age   Often children between the ages of 5 and 10 years, although lesions may arise early in infancy.

Gender   Girls affected 2 to 3 times as frequently as males.

Incidence   Uncommon.

Etiology   Unknown.

HISTORY

Onset   Lesions evolve suddenly and reach their maximum extent within several days to a few weeks.

Duration of Lesions   Regress spontaneously within 6 to 12 months.

Skin Symptoms   Lesions are asymptomatic.

PHYSICAL EXAMINATION

Skin Findings

Type   Discrete and confluent lichenoid papules arranged linearly (Fig. 14-10), involving a width ranging from a few mm up to 2 cm, and displaying a delicate silvery scale.

Color   Pink or light colored in fair skinned individuals; hypopigmented in dark-skinned individuals.

Size and Shape   Small, flat-topped lesions.

Distribution   Extremities, face, neck, trunk, and buttocks.

Sites of Predilection   Often unilateral on an extremity.

DIFFERENTIAL DIAGNOSIS

Characteristic linear appearance of lesions located on an extremity or other common site is indicative of lichen striatus. Histopathology is confirmatory. Lichen striatus needs to be differentiated from other linear disorders such as nevus unius lateris, an epidermal nevus or linear lichen planus.

LABORATORY EXAMINATIONS

Dermatopathology   A dense perivascular or band-like lymphohistiocytic infiltrate appears in the dermis. The epidermis reveals a small lymphocytic invasion with focal areas of acanthosis, parakeratosis, and spongiosis.

COURSE AND PROGNOSIS

An asymptomatic, self-limiting disorder of short duration (6 to 12 months). Pruritic in rare instances.

MANAGEMENT

For symptomatic relief, topical regimens include.

1. Topical steroids:
    a. Low potency steroids (Desowen, 1% hydrocortisone, 2.5% hydrocortisone) should be used on face or groin area, no more than bid × 2 weeks.
    b. Medium potency steroids (Elocon, Dermatop, Cutivate) should be used on the body or extremities no more than bid × 2 weeks.
    c. Strong steroids (Ultravate, Psorcon, Diprolene) are reserved for older children and adults on severely affected areas bid for no more than 2 weeks.
    Patients need to be cautioned about steroid side effects. (See page 48 for more details.)
2. Antihistamines may be somewhat helpful in controlling itching. They are particularly useful at bedtime when itching is usually the worst. Atarax (hydroxyzine, 2 to 4 mg per d divided tid or qid) and Benadryl (diphenhydramine, 5 mg per d divided tid or qid, not to exceed 300 mg per d) can be tried.
3. Antipruritic agents (Pramasone) may also be helpful.

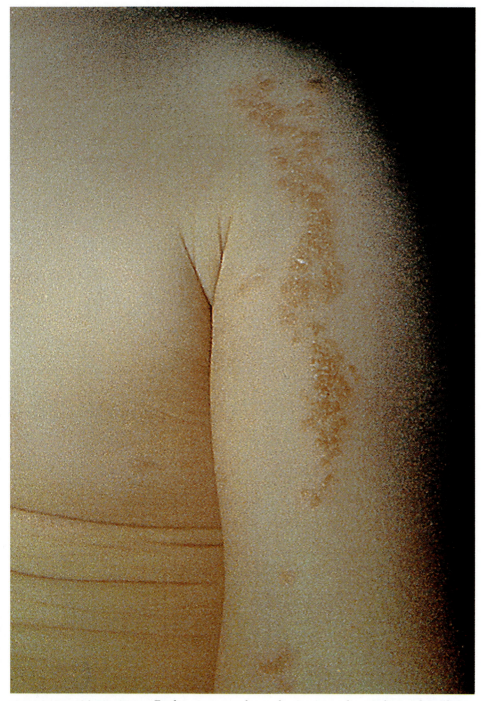

Figure 14-10 Lichen striatus *Erythematous papules coalescing into a linear plaque along the arm of a light-skinned colored child.*

HYPERSENSITIVITY VASCULITIS

Hypersensitivity vasculitis (HV) encompasses a heterogeneous group of vasculitides associated with hypersensitivity to antigens from infectious agents, drugs, or other exogenous or endogenous sources, characterized pathologically by involvement of small blood vessels (principally venules) with segmental inflammation and fibrinoid necrosis. Clinically, skin involvement is characteristic of HV, manifested by "palpable purpura" in the skin; systemic vascular involvement occurs, chiefly in the kidney, muscles, joints, GI tract, and peripheral nerves.

Synonyms   Allergic cutaneous vasculitis, necrotizing vasculitis.

EPIDEMIOLOGY

Age   All ages.

Gender   M = F.

Incidence   Uncommon.

Etiology   Idiopathic 50%.

PATHOPHYSIOLOGY

The most frequently postulated mechanism for the production of necrotizing vasculitis is the deposition in tissues of circulating immune complexes. Initial alterations in venular permeability, which may facilitate the deposition of complexes at such sites, may be due to the release of vasoactive amines from platelets, basophils, and/or mast cells. Immune complexes may activate the complement system or may directly interact with Fc receptors on cell membranes. When the complement system is activated, the generation of anaphylatoxins C3a and C5a could degranulate mast cells. Also, C5a can attract neutrophils that could release lysosomal enzymes during phagocytosis of complexes and subsequently damage vascular tissue.

CLASSIFICATION

Exogenous Stimuli Proved or Suspected
   Henoch-Schönlein purpura Group A streptococci.

Serum sickness/serum sickness-like reactions Sulfonamides, penicillin, serum.
   Other drug-induced vasculitides.
   Vasculititis associated with infectious diseases Hepatitis B virus, group A hemolytic streptococcus, *Staphylococcus aureus, Mycobacterium leprae.*

Endogenous Antigens Likely Involved   Vasculitis associated with:
   Neoplasms Lymphoproliferative disorders, kidney carcinoma.
   Connective tissue diseases SLE, rheumatoid arthritis, Sjögren's syndrome.
   Other underlying diseases Cryoglobulinemia, paraproteinemia, hypergammaglobulinemic purpura.
   Congenital deficiencies of the complement system.

HISTORY

Vasculitic lesions can be acute in onset (days as in drug-induced or idiopathic), subacute (weeks, especially urticarial types), or chronic (recurrent over years). The rash may be pruritic, burning, painful, or asymptomatic. Systemic symptoms include fever, malaise, peripheral neuritis, abdominal pain, arthralgias, myalgias, kidney involvement (microhematuria), and CNS involvement.

PHYSICAL FINDINGS

Skin Findings

Type of Lesion   "Palpable purpura," papules, nodules, vesicles, necrotic ulcers.

Color   Purpuric lesions do not blanch (using a glass slide)

Shape   Round, oval, annular, arciform

Size   2 to 4 mm

Arrangement   Scattered discrete lesions or dense and confluent

Distribution of Lesions   Usually regional localization: lower third of legs, ankles, buttocks, arms. Stasis factor aggravates or precipitates lesions.

General Examination

Should include search for underlying disease and organ involvement (especially a nephritis)

DIFFERENTIAL DIAGNOSIS

Diagnosis   The American College of Rheumatology's 1990 criteria for diagnosis of HV are as follows: a diagnosis of HV is made if at least 3 of these criteria are present:

1. Age at disease onset > 16 years (development of symptoms after age 16).
2. Medication at disease onset (medication was taken at the onset of symptoms that may have been a precipitating factor).
3. Palpable purpura (slightly elevated purpuric rash over one or more areas of the skin; does not blanch with pressure and is not related to thrombocytopenia).
4. Maculopapular rash (flat and raised lesions of various sizes over one or more areas of the skin).
5. Biopsy including arteriole and venule (histologic changes showing granulocytes in a perivascular or extravascular location).

Henoch-Schönlein purpura is a specific subtype of HV; the diagnosis is made if 2 of these 4 criteria are present.

1. Palpable purpura (slightly raised "palpable" hemorrhagic skin lesions, not related to thrombocytopenia).

2. Age < 20 at disease onset (patient 20 years or younger at onset of first symptoms).
3. Bowel angina (diffuse abdominal pain, worse after meals, or the diagnosis of bowel ischemia, usually including bloody diarrhea).
4. Wall granulocytes on biopsy (histologic changes showing granulocytes in the walls of arterioles or venules).

Differential Diagnosis   Palpable purpura due to a hypersensitivity reaction needs to be differentiated from thrombocytopenic purpura, bacteremia, and other non-infectious vasculitides.

LABORATORY EXAMINATIONS

Dermatopathology   Deposition of eosinophilic material (fibrinoid) in the walls of postcapillary venules in the upper dermis, and perivenular and intramural inflammatory infiltrate (neutrophils in those patients with hypocomplementemia, and lymphocytes or neutrophils with normal serum complement). Extravasated RBC and fragmented neutrophils (nuclear "dust") are also present. Frank necrosis of vessel walls. Intramural C3 and immunoglobulin deposition is seen with immunofluorescent techniques.

Other   ESR is elevated. May have hypocomplementemia. UA may show RBC casts or albuminuria.

COURSE AND PROGNOSIS

Depends on underlying etiology for the vasculitis. In the idiopathic variant, multiple episodes can occur over the course of years and each episode is usually self-limited but irreversible damage to kidneys can occur.

MANAGEMENT

Treatment depends on etiology for HV. Antibiotics are used for patients in whom vasculitis follows bacterial infection. Prednisone can be used in patients with severe non-infectious disease. Cytotoxic immunosuppressives (cyclophosphamide, azathioprine) and plasmapheresis has been tried in patients with severe refractory disease.

DRUG HYPERSENSITIVITY REACTION

A drug hypersensitivity reaction is an adverse, allergic response to an ingested or parenterally administered drug characterized by a cutaneous eruption that mimics a viral exanthem.

Synonyms   Morbilliform drug eruption, maculopapular drug eruption.

EPIDEMIOLOGY

Age   Less common in infants, seen in children < adolescents < adults.

Incidence   Most common type of cutaneous drug reaction.

Etiology   *Drugs with high probability of reaction* (10 to 20%): penicillin and related antibiotics, carbamazepine, allopurinol, gold salts. *Medium probability:* sulfonamides (bacteriostatic, antidiabetic, diuretic), nitrofurantoin, hydantoin derivatives, isoniazid, chloramphenicol, erythromycin, streptomycin. *Low probability* (1% or less): pyrazolon derivatives, barbiturates, benzodiazepines, phenothiazines, tetracyclines.

PATHOPHYSIOLOGY

Drug hypersensitivity reactions are likely type III (IgG- or IgM-mediated) or type IV (cell-mediated) immune responses.

HISTORY

Mononucleosis   Up to 100% of patients with Epstein-Barr or cytomegalovirus mononucleosis syndrome given ampicillin or amoxicillin develop an exanthematous drug eruption. They are not actually "allergic" to the medications because this cutaneous response is viral-mediated.

HIV Infection   Up to 50 to 60% of HIV-infected patients who receive sulfa drugs (i.e., trimethoprim-sulfamethoxazole) develop a morbilliform eruption.

Drug History   Increased incidence of reactions in patients on allopurinol given ampicillin/amoxicillin.

Prior Drug Sensitization   Patients with prior history of a drug hypersensitivity reaction will most likely develop a similar or more severe reaction if rechallenged with the same drug. Ten percent of patients sensitive to penicillins given cephalosporins will exhibit cross-drug sensitivity and develop an eruption. Patients sensitized to one sulfa-based drug (bacteriostatic, antidiabetic, diuretic) may cross-react with another category of that drug.

Onset   Sensitization typically occurs during administration or after completing course of drug; peak incidence at 9th day after administration. However, drug eruption may occur at any time between day 1 to day 21 after the beginning of treatment. Reaction to penicillin can begin 2 or more weeks after the drug has been discontinued. After prior sensitization, a re-exposure to the drug will elicit an allergic response 2 to 3 days after administration of the drug.

Systems Review   ± Fever. Usually quite pruritic.

PHYSICAL EXAMINATION

Vital Signs   ± Fever

Skin Findings

Type of Lesion   Macules and/or papules. Purpura may be seen in lesions of lower legs. May progress to generalized exfoliative dermatitis, especially if the drug is not discontinued. Scaling and/or desquamation may occur with healing.

Size   1-mm to 1-cm papules coalescing into plaques.

Color   Pink to bright red at onset fading to purple and brown.

Arrangement of Multiple Lesions   Macules and papules frequently become confluent plaques (Fig. 15-1A).

Distribution of Lesions   Symmetrical. Usually begins on trunk and spreads to face (Fig. 15-1B) and extremities. Confluent lesions

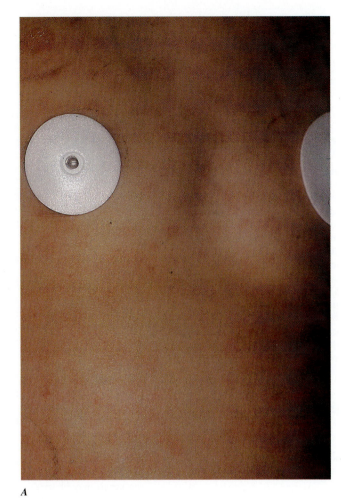

A

Figure 15-1 Drug hypersensitivity reaction *(A) Morbilliform rash on the trunk occuring 1 week after the administration of a systemic cephalosporin.*

in intertriginous areas (i.e., axilla, groin, infra-mammary area). Palms and soles variably involved. In children, may be limited to face and extremities.

Mucous Membranes ± Exanthem on buccal mucosa.

DIFFERENTIAL DIAGNOSIS

A history of drug exposure 1 day to 21 days prior to rash with physical examination of a widespread morbilliform eruption that clears once the drug is stopped is classic for a diagnosis of drug hypersensitivity. The diagnosis can be confirmed by skin biopsy drug rechallenge or allergic testing. Drug rechallenge is not recommended in severe cases of drug hypersensitivity because a rechallenge could elicit a quicker, more severe cutaneous and/or systemic response (i.e., anaphylaxis).

A drug hypersensitivity reaction can be confused with a viral exanthem, widespread allergic contact dermatitis, pityriasis rosea, eczema, psoriasis, or secondary syphilis.

LABORATORY EXAMINATIONS

Blood Work ± Peripheral eosinophils.

Dermatopathology Skin biopsy reveals perivascular inflammation with scattered eosinophils.

COURSE AND PROGNOSIS

Typically, drug hypersensitivity reactions can occur 1 to 21 days after drug exposure. With discontinuation of the drug, the rash begins to fade (often 2- to 3- day lag time after the drug is discontinued). The fiery red rash gradually fades to a dull purple and then desquamates. A rechallenge with the drug often elicits a faster, more severe response.

In rare cases, the morbilliform rash is followed by a more severe hypersensitivity reaction such as serum sickness, Stevens–Johnson syndrome, or toxic epidermal necrolysis, especially in cases where the offending drug has not yet been discontinued.

MANAGEMENT

Correct identification and discontinuation of the offending drug is needed.

Symptomatic relief while the rash fades includes:

1. Baths with colloidal oatmeal (Aveeno).
2. Emollients such as hydrated petrolatum (you must ask the pharmacist to get it), Vaseline, mineral oil, Aquaphor, Lubriderm, Moisturel, and Eucerin creams.
3. Topical steroids are effective if used in appropriate strength. Low potency steroids (Desowen, 1% hydrocortisone, 2.5% hydrocortisone) should be used on face or groin area, no more than bid × 2 weeks. Medium potency steroids (Elocon, Dermatop, Cutivate) should be used on the body or extremities no more than bid × 2 weeks. Strong steroids (Ultravate, Psorcon, Diprolene) are reserved for older children and adults on severely affected areas bid for no more than 2 weeks. Patients need to be cautioned about steroid side effects. (See page 48 for more details.)
4. Antihistamines may be somewhat helpful in controlling itching. They are particularly useful at bedtime when itching is usually the worst. They often have the side effect of producing drowsiness and, in rare instances, hyperactivity. Atarax (hydroxyzine, 2–4 mg/kg per d divided tid or qid) and Benadryl (diphenhydramine, 5 mg/kg per d divided tid or qid, not to exceed 300 mg per d) may be tried.
5. Severe cases may require systemic steroids (prednisone 1–2 mg/kg per d divided qd to bid for 5 to 14 d).

PREVENTION

The patient should be made aware of the possible drug allergen and cross reactants. His or her medical chart should be labeled accordingly. Readministration is not advised with allergic episodes that included urticaria, facial edema, blister, mucosal involvement, purpuric rashes, high fever, or lymphadenopathy. For morbilliform eruptions, the drug can be readminstered. In rare instances, it is even possible to "treat through" a drug hypersensitivity rash in cases where the offending drug is critical and there are no appropriate non-cross-reacting alternative medications.

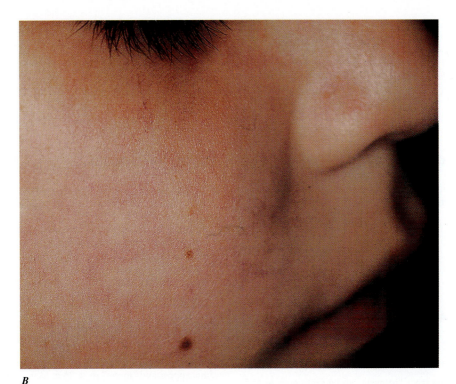

B

Figure 15-1 (continued)   Drug hypersensitivity reaction   *(B) Morbilliform rash eventually spread to the face and extremities of the same child.*

URTICARIA AND ANGIOEDEMA

Urticaria and angioedema are allergic responses characterized by transient edematous plaques (wheals/urticaria/hives) and/or dermal swelling (angioedema). In some cases, urticaria and angioedema are accompanied by respiratory symptoms, vascular collapse, and/or shock (anaphylaxis).

CLASSIFICATION

Urticaria and angioedema are immune-mediated by three mechanisms.

1. IgE (seen especially with antibiotics, radiocontrast).
2. Complement (seen with whole blood or immunoglobulin infusions).
3. Immune complex (seen with penicillin).

EPIDEMIOLOGY

Age Any age.

Gender M = F.

Incidence Urticaria can be seen in up to 15% of population. Angioedema is seen in 1:10,000 courses of penicillin.

Drugs that cause urticaria and angioedema include the following.

1. Antibiotics: penicillins, sulfonamides, and derivatives.
2. Cardiac drugs: amiodarone, procainamide.
3. Immunotheraputics: serum, horse urine.
4. Chemotheraputics: L-asparagine, bleomycin, cisplatin, daunorubicin, 5%-FU, procarbazine, thiotepa.
5. ACE inhibitors: captopril, enalapril, lisinopril.
6. Ca+ channel blockers: nifedipine, diltiazem, verapamil.
7. Histamine-releasers: morphine, radiocontrast dye, muscle relaxants, salicylates, sympathomimetics, hypotensive agents, and antimicrobials.

Foods that cause urticaria and angioedema include milk, eggs, wheat, shellfish, and nuts.

Other things that can cause urticaria include physical urticaria (dermatagraphism, cold; Fig. 15-2), solar, cholinergic, pressure, vibratory; and hereditary angioedema (autosomal dominantly inherited disorder caused by low levels of C1 inactivation or dysfunction inhibitor).

PATHOPHYSIOLOGY

In IgE-mediated disease, IgE sensitizes mast cells or basophilic leukocytes to release vasoactive substances.

In complement-mediated urticaria, activated complement causes anaphylatoxin release which, in turn, induces mast cell degranulation.

In immune-complex mediated urticaria, immune complexes cause mast cell degranulation.

HISTORY

In acute urticaria (< 30 days), transient skin lesions appear and "move" in < 24 h. Skin symptoms can include pruritus, flushing, or burning. In chronic urticaria (> 30 d), skin lesions are transient but clinical course is more relapsing. Systemic symptoms can include respiratory symptoms, arthralgias, fatigue, abdominal pain, fever, and diarrhea.

PHYSICAL EXAMINATION

Urticaria Skin Findings

Type Transient, edematous, well-delineated papule or plaques (Fig. 15-3).

Size 1 mm to 10 cm

Shape Round, oval, annular, polycyclic.

Color Pink to red, with surrounding or central pallor (Fig. 15-4).

Distribution Typically generalized.

Angioedema Skin Findings

Type Diffuse swelling.

Color Pink-red.

Sites of Predilection Face (eyelids, lips, tongue).

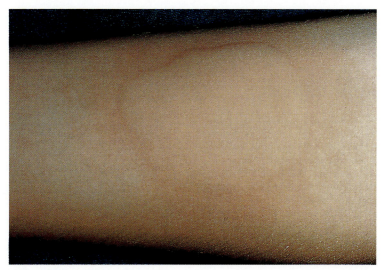

Figure 15-2 Urticaria, cold-induced *Cold urticaria can be reproduced by placing an ice pack on the forearm of an affected child for 2 to 10 mins with a resultant urticarial wheal.*

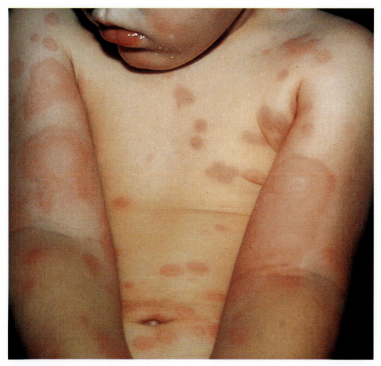

Figure 15-3 Urticaria *Transient, well-circumscribed, erythematous, annular plaques characteristic of urticaria.*

General Findings

Malaise, fever, arthralgias, respiratory symptoms, hypotension, shock.

DIFFERENTIAL DIAGNOSIS

The transient edematous plaques are diagnostic for urticaria, although often parents can mistake blisters or insect bites for urticaria. Urticaria also needs to be differentiated from dermatographism (present in 5% of the normal population), eczema, contact dermatitis, mastocytosis, erythema mulitforme, and allergic vasculitis.

LABORATORY EXAMINATIONS

Dermatopathology Dermal or subcutaneous edema, vascular dilation, and mild perivascular infiltrate.

COURSE AND PROGNOSIS

Urticaria self-resolves in 1 year in 50% of cases. Up to 20% of cases can have a chronic relapsing course.

MANAGEMENT

Identification and elimination of any causative agent is most helpful. In up to 50% of cases, the etiology is unclear. At times, urticaria and angioedema can be precipitated by stress.

Treatment is primarily symptomatic with antihistamines.

1. H_1-blockers
    a. Diphenhydramine (Benadryl, 5 mg/kg/ per d po divided tid or qid).
    b. Hydroxyzine HCl (Atarax, 2 to 4 mg/ kg/per d divided tid or qid).
2. To avoid the sedation effects, a nonsedating H_1-blocker may be preferred.
    a. Cetirizine HCl (Zyrtec 2.5 to 10 mg po qd).
3. In resistant cases, H_2-blockers can used in combination with H_1-blocker.
    a. Cimetidine (Tagamet, 10 to 40 mg/kg/ per d po divided qid).
    b. Ranitidine hydrochloride (Zantac, 2 to 4 mg/dose po bid).
4. A combination H_1- and H_2-blocker antidepressant used in low doses may be helpful, but pediatric use is strictly off label.
    a. Doxepin (Sinequan or Adapin, 5 to 10 mg po qd).

Antihistamines should be continued for 1 to 2 weeks beyond clinical clearance to avoid recurrences or relapses and may need to be tapered slowly over several months.

For severe refractory cases, systemic corticosteroids may be indicated.

1. Prednisone (1 to 2 mg/kg/per d divided bid for 5 d).
2. Prednisolone (1 to 2 mg/kg/per d divided bid for 5 d).

For anaphylactic reactions, epinephrine (0.1 to 0.5 mL of 1:1000 injected subcutaneously) is effective and can be life-saving. Those with anaphylactic reactions or severe urticaria and angioedema should wear a medical alert bracelet and keep an epinephrine pen nearby.

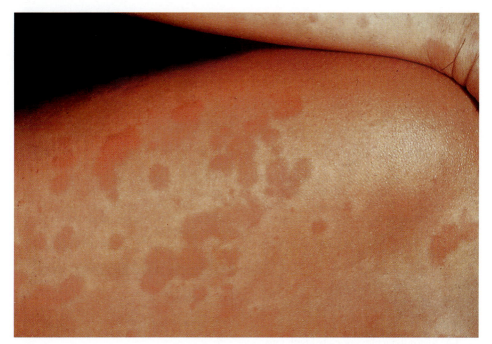

Figure 15-4 Urticaria *Erythematous papules and plaques with surrounding blanched halos characteristic of urticarial lesions on the knee of a child.*

ERYTHEMA MULTIFORME SYNDROME

Erythema multiforme (EM) is a reactive syndrome characterized by "target" vesicobullous lesions of the skin and mucous membranes.

CLASSIFICATION

1. EM minor: mild disease with little to no mucous membrane lesions.
2. EM major (Stevens–Johnson syndrome): more severe disease with two mucous membranes affected and possible systemic symptoms such as fever and prostration.

EPIDEMIOLOGY

Age   50% < 20 years.

Gender   M > F.

Etiologies

1. EM minor: typically associated with infection. Recurrent EM minor is usually associated with herpes simplex outbreaks. Other infections (viral, bacterial, protozoal, fungal, or *Mycoplasma* pneumonia) can also cause EM minor.
2. EM major: typically associated with drugs (sulfonamides, phenytoin, barbiturates, phenylbutazone, penicillin, allopurinol).

Etiology is unknown in up to 50% of cases. Other possible precipitants include vaccination, connective tissue disorders, and rarely, malignancy.

PATHOPHYSIOLOGY

Pathogenesis unclear. Likely a cell-mediated cytotoxic reaction.

HISTORY

Skin lesions may appear 3 to 14 days after insult (infection, drug, etc.) and new lesions can continue to appear for up to 10 days. Skin lesions may be pruritic or painful. Mucous membrane involvement, if present, is painful and debilitating. Fever, malaise, and weakness may also be present.

PHYSICAL EXAMINATION

Skin Lesions

Type   Macules progressing to papules, vesicles and bullae.

Color   Dull red rings alternating with cyanotic or violaceous rings (Fig. 15-5).

Size   1 to 2 cm.

Shape   Target or iris lesions are typical.

Distribution   Symmetric and bilateral, any part of the body.

Sites of Predilection   Palms, soles, dorsa of hands and feet, extensor surfaces of the arms/legs.

Mucous Membranes   Oral (Fig. 15-6A), ocular (Fig. 15-6B), and genital blistering and ulceration may be present.

Other Organs   Pulmonary and renal involvement may also occur.

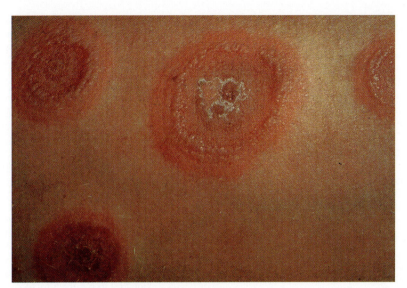

Figure 15-5   Erythema multiforme minor (EM minor)   *Polycyclic target lesions with alternating rings of erythema and dusky desquamation on the arm.*

DIFFERENTIAL DIAGNOSIS

Erythema multiforme can be confused with viral exanthems, bullous diseases, urticaria, secondary syphilis, psoriasis, or pityriasis rosea. The "target lesions" are classic for EM, but may be confused with erythema annulare centrifugum or other annular eruptions.

LABORATORY EXAMINATIONS

Dermatopathology Skin biopsy reveals dermal edema with a perivascular lymphocytic infiltrate, leukocytoclasis, and extravasated red blood cells. Necrotic kertinocytes leads to subepidermal bullae formation.

COURSE AND PROGNOSIS

1. **EM minor:** rash appears 3 to 14 days after precipitating infection or drug. Mucous membrane involvement is mild if present at all. No systemic symptoms. Each episode resolves in 2 to 4 weeks, but recurrences can be frequent, especially in cases where herpes simplex is the precipitating cause.
2. **EM major:** (Stevens–Johnson syndrome): rash appears and worsens until precipitating cause is removed (i.e., discontinuation of drug). Rash is extensive with bullous lesions and > two mucous membranes are involved with systemic complications. Cheilitis and stomatitis interfere with eating, vulvitis and balanitis complicate micturition, conjunctivitis and keratitis can lead to ocular impairment, and lesions in the pharynx, larynx, and trachea can occlude the airway. Fever and prostration are seen.

MANAGEMENT

1. **EM minor:** rash self-resolves in 5 to 15 days. Symptomatic relief can be obtained with the following.
   a. Baths with colloidal oatmeal (Aveeno).
   b. Emollients such as hydrated petrolatum, Vaseline, mineral oil, Aquaphor, Lubriderm, Moisturel, and Eucerin creams.
   c. Topical steroids are effective if used in appropriate strengths. Low potency steroids (Desowen, 1% hydrocortisone, 2.5% hydrocortisone) should be used on face or groin area, no more than bid × 2 weeks. Medium potency steroids (Elocon, Dermatop, Cutivate) should be used on the body or extremities no more than bid × 2 weeks. Strong steroids (Ultravate, Psorcon, Diprolene) are reserved for older children and adults on severely affected areas bid for no more than 2 weeks. (See page 48 for more details.)
   d. Antihistamines may be somewhat helpful in controlling itching. Atarax (hydroxyzine, 2 to 4 mg/kg/ per d divided tid or qid) or Benadryl (diphenhydramine, 5 mg/kg/per d divided tid or qid, not to exceed 300 mg per d may be tried.
   e. Severe cases may require systemic steroids (prednisone 1 to 2 mg/kg/d divided qd to bid for 5 to 14 d).
   f. Control of herpes outbreaks in recurrent cases of EM minor with prophylactic acyclovir is indicated.
2. **EM major:** identification and elimination of the precipitating agent is critical. Supportive care includes:
   a. Wound care includes baths with gentle cleansers (Aquanil or Cetaphil liquid cleansers) and topical petrolatum-impregnated gauze (Xeroform) can help reduce chance of secondary infection and will also help healing. Topical emollients (Vaseline petroleum jelly, hydrated petrolatum, or Aquaphor healing ointment) can reduce friction on the healing area. Topical antibiotics (Bactroban, bacitracin, neosporin, or polysporin) can be used if evidence of bacterial superinfection is present (yellow exudate, frank pus, crusting). A water mattress with fleece covering may be necessary to limit trauma to the skin.
   b. Topical steroids (see above for details).
   c. Widespread denudation of the skin requires hospitalization for thermoregulation and food administration (especially in cases with extensive oral involvement). Systemic corticosteroids are of questionable efficacy. Constant cultures and local debridement should be done to prevent infection and risk of sepsis until skin fully heals.

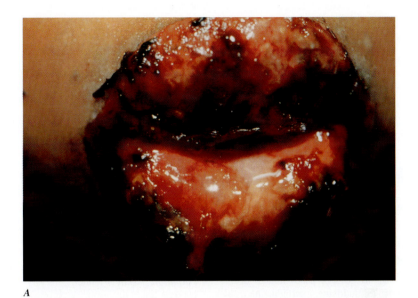

A

B

Figure 15-6 **Erythema multiforme major (EM major)** *(A) Debilitating mucosal involvement with hemorrhagic ulcerations and crusting requiring hospital admission for IV fluids and supportive care. (B) Ocular involvement with erosions and ulcerations in the same child.*

TOXIC EPIDERMAL NECROLYSIS

Toxic epidermal necrolysis (TEN) is a cutaneous drug-induced or idiopathic reaction pattern characterized by skin tenderness and erythema of skin and mucosa, followed by extensive (> 30% body surface area) cutaneous and mucosal exfoliation. It is potentially life-threatening due to multisystem involvement.

Synonym   Lyell's syndrome.

EPIDEMIOLOGY

Age   Older children. More common in adults > 40 years old.

Gender   M = F.

Incidence   1:1,000,000 person-years.

Etiology   Up to 80% of cases due to drugs: sulfa drugs (sulfadoxine, sulfadiazine, sulfasalazine, clotrimazole), allopurinol, antibiotics, barbiturates, hydantoins, carbamazepine, phenylbutazones (and other NSAIDs), piroxicam, chlormezanone, amithiozone, aminopenicillins, cephalosporins, fluroquinolones, vancomycin, rifampin, ethambutol, barbiturates, salicylates, phenytoin, and griseofulvin. Other precipitants include: infections (viral, fungal, bacterial septicemia), vaccinations, leukemia, lymphoma, graft-versus-host reaction.

PATHOPHYSIOLOGY

Pathogenesis unclear but thought to be a cell-mediated cytotoxic reaction against the basal cell keratinocytes.

HISTORY

One to 3 weeks after drug exposure, rash begins with diffuse tender erythema. Small blisters then form, becoming irregularly confluent. Entire thickness of epidermis becomes necrotic and shears off in large sheets (Nikolsky's sign). Regrowth of epidermis takes 1 to 3 weeks. Pressure points and perioral areas heal more slowly. Systemic symptoms include fever, malaise, myalgia, arthralgias, nausea and vomiting, diarrhea, and conjunctival burning.

PHYSICAL EXAMINATION

Skin Findings

Type   Papules coalescing into plaques, bullae (rare), diffuse desquamation (Fig. 15-7).

Color   Pink-red to dusky cyanotic.

Palpation   Skin is tender.

Distribution   Generalized.

Mucous Membranes   Oral and genital lesions (painful erosions, bullae) in 90%.

Ocular Involvement   Conjunctival hyperemia, keratitis, pseudomembrane formation, or erosions in 85%.

General Findings   Fever (usually > 38°C). Renal involvement with tubular necrosis and resultant renal failure. Erosions in respiratory and GI tract as well.

DIFFERENTIAL DIAGNOSIS

TEN can be confused with staphylococcus scalded skin syndrome (SSSS). A "jelly roll" of the skin in TEN will show a subepidermal split in the skin, whereas in SSSS, a more superficial intradermal separation is noted. TEN can also be confused with graft-versus-host disease (GVHD), phototoxic eruptions, or generalized erythroderma (from severe psoriasis, atopic dermatitis, mycosis fungoides, etc.).

LABORATORY EXAMINATIONS

Dermatopathology   Skin biopsy reveals necrosis of the basal cell layer with subepidermal

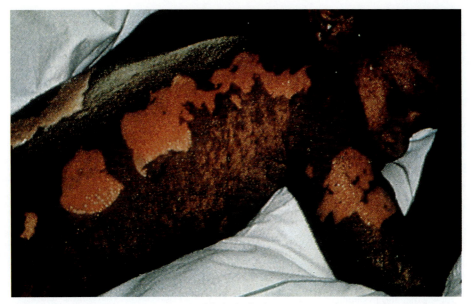

Figure 15-7 Toxic epidermal necrolysis *Whole body desquamation characteristic of toxic epidermal necrolysis.*

bullae formation. Severe TEN can show full-thickness epidermal necrosis.

Hematology Neutropenia correlates with poor prognosis. Anemia, lymphopenia uncommon.

COURSE AND PROGNOSIS

Course is similar to that of severe widespread thermal burns. Patient demise often secondary to sepsis or fluid and electrolyte imbalances. Mortality rate is 30%.

MANAGEMENT

Management consists of elimination of causative agent. Patient best cared for in a burn or intensive care unit with IV fluid and electrolyte replenishment, temperature control, and vigilant wound care. Systemic steroids are probably <u>not</u> helpful. High-dose IV immunoglobulins may be of some benefit if administered early. Ocular care and ophthalmologic consultation are needed. Liquid diets and parenteral nutrition may be needed.

PREVENTION

Those who do recover from TEN need to be aware of their drug sensitivity and possible cross-reactants. Re-exposure to the offending agent can lead to a faster, more severe TEN episode, thus drugs should not be readministered and the patient should wear a medical alert bracelet.

FIXED DRUG ERUPTION

A fixed drug eruption (FDE) is a recurrent cutaneous reaction to an ingested drug characterized by the formation of a fixed plaque, bulla, or erosion at the same site, hours after the offending drug is ingested.

EPIDEMIOLOGY

Age   Any age.

Gender   M = F.

Incidence   Uncommon.

Etiology   The drugs most commonly implicated are the following.

1. Phenolphthalein.
2. Antimicrobial agents: tetracyclines (tetracycline, minocycline), sulfonamides, metronidazole, and nystatin.
3. Anti-inflammatory agents: salicylates, NSAIDs, phenylbutazone, and phenacetin.
4. Psychoactive agents: barbituates.
5. Quinine, quinidine.

The foods most commonly implicated are peas, beans, and lentils.

PATHOPHYSIOLOGY

Unknown.

HISTORY

Patients will report a recurrent erythematous to violaceous plaque that recurs at the same site at seemingly random intervals. Careful history will usually elicit the sporadic use of an over-the-counter or PRN medication that is causing the recurrent rash (i.e., Advil, aspirin, eyedrops, laxatives, etc.).

PHYSICAL EXAMINATION

Skin Findings

Type   Macule or plaque. Occasionally bullae.

Shape   Round to oval.

Color   Initially erythema, then dusky-red to violaceous (Fig. 15–8). After healing, dark brown with violet hue of postinflammatory hyperpigmentation.

Size   0.5 to 20 cm in diameter.

Number   Usually a solitary lesion. With repeated attacks, multiple lesions may occur.

Palpation   Eroded lesions, especially on genital or oral mucosa, are quite painful.

Distribution   Any skin site.

Sites of Predilection   The genital skin is the most commonly involved site.

Mucous Membranes   Lesions may rarely occur within the mouth or on the conjunctiva.

DIFFERENTIAL DIAGNOSIS

The diagnosis of fixed drug eruption can be made on clinical findings and history. Readministration of the drug or skin biopsy of the lesion will help to confirm the diagnosis. Fixed drug eruption can be confused with recurrent herpetic lesions, other drug reactions, a contact dermatitis, or other eczematous processes.

LABORATORY EXAMINATIONS

Dermatopathology   Skin biopsy will show dyskeratosis, basal cell vacuolization, dermal edema, perivascular and interstitial lymphohistiocytic infiltrate, at times with eosinophils and/or subepidermal vesicles and bullae with overlying epidermal necrosis. Between outbreaks, the site of the fixed drug eruption shows marked pigmentary incontinence with melanin in macrophages in upper dermis.

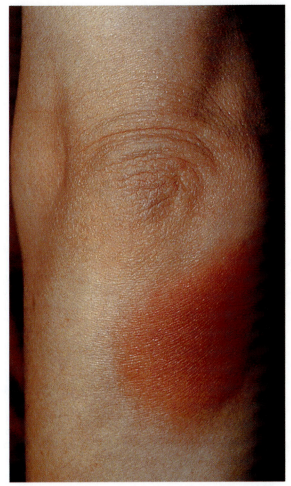

Figure 15-8 **Fixed drug eruption** *A large red-violet plaque on the arm of a child.*

COURSE AND PROGNOSIS

The cutaneous lesions of fixed drug eruption resolve within a few weeks of withdrawing the offending agent. The rash recurs within hours following ingestion of a single dose of the drug.

MANAGEMENT

The management for a fixed drug eruption is to identify and withhold the offending drug. The hyperpigmented postinflammatory changes will slowly resolve with time.

SERUM SICKNESS

Serum sickness is an allergic reaction characterized by urticaria, malaise, fever, lymphadenopathy, splenomegaly, and arthralgias. It originally was seen most in treatment with horse or rabbit antiserum; it is now seen with drugs or vaccinations.

EPIDEMIOLOGY

Age   Any age.

Gender   M = F.

Incidence   Uncommon.

Etiology   Immune-mediated reaction.

PATHOPHYSIOLOGY

Serum sickness is mediated by circulating antigen-antibody complexes (type III-Arthus reaction), in which IgG is the predominant immunoglobulin.

HISTORY

Urticarial rash and low-grade fever, usually 7 to 21 days following administration of offending agent, or earlier in individuals previously sensitized to the agent.

PHYSICAL EXAMINATION

Skin Findings

Type   90% have urticarial wheals, and localized or generalized edema (Fig. 15-9). Less commonly, exanthematous (morbilliform/scarlatiniform) eruption or erythema nodosum-erythema multiforme-like lesions can be seen.

Color   Pink with central pallor, bright red.

Shape   Round, oval, and polycyclic.

Arrangement   Scattered, discrete lesions or dense, confluent areas.

Distribution   Trunk, extremities, face.

Mucous Membranes   May be involved.

General Findings

Regional or generalized lymphadenopathy (often presenting in epitrochlear region), joint symptoms in 50% of patients (ranging from mild arthralgia to severe polyarthritis), neurologic manifestations (peripheral neuritis, radiculitis, optic neuritis, cerebral edema), renal glomerulonephritis.

DIFFERENTIAL DIAGNOSIS

Diagnosis is made by taking a detailed history of all recent immunizations and medications including over-the-counter preparations. Serum sickness can be confused with urticaria, angioedema, urticarial vasculitis, a viral exanthem, toxic epidermal necrolysis, or subacute bacterial endocarditis.

LABORATORY EXAMINATIONS

Dermatopathology   Skin biopsy findings would be identical to urticaria (engorged blood vessels with edema and perivascular inflammation).

Hematology   ± Eosinophilia, elevated ESR, hypocomplementemia.

COURSE AND PROGNOSIS

Serum sickness has a self-limited course, progression may continue for a while, and then disappear within 2 to 3 weeks. Most cases resolve with no permanent sequelae. In rare instances, coronary artery vasculitis or neuropathy may persist.

MANAGEMENT

Symptomatic treatment of serum sickness includes analgesics and antihistamines.
   Antihistamines include the following.

1. H$_1$-blockers
   a. Diphenhydramine (Benadryl, 5 mg/kg per d po divided tid or qid).
   b. Hydroxyzine HCl (Atarax, 2 to 4 mg/kg per d divided tid or qid).
2. To avoid the sedation effects, a nonsedating H-blocker may be preferred.
   a. Cetirizine HCl (Zyrtec 2.5 to 10 mg po qd).
3. In resistant cases, H$_2$-blockers can be used in combination with H$_1$-blockers.
   a. Cimetidine (Tagamet, 10 to 40 mg/kg per d po divided qid).
   b. Ranitidine hydrochloride (Zantac, 2 to 4 mg/dose po bid).
4. A combination H$_1$- and H$_2$-blocker antidepressant used in low doses may be helpful, but pediatric use is strictly off-label.
   a. Doxepin (Sinequan or Adapin, 5 to 10 mg po qd).

Antihistamines should be continued for 1 to 2 weeks beyond clinical clearance to avoid recurrences or relapses and may need to be tapered slowly over several months.

Although their efficacy has not been proven, systemic steroids are used if common measures fail to comfort patient, including prednisone (1 to 2 mg/kg per d divided bid for 5 d) and prednisolone (1 to 2 mg/kg per d divided bid for 5 d).

For anaphylactic or life-threatening situations (individuals with facial edema or respiratory symptoms), epinephrine (0.1 to 0.5 mL of 1:1000 injected subcutaneously) is effective.

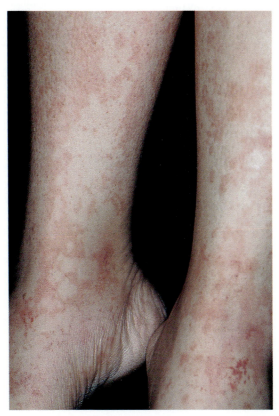

Figure 15-9 Serum sickness *Urticarial, coalescing plaques on the lower legs of an adolescent with serum sickness.*

ERYTHEMA ANNULARE CENTRIFUGUM

Erythema annulare centrifugum (EAC) is a cutaneous eruption characterized by migratory erythematous annular lesions with raised borders and central clearing. The etiology of EAC is unknown but it has been speculated that it occurs as a hypersensitivity reaction to an underlying infectious, inflammatory, or neoplastic process.

Synonyms Erythema perstans, gyrate erythema.

EPIDEMIOLOGY

Age Any age.

Gender M = F.

Etiology Unknown. Possible hypersensitivity reaction to drugs, foods, infections (dermatophytes, *Candida albicans,* EBV, molluscum contagiosum), blood dyscrasias, immunologic disorders (neonatal lupus, Sjögren's syndrome), liver disease, hyperthyroidism, or neoplasms.

HISTORY

Rash appears and spreads centrifugally. It is typically asymptomatic or mildly pruritic and can recur for months to years depending upon its etiologic process.

PHYSICAL EXAMINATION

Skin Findings

Type Single or multiple edematous papules that expand centrifugally forming large rings with a cleared center and a raised thin-wall-like border with or without scale.

Size 1 cm, may expand slowly (3 mm per d) and may reach a size of 10 cm or more in diameter.

Color Pink to red.

Shape Irregular, oval, circinate, semiannular, target-like, or polycyclic lesions (Fig. 15-10).

Distribution Trunk, buttocks, thighs, and lower legs.

DIFFERENTIAL DIAGNOSIS

The diagnosis of EAC is made by history, examination and/or skin biopsy. Other annular rashes include: pityriasis rosea, erythema multiforme, erythema chronicum migrans, dermatophyte infections (more pronounced epidermal changes, scaling on both edges of the border, positive KOH scraping, or fungal culture), or annular lupus erythematosus.

LABORATORY EXAMINATIONS

Dermatopathology Skin biopsy shows parakeratosis and focal infiltration of lymphocytes around dermal blood vessels and adnexal structures in a "coat-sleeve" pattern. There is minimal papillary edema and no spongiosis.

COURSE AND PROGNOSIS

The duration of EAC is extremely variable; new lesions may continue to form for months or even years, appearing in successive forms.

MANAGEMENT

The treatment of EAC depends on the etiology. Antihistamines are recommended for symptomatic relief.

1. Atarax (hydroxyzine, 2 to 4 mg/kg per d divided tid or qid).
2. Benadryl (diphenhydramine, 5 mg/kg per d divided tid or qid, not to exceed 300 mg per d).

Empirical therapy with antifungal or antibiotic agents can help if cause has not been identified.

Systemic steroids may suppress EAC but the disorder frequently recurs after cessation.

1. Prednisone (1 to 2 mg/kg per d divided bid for 5 d).
2. Prednisolone (1 to 2 mg/kg per d divided bid for 5 d).

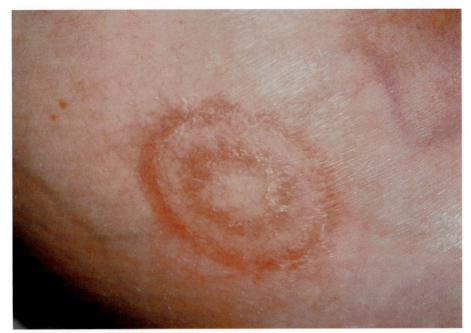

Figure 15-10 Erythema annulare centrifugum *Polycyclic lesion on the thigh of a child with a tinea capitis infection.*

GRAFT-VERSUS-HOST DISEASE

Graft-versus-host disease (GVHD) is an immune disorder caused by the response of histoincompatible, immunocompetent donor cells against the tissues of an immunoincompetent host. The disorder is characterized by acute cutaneous changes ranging from a maculopapular eruption to toxic epidermal necrolysis and systemic symptoms such as diarrhea and liver dysfunction. The chronic skin changes range from lichenoid eruptions to sclerodematous changes.

EPIDEMIOLOGY

Age Any age.

Gender M = F.

Incidence Varies between 60 and 80% of successful engraftment with allogeneic marrow. Mild GVHD occurs in 8% of autologous bone marrow transplants. Low incidence in blood transfusions to immunosuppressed patients or maternal–fetal transfer in immunodeficient infants.

Etiology

Host Recipients of marrow transplants include aplastic anemia, acute leukemia, some immunodeficiency disorders. Immunosuppressed patients receiving blood transfusions containing immunocompetent leukocytes. Immunodeficient fetus with maternal–fetal transfer of leukocytes.

Donor Bone marrow transplantation.

Clinical Grading of Acute Cutaneous GVHD

1. Erythematous maculopapular eruption involving < 25% of body surface.
2. Erythematous maculopapular eruption involving 25 to 50% of body surface.
3. Erythroderma.
4. Bulla formation.

PATHOPHYSIOLOGY

GVHD is an inflammatory reaction mounted by the donor cells against specific host organs (skin, liver, or GI tract). Severity of GVHD is related to histocompatibility match between donor and recipient and preparatory regimen used. With successful engraftment, there is replacement of host marrow by immunocompetent donor cells capable of reacting against the "foreign" tissue antigens of the host.

HISTORY

History *Acute:* Rash and pruritus occur during first 3 months after bone marrow transplantation (usually between 14 to 21 d).

Chronic: Rash appears > 100 days after bone marrow transplantation, either evolving from acute GVHD or arising de novo. Acute GVHD is not always followed by chronic GVHD.

Systemic Symptoms Nausea and vomiting, right upper quadrant pain and tenderness, cramping abdominal pain, watery diarrhea, jaundice, dark urine.

PHYSICAL EXAMINATION

Skin Findings

Types of Lesions *Acute:* Initially, subtle, discrete macules and/or papules; mild edema/violaceous hue, in periungual region and pinna (Fig. 15-11). If controlled or resolves, erythema diminishes with subsequent desquamation and postinflammatory hyperpigmentation. If progresses, macules and papules become confluent and patient appears erythrodermic. Subepidermal bullae can ensue especially over pressure and trauma sites with toxic epidermal necrolysis-like (TEN-like) skin findings (Fig. 15-12).

Chronic: Flat-topped papules, lichen planuslike (Fig. 15-13). Confluent areas of dermal sclerosis with overlying scale. Hair loss; anhidrosis, vitiligo-like hypopigmentation; lichen planus-like lesions in oral mucosa; erosive stomatitis, oral and ocular sicca-like syndrome; esophagitis, serositis. More common are severe sclerodermoid changes with necrosis and ulceration on acral and pressure sites.

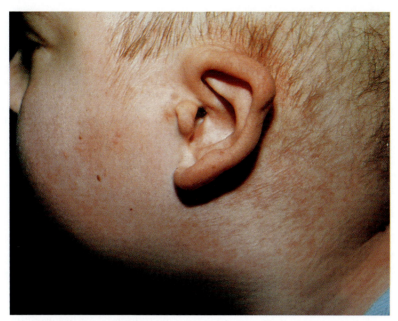

Figure 15-11   Graft-versus-host disease, acute   *Erythematous-to-violaceous hue to the pinna of the ear in acute GVHD.*

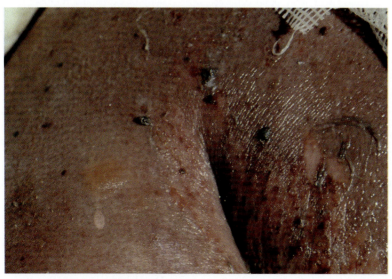

Figure 15-12   Graft-versus-host disease, acute   *Epidermal sloughing in acute GVHD resembling TEN-like changes.* (Reproduced with permission from TB Fitzpatrick et al., Color Atlas and Synopsis of Clinical Dermatology, 4th edition. New York: McGraw-Hill, 2001).

Color   *Acute:* Erythematous to violaceous hue.

Palpation   Pain with pressure.

Distribution of Lesions   *Acute:* Earliest findings—upper trunk, hands and feet especially palms and soles.
Chronic: Distal extremities. Diffuse sclerosis on trunk, buttocks, hips, thighs.

General Examination

Acute: Fever, jaundice, diarrhea, serositis, pulmonary insufficiency.
Chronic: Chronic liver disease, wasting.

DIFFERENTIAL DIAGNOSIS

Acute GVHD can be confused with an exanthematous drug reaction, viral exanthem, or TEN. Chronic GVHD can be confused with lichen planus, lichenoid drug reaction, scleroderma, or poikiloderma. The diagnosis can be confirmed by skin biopsy.

LABORATORY EXAMINATIONS

Dermatopathology
Acute: Skin biopsy will show basal cell vacuolization and *necrosis of individual keratinocytes* with a mild perivenular mononuclear cell infiltrate. Aposition of lymphocytes to necrotic keratinocytes can be seen and vacuoles coalesce forming subepidermal clefts.
Chronic: Skin biopsy will show hyperkeratosis, mild hypergranulosis, mild irregular acanthosis, moderate basal vacuolization, mild perivascular mononuclear cell infiltrate, melanin incontinence, loss of hair follicles, entrapment of sweat glands, and dense dermal sclerosis.

COURSE AND PROGNOSIS

Mild to moderate acute GVHD responds well to treatment. Severe GVHD patients are susceptible to infections (bacterial, fungal, or viral) and those with TEN-like skin changes have a very poor prognosis. Acute GVHD has mortality rate of 45% in transplant patients.

Chronic GVHD with sclerodermoid changes and tight skin and joint contractures may result in impaired mobility and ulcerations. There is also associated hair loss, xerostomia, and xerophthalmia resulting in corneal ulcers and blindness. GI disease leads to malabsorption. Mild chronic cutaneous GVHD may resolve spontaneously. Severe changes are usually permanent and debilitating. Chronic GVHD has an overall survival rate of 42% at 10 years.

MANAGEMENT

Supportive measures include:

1. Hyperalimentation.
2. Protective isolation.
3. Antibiotics.
4. Physical therapy.

Topical corticosteroids can give symptomatic relief.

1. Low potency steroids (Desowen, 1% hydrocortisone, 2.5% hydrocortisone) should be used on face or groin area, no more than bid × 2 weeks.
2. Medium potency steroids (Elocon, Dermatop, Cutivate) should be used on the body or extremities no more than bid × 2 weeks.
3. Strong steroids (Ultravate, Psorcon, Diprolene) are reserved for older children and adults on severely affected areas bid for no more than 2 weeks.

In more extensive disease, high dose systemic steroids may be required if GI or liver disease is present, and cyclosporine A may be added. Both systemic medications can be discontinued once skin, GI, and liver disease is under control.

Other possible therapies include:

1. PUVA for subacute and chronic GVHD in older children (> 10 years old).
2. Extracorporeal photophoresis.
3. Antithymocyte globulin and pan-T lymphocyte antibody-ricin A chain immunotoxin.
4. Azathioprine.
5. Thalidomide.

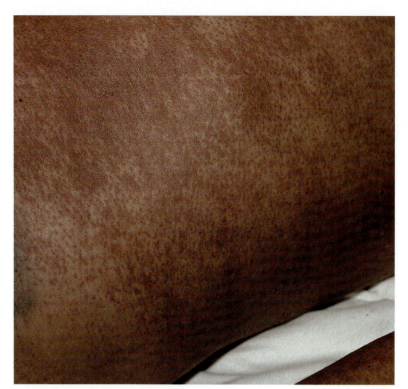

Figure 15-13 **Graft-versus-host- disease, chronic** *Lichenoid papules coalescing into plaques 3 months after an allogeneic bone marrow transplant.* (Reproduced with permission from TB Fitzpatrick et al., Color Atlas and Synopsis of Clinical Dermatology, 4th edition. New York: McGraw-Hill, 2001).

ERYTHEMA NODOSUM

Erythema nodosum (e. nodosum) is a cell-mediated hypersensitivity reaction character-ized by tender red nodules on the pretibial area.

EPIDEMIOLOGY

Age   Any age. Most commonly seen in pa-tients ages 15 to 30 years.

Gender   F > M, 3:1.

Incidence   Uncommon.

Season   Spring and fall prevalence.

Etiology   Up to 40% or more cases are idio-pathic. Other possible etiologies include:

1. Infections:
   a. Primary tuberculosis.
   b. Beta-hemolytic streptococcus.
   c. Coccidioidomycosis.
   d. Histoplasmosis.
   e. Leprosy.
   f. Leishmaniasis.
   g. Cat-scratch disease.
   h. *Mycobacterium marinum.*
   i. *Yersinia.*
   j. Lymphogranuloma venereum.
2. Drugs:
   a. Sulfonamides.
   b. Oral contraceptives with ethinyl estra-diol or norethynodrel.
   c. Phenytoin.
3. Other:
   a. Sarcoidosis.
   b. Ulcerative colitis.
   c. Behçet's disease.
   d. Regional ileitis.
   e. Internal malignancy.

PATHOPHYSIOLOGY

Erythema nodosum represents a delayed-type hypersensitivity reaction to a variety of differ-ent stimuli.

HISTORY

Skin lesions appear over a few days as warm tender red nodules on the pretibial area. The skin lesions slowly heal over 3 to 6 weeks but can recur, especially with recurrent infection.

Associated arthralgias (50%), fever, and malaise may be present.

PHYSICAL EXAMINATION

Skin Findings

Type   Deep seated nodules (Fig. 15-14).

Color   Bright to deep red followed by purple to brown.

Size   1 to 5 cm.

Shape   Round, oval.

Palpation   Indurated, tender.

Arrangement   Scattered discrete lesions.

Distribution   Bilateral lower legs, symmetri-cally. Can also be on arms, face, neck, knees, thighs.

Sites of Predilection   Pretibial area.

DIFFERENTIAL DIAGNOSIS

Erythema nodosum is a clinical diagnosis that can be confirmed with skin biopsy. The differ-ential diagnosis includes ecchymoses, cellulitis, erysipelas, deep fungal infections, insect bites, thrombophlebitis, erythema induratum, and other panniculitides.

LABORATORY EXAMINATIONS

Dermatopathology   Skin biopsy shows acute and chronic inflammation (lymphocytes, neu-trophils, giant cells, histiocytes, and at times, plasma cells) in the deep dermis and subcuta-neous fat, especially around blood vessels in the septum and adjacent fat.

Work-up for an etiologic agent includes:

1. Careful drug history.
2. Throat culture to rule out streptococcus.
3. Chest x-ray to rule out sarcoidosis.
4. Tuberculin test to rule out primary tuber-culosis.

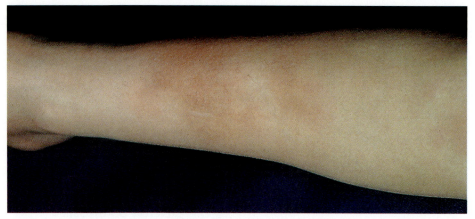

Figure 15-14 Erythema nodosum *Tender, red nodules on the pretibial area of an adolescent.*

5. Other tests as deemed necessary by history (i.e., stool culture to rule out *Yersinia*).

COURSE AND PROGNOSIS

Most cases of e. nodosum resolve spontaneously in 3 to 6 weeks, especially with rest and leg elevation. Ultimately, the course depends upon the underlying etiology and elimination of the precipitant when possible (i.e., discontinue oral contraceptives, treat infection, etc.). Recurrences are also dependent on etiology and recurrent e. nodosum in children is primarily seen with recurrent streptococcal infection.

MANAGEMENT

Identification and elimination of the etiologic agent is most helpful. Symptomatic includes:

1. Bed rest, leg elevation, and compressive bandages.
2. Salicylates and other nonsteroidal anti-inflammatory drugs such as indomethacin or naproxen.
3. Intralesional or systemic steroids can be used only if the etiologic agent is known (and infectious agents have been excluded).

Other possible treatments include:

1. Potassium iodide (SSKI solution, 0.15 to 0.3 mL po tid–qid).
2. Colchicine.

COLD PANNICULITIS

Cold panniculitis is characterized by erythematous plaques or nodules that appear on exposure to the cold.

Synonym Popsicle panniculitis.

EPIDEMIOLOGY

Age Any age, much more common in infants.

Gender M = F.

Etiology Exposure to the cold (weather or cold foods, e.g., popsicles) causes the fat to solidify with resultant plaque or nodule formation.

PATHOPHYSIOLOGY

Cold panniculitis occurs when the body fat solidifies and then liquefies on rewarming, with resulting inflammatory changes. The higher prevalence in infants and children is thought to be related to the fact that the subcutaneous fat in young children solidifies more easily than it does in adults.

HISTORY

Erythematous plaques or nodules develop on the exposed area hours after exposure to the cold. The areas may be painful or asymptomatic.

PHYSICAL EXAMINATION

Skin Findings

Type Erythematous plaques or nodules resolving to macular hyperpigmentation.

Color Pink to red.

Shape Round to oval.

Distribution Bilateral and symmetric.

Sites of Predilection Bilateral cheeks (Fig. 15-15).

DIFFERENTIAL DIAGNOSIS

The diagnosis of cold panniculitis is made clinically by eliciting a history of antecedent cold exposure. The differential diagnosis includes other forms of panniculitis, cellulitis, erysipelas, insect bites, or ecchymoses.

LABORATORY EXAMINATIONS

Dermatopathology Skin biopsy shows nonspecific inflammation in the deep dermis and subcutaneous fat.

COURSE AND PROGNOSIS

Cold panniculitis lesions can appear 5 minutes to 3 days after cold exposure, and regress over a period of weeks to months with postinflammatory pigmentation changes that can persist for up to 1 year.

MANAGEMENT

Cold panniculitis self-resolves and treatment is unnecessary.

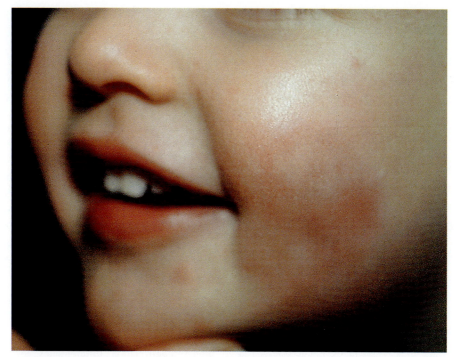

Figure 15-15 Cold panniculitis *Erythematous nodule on the cheeks of a child a few days after cold exposure.*

SWEET'S SYNDROME

Sweet's syndrome (SS) is a rare, recurrent skin disease characterized by painful papules, plaques, and nodules on the limbs, face, and trunk, accompanied by fever and leukocytosis.

Synonym   Acute febrile neutrophilic dermatosis.

EPIDEMIOLOGY

Age   Any age, but uncommon in children.

Gender   F > M.

Incidence   Rare.

Etiology   Unknown. Possibly hypersensitivity reaction to viral or bacterial infection. In adults, SS can be seen as an immunologic response to a leukemic state or other malignancy.

PATHOPHYSIOLOGY

SS is thought to represent a hypersensitivity reaction to either an infectious or malignant process. Some cases of SS follow bacterial or *Yersinia* infections. Other cases have been associated with acute myeloid leukemia, transient myeloid proliferation, various malignant tumors, ulcerative colitis, or benign monoclonal gammopathy.

HISTORY

Spiking fevers and upper respiratory tract infection symptoms precede the skin lesions by 1 to 3 weeks. Then there is a sudden appearance of tender and painful papules and plaques on the face, neck, and limbs (usually spares torso), associated with a leukocytosis and polyarthritis.

PHYSICAL EXAMINATION

Skin Findings

Types of Lesions   Papules or nodules which coalesce. Inflammatory plaques may lead to vesiculation (Fig. 15–16).

Color   Red, bluish red.

Size   1 to 2 cm.

Palpation   Lesions are tender.

Shape of Individual Lesion   As lesions evolve, central clearing may lead to annular or arcuate patterns.

Arrangement   May present as single lesion or multiple lesions, asymmetrically distributed.

Distribution of Lesions   Most commonly, face, neck, and extremities. Spares the torso.

Mucous Membranes   ± Conjunctivitis, episcleritis.

General Examination   Patient may appear ill.

DIFFERENTIAL DIAGNOSIS

History, physical examination, and skin biopsy confirmation differentiates Sweet's syndrome from erythema multiforme, erythema nodosum, pre-vesicular herpes simplex infection, pre-ulcerative pyoderma gangrenosum, bowel-bypass syndrome, urticaria, serum sickness, other vasculitides, SLE, and panniculitis.

The diagnosis should be made in patients with an abrupt onset of erythematous-to-violaceous nodules with predominantly a neutrophilic infiltration in the dermis. Other findings include fever, arthralgias, leukocytosis ($> 10,000/ \text{mm}^3$), and a good response to systemic steroids.

LABORATORY EXAMINATIONS

Dermatopathology   Skin biopsy shows edema and a dense, perivascular infiltration with polymorphonuclear leukocytes in the upper and mid dermis without vasculitis.

Hematology   Leukocytosis ($> 10,000/ \text{mm}^3$).

COURSE AND PROGNOSIS

Untreated, SS lesions enlarge over a period of days or weeks, and eventually resolve without scarring after 1 to 12 months. When treated with

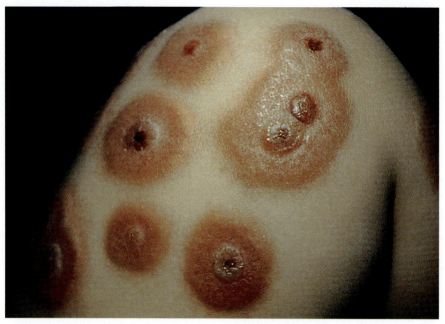

Figure 15-16 Sweet's syndrome *Erythematous plaques and nodules with central bullous changes on a child's knee.*

systemic steroids, the skin lesions resolve within a few days. Recurrences are seen in 50% of patients, often in previously involved sites.

MANAGEMENT

After infection has been ruled out, Sweet's syndrome responds dramatically to steroids.

1. Prednisone (1 to 2 mg/kg per d PO × 10 d followed by a 2- to 3-week taper).

2. Prednisolone (1 to 2 mg/kg per d PO × 10 d followed by a 2- to 3-week taper).

Other treatments include potassium iodide (SSKI, 0.3 to 0.6 mL PO tid–qid), clofazimine, colchicine, indomethacin, and dapsone.

In chronic or relapsing cases, pulsed steroids with chlorambucil has been used. Appropriate antibiotic therapy clears eruption in *Yersinia*-associated cases; in other cases antibiotics are typically ineffective.

PYODERMA GANGRENOSUM

Pyoderma gangrenosum (PG) is a rapidly evolving, chronic, and severely debilitating skin disease characterized by painful ulcers with undermined borders and a purulent necrotic base. It occurs most commonly in association with systemic disease, especially ulcerative colitis.

EPIDEMIOLOGY

Age   Adolescents and adults.

Gender   M = F.

Incidence   Rare.

Etiology   Unknown.

HISTORY

Acute onset with painful hemorrhagic pustule or nodule either de novo or following minimal trauma, typically on the lower legs. Lesions slow to heal and gentle debridement is needed to avoid the development of new lesions at sites of minimal trauma.

PHYSICAL EXAMINATION

Skin Findings

Type of Lesion   Primary lesion: deep-seated nodule, or superficial hemorrhagic pustule. Breakdown of this lesion occurs with ulcer formation. Ulcer borders: irregular and raised, undermined, boggy, with perforations that drain pus (Fig. 15-17). Ulcer base: purulent, hemorrhagic exudate; partially covered by necrotic eschar; ± granulation tissue. Healing of ulcers results in thin, atrophic, ± cribriform scars.

Size   1 to 10 cm.

Color   Ulcer border: dusky red or purple. Halo of erythema spreads centrifugally at the advancing edge of ulcer.

Palpation   Primary nodule and ulcer are painful.

Shape of Individual Lesion   Ulcer margin may be irregular or serpiginous.

Arrangement of Lesions   Usually solitary. May form in clusters that coalesce.

Distribution of Lesions   Most common sites: lower extremities > buttocks > abdomen > face.

Mucous Membranes   Rarely, aphthous stomatitis-like lesions; massive ulceration of oral mucosa and conjunctivae.

General Examination   Patient may appear ill.

Associated Systemic Diseases   Up to 50% occur without associated disease. Remainder of cases associated with large- and small-bowel disease, arthritis, paraproteinemia, multiple myeloma, leukemia, active chronic hepatitis, and Behçet's syndrome

DIFFERENTIAL DIAGNOSIS

The diagnosis of PG is a clinical diagnosis based on course of illness. The histology is not diagnostic. Differential diagnoses include: gangrene, ecthyma gangrenosum, atypical mycobacterial infection, clostridial infection, deep mycoses, amebiasis, bromoderma, pemphigus vegetans, stasis ulcers, and Wegener's granulomatosis.

LABORATORY EXAMINATIONS

Dermatopathology   Skin biopsy is not diagnostic. Massive neutrophilic inflammation, engorgement, and thrombosis of the small and medium vessels. Necrosis and hemorrhage may be present.

COURSE AND PROGNOSIS

Untreated, PG may last months to years. Ulceration may extend rapidly within a few days, or slowly and new ulcers may appear as older lesions resolve.

MANAGEMENT

PG is best managed by identification and treatment of any associated underlying disease.
   Topical symptomatic measures include:

1.   Gentle cleansing.
2.   0.25% acetic acid soaks.

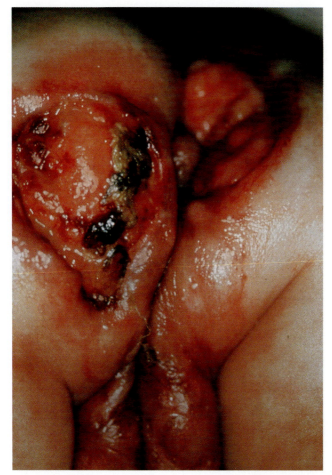

Figure 15-17   Pyoderma gangrenosum   *Necrotic ulcers with undermined borders on the buttocks of an infant with pyoderma gangrenosum.*

3. Wet dressings with potassium permanganate.
4. Whirlpool baths.
5. Silver sulfadiazine cream.
6. Sodium cromoglycate solution.
7. Topical or intralesional steroids.

Severe or refractory cases may require systemic therapy with:

1. Prednisone (1-2 mg/kg per d po divided bid for 10 d followed by a 2- to 3-week taper).

2. Prednisolone (1 to 2 mg/kg/d po divided bid for 10 d followed by a 1 week taper).

Surgical debridement and excision of the ulcers should be avoided because PG is subject to pathergy in 20% of cases.

Other reported treatment modalities include: dapsone, sulfapyridine, minocycline, clofazimine, rifampin, thalidomide, cyclophosphamide, cyclosporine, and hyperbaric oxygen.

SARCOIDOSIS

Sarcoidosis is a chronic granulomatous inflammatory process of unknown etiology that affects the skin, eye, lungs, and reticuloendothelial system.

EPIDEMIOLOGY

Age   Adolescents and adults (commonly seen between ages 20 and 40 years.

Gender   M = F.

Incidence   Uncommon.

Race   Affects all races but most common in Scandinavians, American blacks, and Southeastern whites.

Geography   Seen most in the Southeast states, the "sarcoid belt" of the United States.

Etiology   Unknown. Multifactorial with host response/delayed hypersensitivity and abnormal immunoregulation all playing a role.

Genetics   Familial cases have been reported.

HISTORY

Children with sarcoidosis develop asymptomatic eczematous or infiltrated plaques and pustules. Preschool children tend to have polyarthritis, uveitis, and not as many pulmonary symptoms. Older children and adolescent symptoms resemble the adult form of sarcoidosis with fever, cough, weight loss, abdominal pain, adenopathy, lung disease, hypergammaglobulinemia, and hypercalcemia.

PHYSICAL EXAMINATION

Skin Lesions

Type   Infiltrated plaques and scattered multiple maculopapular lesions.

Size   0.5- to 1.0-cm papules, larger plaques and nodules.

Color   Red to violaceous in hue. Upon blanching with glass slide (diascopy), cutaneous lesions of sarcoidosis reveal "apple-jelly" yellowish-brown color.

Shape   Annular, polycyclic, serpiginous (Fig. 15-18A).

Arrangement   Scattered discrete lesions (maculopapular and nodular types) and diffuse infiltration.

Distribution   Extremities, buttocks, trunk and face (Fig. 15-18B).

Special Types

1. *Lupus pernio:* Soft, violaceous plaques on the nose, cheek, and earlobes.
2. *Scar sarcoidosis:* Purple nodules occurring in an old scar.
3. *Angiolupoid:* Purple plaques with telangiectasia on the nose, especially the nasal rim, suggestive of pulmonary involvement.

General Findings

Arthralgias, low-grade fever, and abdominal pain are seen with sarcoid in children. Pulmonary involvement will lead to coughing and characteristic bilateral hilar adenopathy detection on chest x-ray. Ocular involvement includes uveitis and iritis. Parotid gland enlargement and peripheral adenopathy are common in children. Facial nerve paralysis and CNS involvement is rare.

DIFFERENTIAL DIAGNOSIS

The diagnosis of sarcoid is best made by tissue biopsy of skin or lymph nodes.

LABORATORY EXAMINATIONS

Dermatopathology   Skin biopsy shows large islands of epithelioid cells with a few giant cells, and lymphocytes, so-called "naked" tubercles. Asteroid bodies in large histiocytes; occasionally fibrinoid necrosis.

Skin Tests   Intracutaneous tests for recall antigens usually but not always negative.

Internal Organs   Systemic sarcoidosis is verified radiologically by gallium scan and transbronchial, liver, or lymph-node biopsy.

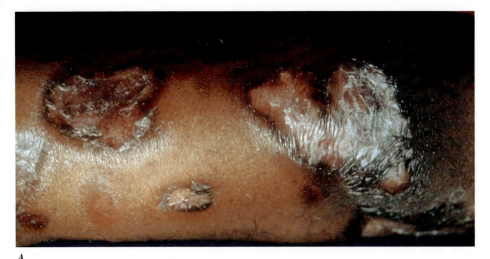

A

Figure 15-18 Sarcoidosis *(A) Violaceous annular plaques on the elbow of a child.*

Blood Chemistry

1. Increase in serum angiotensin-converting enzyme (ACE) is seen in up to 80% of children with active sarcoidosis.
2. Hypergammaglobulinemia.
3. Hypercalcemia.

COURSE AND PROGNOSIS

Sarcoidosis in children tends to regress completely over several years. Mortality is less than 5%.

MANAGEMENT

Cutaneous Sarcoidosis Topical corticosteroids under plastic dressings or intralesional steroids can be used with moderate improvement.

Systemic Sarcoidosis Systemic corticosteroids for active ocular disease, active pulmonary disease, cardiac arrhythmia, CNS involvement, facial palsy, or hypercalcemia.

1. Prednisone (1 to 2 mg/kg per d po divided bid until symptoms improve and then taper).
2. Prednisolone (1 to 2 mg/kg per d po divided bid until symptoms improve and then taper).

Other drugs used in adults with sarcoidosis have not yet been studied in children. These include oxyphenbutazone, chloroquine, potassium p-aminobenzoate, azathioprine, and chlorambucil.

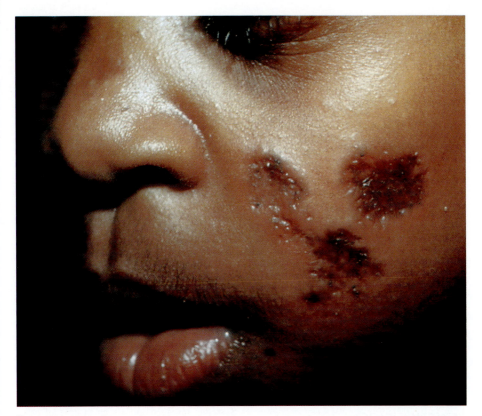

B

Figure 15-18 (continued)   **Sarcoidosis**   *(B) Violaceous scarred plaques on the cheek of the same child.*

CUTANEOUS VASCULITIS

HENOCH-SCHÖNLEIN PURPURA

Henoch-Schönlein purpura (HSP) is an inflammatory disorder of children and young adults characterized by a diffuse vasculitis of the skin, joints, GI tract, CNS, and kidneys in response to a variety of etiologic factors.

Synonym Anaphylactoid purpura.

EPIDEMIOLOGY

Age Children and adolescents (especially between ages 3 and 10 years old).

Gender M = F. Intussusception in M > F.

Incidence Uncommon.

Etiology IgA-mediated hypersensitivity reaction to bacterial infections (betahemolytic streptococcus), viral syndromes (hepatitis B), medications, food, insect bites, immunizations, cold exposure, or chemical toxins.

PATHOPHYSIOLOGY

HSP vasculitis is caused by deposition of immune complexes of lgA class in the capillaries, pre- and postcapillary venules of the upper dermis, GI tract, glomeruli, and synovial membrane, lungs, and CNS. The immune complex deposition results in release of vasoactive amines from platelets, basophils, mast cell interaction with the Fc receptor on cell membranes, and activation of complement (C3a, C5a), with subsequent chemotaxis of neutrophils and release of lysosomal enzymes that further contribute to tissue damage.

HISTORY

A distinctive rash (erythematous papules followed by purpura) is accompanied by joint pain and abdominal symptoms. Renal involvement may or may not occur.

PHYSICAL EXAMINATION

Skin Findings

Type Macules (petechiae), patches (ecchy-moses), and papules (palpable purpura) that resolve with hyperpigmentation (Fig. 15-19).

Size 2 to 10 mm.

Color Red to violaceous, then brown.

Shape Annular, oval, arciform.

Arrangement Discrete or confluent.

Distribution Purpura: symmetrically on extensor surfaces of extremities (especially lower legs, ankles, knees, elbows) and buttocks.

General Findings

Systemic involvement is seen in 85% of cases of HSP with involvement of GI tract (abdominal pain, vomiting, visceral infarction, perforation, pancreatitis, cholecystitis, colitis, protein-losing enteropathy, chronic intestinal obstruction and intussusception in 2% of patients, joints (warm and painful swelling of the ankles and knees), kidneys (gross or micro hematuria and proteinuria), CNS (headache, diplopia, subarachnoid hemorrhage), lungs (pulmonary infiltrates, hemorrhage), and testicles (hemorrhage).

DIFFERENTIAL DIAGNOSIS

The diagnosis of HSP is made by the clinical finding of palpable purpura over lower extremities in children or young adults. Histologic and immunofluorescence findings confirm the diagnosis.

The **American College of Rheumatology** 1990 criteria for diagnosis of HSP is made if two of these four criteria are present.

1. *Palpable purpura:* slightly raised "palpable" hemorrhagic skin lesions, not related to thrombocytopenia.
2. *Age-20 or less at disease onset:* patient 20 years or younger at onset of first symptoms.

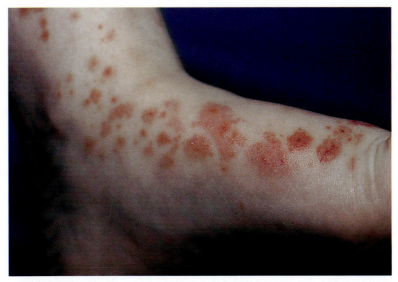

Figure 15-19   Henoch-Schönlein purpura   *Hemorrhagic macules, papules, and urticarial lesions on the foot of a child.*

3. *Bowel angina:* diffuse abdominal pain, worse after meals, or the diagnosis of bowel ischemia, usually including bloody diarrhea.
4. *Wall granulocytes on biopsy:* histologic changes showing granulocytes in the walls of arterioles or venules.

The differential diagnosis for HSP include: acute rheumatic fever, disseminated intravascular coagulation, meningococcal septicemia, Rocky Mountain spotted fever, pigmented purpuric dermatoses.

LABORATORY EXAMINATIONS

Dermatopathology   Skin biopsy shows leukocytoclastic vasculitis with fibrinoid degeneration of vessel walls, perivascular and intramural infiltrate of neutrophils and/or lymphocytes, nuclear dust (from disintegrated polymorphonuclear leukocytes), and RBC extravasation with deposits of hemosiderin.

Immunofluorescence   Deposition of IgA and C3 in dermal vessels.

Chemistry   ASLO titer.

Urinalysis   Hematuria, proteinuria, red cell casts. Guaiac positive stools.

Immunology   Complement may be reduced or normal.

Hematology   Leukocytosis, anemia, thrombocytosis, elevated sedimentation rate.

Bacteriology   Throat culture to rule out streptococcus.

COURSE AND PROGNOSIS

The prognosis is excellent for most patients. Full recovery without permanent sequelae is usually seen. Recurrent attacks may occur. Younger children tend to have a milder disease course of shorter duration with less GI and renal involvement and reduced recurrence rate. Up to 5% of patients with HSP-associated nephritis will progress to ESRD. Mortality is estimated to be less than 1 to 3%, usually due to renal or GI complications.

MANAGEMENT

Treatment consists of bedrest and supportive care. Antibiotics may be given if an upper respiratory infection is suspected. Systemic steroids may be useful for complicated noninfectious cases of HSP with GI, renal, CNS, or pulmonary manifestations. For chronic glomerulonephritis, steroids, immunosuppressive agents, and anticoagulants are helpful. Factor XIII concentrate may benefit some patients with severe abdominal pain and low factor XIII.

POLYARTERITIS NODOSA

Polyarteritis nodosa (PAN) is a multisystem, necrotizing vasculitis of small- and medium-sized muscular arteries characterized by its involvement of the renal and visceral arteries. There is a severe life-threatening pediatric form, and a less severe adult form.

Synonym Periarteritis nodosa.

EPIDEMIOLOGY

Age *Pediatric PAN:* children < 2 years old. *Adult PAN:* Older children and adults.

Gender *Pediatric PAN:* M = F. *Adult PAN:* M > F, 2.5:1.

Incidence Rare.

Etiology Unknown. Presumed to represent a hypersensitivity reaction that leads to IgM, C3 deposition in affected vessel walls.

PATHOPHYSIOLOGY

Necrotizing inflammation of small- and medium-sized muscular arteries; may spread circumferentially to involve adjacent veins. Lesions segmental, tend to involve bifurcations of arteries. Up to 30% of cases associated with hepatitis B antigenemia (i.e., immune complex formation).

HISTORY

Pediatric PAN: begins as a febrile illness and cardiac arteritis leads to fatal coronary disease. Renal and CNS arteries are also diseased with severe sequelae. Many people think pediatric PAN may be a severe form of Kawasaki's disease.
Adult PAN: characterized by painful nodules, fever, arthritis, abdominal pain, hypertension, peripheral neuropathy, and myocardial infarction.

PHYSICAL EXAMINATION

Skin Findings

Occur in 15% of cases.

Type of Lesion Subcutaneous nodules that follow the course of involved arteries; may ulcerate. Palpable purpura. Violaceous

macules, with diffuse livedo reticularis pattern (Fig. 15-20).

Size 0.5 to 2 cm.

Color Nodules bright red turning violaceous.

Palpation Nodules often more palpable than visible. Tender.

Distribution of Lesions Palpable purpura, lower extremities. Nodules: usually bilateral. Lower legs > thighs. Other: arms > trunk > head and neck > buttocks.

General Examination

Neurologic Examination CNS: cerebrovascular accident. Peripheral nerves: mixed motor and sensory involvement with mononeuritis multiplex pattern.

Eye Hypertensive changes, ocular vasculitis, retinal artery aneurysm, optic disc edema and atrophy.

Other Hypertension.

DIFFERENTIAL DIAGNOSIS

American Rheumatologic Association's 1990 criteria for the classification of polyarteritis nodosa states that PAN is present if 3 out of 10 of the following are present.

1. Weight loss > 4 kg.
2. Livedo reticularis.
3. Testicular pain or tenderness.
4. Myalgias, weakness, or leg tenderness.
5. Mono- or polyneuropathy.
6. Diastolic BP > 90 mm Hg.
7. Elevated BUN or creatinine.
8. Hepatitis B virus.
9. Arteriographic abnormality.
10. Biopsy of small or medium-sized artery containing polymorphonuclear neutrophils.

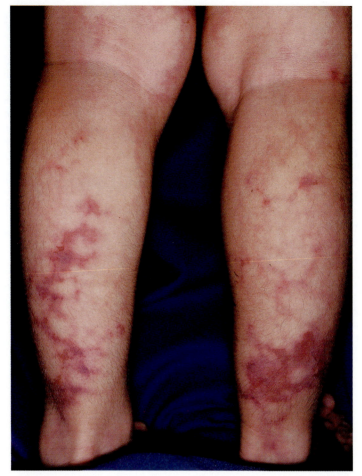

Figure 15-20 Polyarteritis nodosa *Livedo pattern of the lower legs with purpura and subcutaneous nodules on the bilateral legs.*

PAN needs to be differentiated from other vasculitic disorders or panniculitis.

LABORATORY EXAMINATIONS

Dermatopathology A deep wedge biopsy will show polymorphonuclear neutrophils infiltrating all layers of the vessel wall and perivascular areas. Fibrinoid necrosis of vessel wall occurs with occlusion of lumen, thrombosis, and infarction of tissues supplied by involved vessel. Skin pathology is identical in both systemic and cutaneous PAN.

CBC Commonly neutrophilic leukocytosis; rarely eosinophilia; anemia of chronic disease. ± Elevated ESR.

Serology Antineutrophil cytoplasmic antibodies (ANCA) in serum. Hepatitis B surface antigenemia in 30% of cases.

Chemistry Elevated creatinine, BUN.

Arteriography Aneurysms in small- and medium-sized muscular arteries of kidney, hepatic, and visceral vasculature.

COURSE AND PROGNOSIS

The prognosis for pediatric PAN is poor with death related to cardiac failure. Untreated, adult PAN also has a very high morbidity and mortality characterized by fulminant deterioration or by relentless progression associated with intermittent acute exacerbations. Mortality results from renal failure, bowel perforation, cardiovascular failure, or intractable hypertension. Effective treatment reduces mortality to 50%.

MANAGEMENT

Pediatric PAN

1. Management consists of aspirin or NSAIDs (indomethacin or naproxen), IV gamma-globulin.
2. Other theraputic modalities used in adults include systemic corticosteroids, immunosuppressive agents (azathioprine or cyclophosphamide).

URTICARIAL VASCULITIS

Urticarial vasculitis is a multisystem disease characterized by cutaneous lesions resembling urticaria and biopsy findings of a leukocytoclastic vasculitis, accompanied by varying degrees of arthritis, arthralgia, angioedema, uveitis, myositis, abdominal or chest pain.

Synonym Hypocomplementemic vasculitis.

EPIDEMIOLOGY

Age Any age, typically affects young adults (30 to 50 years old).

Gender F > M, 3:1.

Etiology Unknown. Likely an immune complex disorder or nonspecific reaction pattern to different etiologic agents.

PATHOPHYSIOLOGY

Thought to be an immune complex disease, similar to cutaneous vasculitis with deposition of antigen-antibody complexes in cutaneous blood vessel walls leading to complement activation and neutrophil chemotaxis. Collagenase and elastase released from neutrophils cause vessel wall and cell destruction.

HISTORY

Skin lesions are transient (24 to 72 h) papules, plaques or wheals that may itch, burn, sting. Systemically, it is associated with fever (10 to 15%), arthralgias ± arthritis in one or more joints (ankles, knees, elbows, wrists, small joints of fingers), GI involvement (nausea, abdominal pain), pulmonary involvement (cough, dyspnea, hemoptysis), pseudotumor cerebri, cold sensitivity, and renal involvement (diffuse glomerulonephritis).

PHYSICAL EXAMINATION

Skin Findings

Type of Lesion Urticaria-like (i.e., edematous) lesions: raised, occasionally indurated, erythematous, circumscribed wheals; macular erythema; angioedema ± resolve with purpura; hyperpigmentation. Less commonly: cold urticaria, Raynaud's phenomenon, palpable purpura, bullae, erythema-like lesions.

Color Pink to red, blanch when pressed, but purpura remains (Fig. 15-21). Resolving lesions leave a yellow-green stain.

Palpation Indurated.

General Examination

Extracutaneous manifestations: joints (70%), GI tract (20 to 30%), CNS (> 10%), ocular system (> 10%), kidneys (10 to 20%), lymphadenopathy (5%).

DIFFERENTIAL DIAGNOSIS

Urticarial vasculitis is suspected with a clinical history of urticarial lesions of 1 to 3 days duration and confirmed by skin biopsy. It may be confused with urticaria, serum sickness, other vasculitides, SLE, and urticaria in acute hepatitis B infection.

LABORATORY EXAMINATIONS

Dermatopathology Biopsy of early lesions shows features of a leukocytoclastic vasculitis: perivascular infiltrate consisting primarily of neutrophils; leukocytoclasia; fibrinoid deposition in and around vessel walls; endothelial cell swelling and extravasation of RBC. In contrast, common urticaria exhibits dermal edema; sparse perivascular lymphohistiocytic infiltrate ± eosinophils.

Urinalysis Microhematuria, proteinuria in 10% of patients.

Serologic Findings Hypocomplementemia (70%); circulating immune complexes, elevated sedimentation rate.

COURSE AND PROGNOSIS

Urticarial vasculitis has a chronic (months to years) but benign course. Episodes recur over

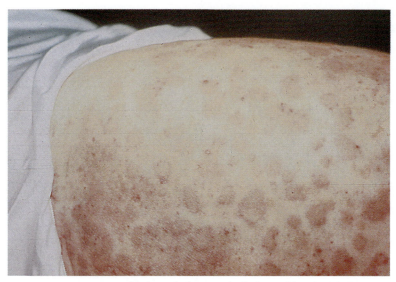

Figure 15-21 **Urticarial vasculitis** *Urticarial plaques which do not blanch with diascopy (gentle pressure with a glass slide).* (Slide courtesy of Lisa Cohen, MD.)

periods ranging from months to years. Renal disease occurs only in hypocomplementemic patients.

MANAGEMENT

First-line treatment includes H_1- and H_2-blockers plus NSAIDs.

1. H_1-blockers
   a. Diphenhydramine (Benadryl, 5 mg/kg per d PO divided tid or qid).
   b. Hydroxyzine HCl (Atarax, 2 to 4 mg/kg per d divided tid or qid).
2. To avoid the sedation effects, a nonsedating H_1-blocker may be preferred.
   a. Cetirizine HCl (Zyrtec 2.5 to 10 mg PO qd).
3. In resistant cases, H_2-blockers can be used in combination with H_1-blockers.
   a. Cimetidine (Tagamet, 10 to 40 mg/kg per d PO divided qid).
   b. Ranitidine hydrochloride (Zantac, 2 to 4 mg/dose PO bid).
4. A combination H_1- and H_2-blocker antidepressants used in low doses may be helpful, but pediatric use is strictly off-label.
   a. Doxepin (Sinequan or Adapin, 5 to 10 mg PO qd).
5. NSAIDs: ibuprofen (Motrin, Advil), indomethacin (Indocin), naproxen (Naprosyn).

Second-line treatment includes colchicine, dapsone.

Third-line treatment includes:

1. Prednisone (1–2 mg/kg per d divided bid).
2. Prednisolone (1 to 2 mg/kg per d divided bid).

Fourth-line treatment would be cytotoxic immunosuppressives:
   a. Azathioprine.
   b. Cyclophosphamide.

IDIOPATHIC THROMBOCYTOPENIC PURPURA

Idiopathic thrombocytopenic purpura (ITP) is a common autoimmune disorder of child-hood resulting in increased destruction of platelets.

Synonym   Immune thrombocytopenic purpura.

EPIDEMIOLOGY

Age   Age 2 months to adulthood, mean age of onset: 6 years old.

Gender   M = F.

Etiology   Increased platelet destruction thought to be autoimmune and frequently fol-lows illness (varicella, rubella, rubeola, and res-piratory infections).

PATHOPHYSIOLOGY

Autoimmune destruction of platelets caused by antibodies against platelets.

HISTORY

Acute presentation of bleeding into the skin (from petechiae to ecchymoses) usually fol-lowing a febrile illness.

PHYSICAL EXAMINATION

Skin Findings

Type of Lesion   *Petechiae:* small (pinpoint to pinhead) red nonblanching macules (Fig. 15-22). *Ecchymoses:* black-and-blue spots; larger area or hemorrhage.

Size   1 mm to several cm.

Color   Fresh areas of hemorrhage: red to dark brown. Older lesions: yellowish-green tinge

Palpation   Nonpalpable. Lesions do not blanch with pressure.

Distribution of Lesions   Random sites of predilection increased at pressure points (face and neck from crying, under elastic socks).

Mucous Membranes   Petechiae, gingival bleeding.

General Examination

Possible CNS hemorrhage.

DIFFERENTIAL DIAGNOSIS

History, clinical presentation, CBC and coagulation screening tests help differentiate ITP from telangiectasia, palpable purpura (vasculitis) purpura of scurvy, progressive pigmentary purpura (Schamberg's disease), purpura following severe Valsalva maneuver (tussive, vomiting and retching), traumatic purpura, factitial or iatrogenic purpura, and Gardner–Diamond syndrome (autoerythrocyte sensitization syndrome).

LABORATORY EXAMINATIONS

Dermatopathology   May be contraindicated due to postsurgical hemorrhage.

Hematology   Thrombocytopenia (platelets be-low 50,000/mm^3) coagulation studies are nor-mal (PT, PTT, fibrin split products) and exclude a consumptive process.

COURSE AND PROGNOSIS

ITP of childhood is an acute, self-limited dis-order. Up to 80% of cases resolve in 4 weeks; 90% resolve in 6 months. Rarely, thrombocy-topenia can last for months with a prolonged risk of hemorrhage. Only 10% of children have a more chronic course (> 6 months) but these cases usually self-resolve as well.

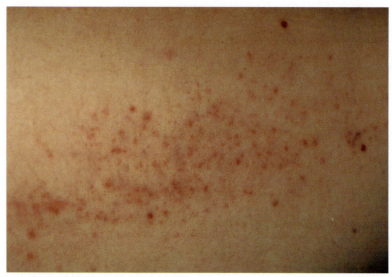

Figure 15-22   Idiopathic thrombocytopenic purpura *Numerous petechial lesions on the leg of a child.*

MANAGEMENT

Treatment is not usually needed given the high rate of spontaneous recovery. Conservative management includes:

1. Avoiding platelet inhibitors (i.e., aspirin).
2. Limiting strenuous physical activities (injury might lead to severe hemorrhage).
3. Bedrest.

Persistent severe thrombocytopenia (platelets $< 20,000/mm^3$) may warrant treatment with:

1. IV immunoglobulin.
2. Prednisone (before prednisone, a bone marrow biopsy is prudent to rule out an occult leukemia).
3. Platelet transfusion (for platelets $< 10,000/mm^3$).
4. Splenectomy for chronic cases.

DISSEMINATED INTRAVASCULAR COAGULATION

Disseminated intravascular coagulation (DIC) is a life-threatening bleeding disorder resulting from widespread blood clotting within blood vessels, associated with a wide range of clinical circumstances (bacterial sepsis, massive trauma) and manifested by purpura fulminans (cutaneous infarctions and/or acral gangrene) or bleeding from multiple sites.

Synonyms Purpura fulminans, consumption coagulopathy, defibrination syndrome, coagulation-fibrinolytic syndrome.

EPIDEMIOLOGY

Age Purpura fulminans most commonly in children.

Gender M = F.

Etiology
Events that predispose one to DIC:

1. Acquired or congenital protein C and protein S deficiency.
2. *Massive tissue destruction:* tumor products, crushing trauma, extensive surgery, severe intracranial damage; retained contraception products, placental abruption, amniotic fluid embolism; certain snake bites; hemolytic transfusion reaction; acute promyelocytic leukemia; burn injuries.
3. *Extensive destruction of endothelial surfaces, exposure to foreign surfaces:* vasculitis (Rocky Mountain spotted fever, meningococcemia or occasionally, gram-negative septicemia); heat stroke, malignant hyperthermia; extensive pump-oxygenation (repair of aortic aneurysm); eclampsia, preeclampsia; giant hemangioma (Kasabach–Merritt syndrome); immune complexes; postvaricella purpura gangrenosa.

Events that complicate and propagate DIC: Shock; complement pathway activation.

PATHOPHYSIOLOGY

Uncontrolled activation of coagulation results in thrombosis and consumption of platelets/clotting factors II, V, VIII. If the activation occurs slowly, excess activated products produced, predisposing to vascular infarctions/venous thrombosis. If the picture is brisk and explosive, the clinical picture is dominated by hemorrhage surrounding wound sites, IV lines and catheters, bleeding into deep tissues.

HISTORY

DIC typically has its onset 3 to 30 days after a resolving infection. Hemorrhagic lesions appear rapidly and systemic symptoms include fever, tachycardia, anemia, and prostration. The prognosis is grave but can be improved with therapy.

PHYSICAL EXAMINATION

Skin Findings

Type of Lesion *Hemorrhage* from multiple cutaneous sites (i.e., surgical incisions, venipuncture, or catheter sites). *Preinfarction:* peripheral acrocyanosis. *Infarction (purpura fulminans):* massive ecchymoses (Fig. 15-23) with sharp, irregular ("geographic") borders and erythematous halos ± evolution to hemorrhagic bullae and blue to black gangrene; peripheral gangrene on hands, feet, tip of nose with subsequent autoamputation if patient survives.

Color Infarctive lesions are deep purple to black.

Arrangement of Multiple Lesions Often symmetrical.

Distribution of Lesions *Infarctive lesions:* distal extremities; areas of pressure; lips, ears, nose, trunk.

Mucous Membranes Hemorrhage from gingiva.

General Findings

High fever, ± shock. Multitude of findings depending on the associated medical/surgical problem.

DIFFERENTIAL DIAGNOSIS

The diagnosis of DIC is made by clinical suspicion confirmed by coagulation studies. Other diffuse hemorrhagic entities include coumarin or heparin necrosis.

LABORATORY EXAMINATIONS

Dermatopathology   Skin biopsy reveals occlusion of arterioles with fibrin thrombi and a dense polymorphonuclear infiltrate around the infarct with massive hemorrhage.

Hematologic Studies   *CBC:*   schistocytes (fragmented RBC) arising from RBC entrapment and damage within fibrin thrombi, seen on blood smear; thrombocytopenia. *Coagulation studies:* reduced plasma fibrinogen; elevated fibrin degradation products; prolonged PT, PTT, and thrombin time.

COURSE AND PROGNOSIS

The mortality rate from DIC is high. Surviving patients require skin grafts or amputation for gangrenous tissue. Common complications include severe bleeding, thrombosis, tissue ischemia and necrosis, hemolysis, organ failure. Mortality without therapy is 90% and occurs within 48 to 72 hours. Prompt therapy can improve the prognosis and reduce mortality to as low as 18%.

MANAGEMENT

Treatment of DIC requires prompt recognition and appropriate antibiotics, clotting factors, and/or supportive care.

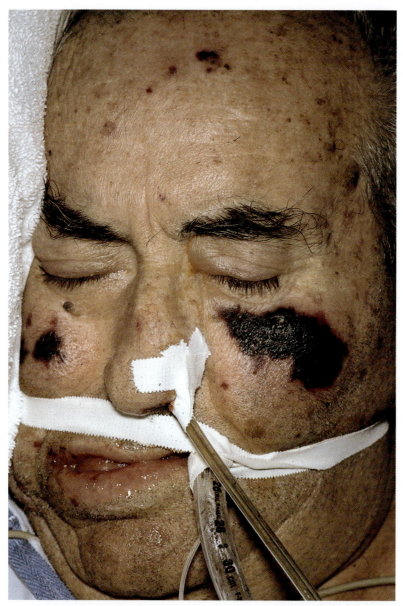

Figure 15-23 Disseminated intravascular coagulation, purpura fulminans Geographic areas of infarction on the cheeks of a diabetic patient with *Staphylococcus aureus* sepsis. (Reproduced with permission from TB Fitzpatrick et al., Color Atlas and Synopsis of Clinical Dermatology, 4th edition. New York: McGraw-Hill, 2001).

KAWASAKI'S DISEASE

Kawasaki's disease (KD) is an acute febrile illness of infants and children, characterized by cutaneous and mucosal erythema and edema with subsequent desquamation and cervical lymphadenitis. The disease is later complicated by coronary artery aneurysms in up to 20% of patients.

Synonyms   Mucocutaneous lymph node syndrome, juvenile periarteritis nodosa.

EPIDEMIOLOGY

Age   Up to 35% of patients < 5 years old; 50% less than 2½ years old.

Gender   Male predominance, 1.5:1.

Race   Japanese > Afro-American > white children.

Etiology   Unknown. Probably infectious with winter and spring epidemics.

Genetics   Possible genetic susceptibility since it is much more prevalent in the Japanese population.

PATHOPHYSIOLOGY

Kawasaki's disease is thought to be an immunologic disorder triggered by an infectious or toxic agent. This leads to a generalized aneurysm vasculitis.

HISTORY

Children present with high fever for 5 days followed by conjunctivitis, infection, changes on lips and mouth, body rash, and lymphadenopathy. Constitutional symptoms include: diarrhea, arthralgias, arthritis, tympanitis, and photophobia.

PHYSICAL EXAMINATION

Skin Findings

Type of Lesion   Scarlatiniform, morbilliform, body rash (Fig. 15-24). Erythema on the palms and soles. Edema on the hands and feet. Subsequent desquamation. Perineal: confluent macules to plaque-type erythema, followed by desquamation (Fig. 15-25A).

Palpation   Lesions may be tender.

Distribution   Hands and feet, striking erythema ± indurative edema; truncal erythema.

Mucous Membranes   Bulbar conjunctiva are hyperemic; lips are red, dry, and fissured; pharynx is injected, and there is a "strawberry" appearance to the tongue (Fig. 15-25B).

General Findings

Meningeal irritation, pneumonia, lymphadenopathy (usually >1.5 cm cervical node), arthritis and arthralgias (knees, hips, elbows), and cardiac problems (pericardial tamponade, dysrhythmias, rubs, congestive heart failure, left ventricular dysfunction).

DIFFERENTIAL DIAGNOSIS

Diagnosis   Diagnostic criteria: fever spiking to > 39.4°C lasting for 5 days without other cause, associated with 4 of 5 criteria.

1.   Bilateral conjunctival injection.
2.   At least one of following mucous membrane changes: injected/fissured lips, injected pharynx, "strawberry" tongue.
3.   At least one of the following extremity changes: erythema of palms and soles, edema of hands and feet, desquamation, generalized/periungual desquamation.
4.   Diffuse scarlatiniform erythroderma, diffuse centrally/sharply demarcated borders on extremities; deeply erythematous maculopapular rash; iris lesions.
5.   Cervical lymphadenopathy (at least one lymph node > 1.5 cm in diameter).

Differential Diagnosis   The diagnosis of Kawasaki's disease is based on the above criteria. Kawasaki's can be mistaken for juvenile rheumatoid arthritis, infectious mononucleosis, viral exanthems, leptospirosis, Rocky Mountain spotted fever, toxic shock syndrome, staphylococcal scalded-skin syndrome, erythema multi-

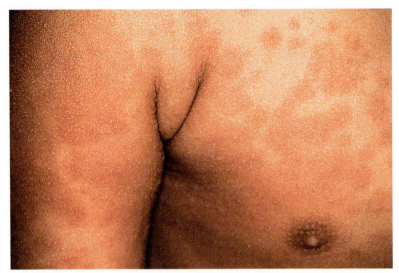

Figure 15-24   Kawasaki's disease   *Blotchy erythema on the trunk of a child with Kawasaki's disease.* (Reproduced with permission from TB Fitzpatrick et al., Color Atlas and Synopsis of Clinical Dermatology, 4th edition. New York: McGraw-Hill, 2001).

forme, serum sickness, SLE, and Reiter's syndrome.

LABORATORY EXAMINATIONS

Echocardiography Kawasaki's disease can lead to the formation of coronary aneurysms.

COURSE AND PROGNOSIS

The actual acute episode of Kawasaki's disease self-resolves in the majority of children with no sequelae. Up to 20% of Kawasaki's patients will go on to develop cardiovascular complications; coronary artery aneurysms can occur in 2 to 8 weeks after febrile episode. This can result in myocarditis, myocardial ischemia and infarction, pericarditis, peripheral vascular occlusion, small bowel obstruction, and stroke. Mortality rate is 1%.

MANAGEMENT

Treatment is directed at prevention of the cardiovascular complications and includes aspirin and high-dose IV gammaglobulin.

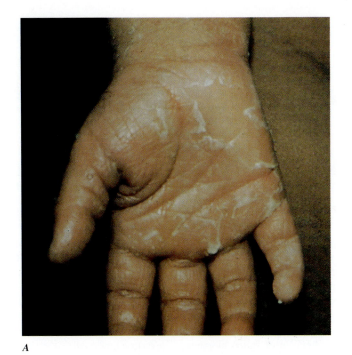

A

B

Figure 15-25   Kawasaki's disease   *(A) Palmar desquamation on the hands of a child with Kawasaki's disease. (B) Red "strawberry tongue" and perioral erythema in the same child.*

PHOTOSENSITIVITY AND PHOTOREACTIONS

PHOTOSENSITIVITY: IMPORTANT REACTIONS TO LIGHT

The term photosensitivity describes an abnormal response to light—usually sunlight. Two broad types of acute photosensitivity are:

1. A "*sunburn*" type response with the development of morphologic skin changes simulating a normal sunburn: erythema, edema, vesicles, and bullae—examples are porphyria cutanea tarda, phytophotodermatitis.
2. A "*rash*" response to light exposure with development of varied morphologic expressions: macules, papules, plaques, eczematous dermatitis, urticaria—examples are polymorphous light eruption, urticaria, eczematous drug reaction to sulfonamides.

The skin response to light exposure is strictly limited to the areas that have been exposed, and sharp borders are usually noted.

It should be emphasized that *sparing* of certain skin areas may provide the clue to photosensitivity: the upper eyelids (which are closed, normally), the skin on the upper lip and under the chin (submental area), a triangle behind the ears, under a watchband, or in the area covered by a bathing suit, in body creases on the back and sides of the neck, or on the abdomen.

ACUTE SUN DAMAGE (SUNBURN)

A sunburn is an acute, delayed, and transient erythema of the skin following exposure to ultraviolet radiation (UVR) obtained from sunlight or artificial sources. Sunburn is characterized by erythema, and, if severe, by vesicles and bullae, edema, tenderness, and pain. UVR is divided into two principal types: UVB (290 to 320 nm) the "sunburn" spectrum and UVA (320 to 400 nm). UVB erythema develops in 12 to 24 h and fades within 72 to 120 h. UVA erythema peaks between 4 and 16 h and fades within 48 to 120 h.

EPIDEMIOLOGY

Age Infants have an increased susceptibility to sunburn.

Gender M = F.

Phototypes Sunburn is most frequently seen in individuals who have lighter skin and a limited capacity to develop *facultative* melanin pigmentation (tanning) following exposure to UVR. Skin color (*constitutive* melanin pigmentation) is divided into white, brown, and black.

Not all persons with white skin have the same capacity to develop tanning and this is the principal basis for the classification of individuals into *Skin Phototypes* (SPT) (Table 16-1).

Race White skin types sunburn the most. Persons with brown and black skin color can sunburn following long exposures.

Etiology UVB (290 to 320 nm) overexposure leads to erythema and edema. The skin reaction can be augmented by photosensitization drugs or chemicals (psoralens, sulfonamides, tetracyclines, doxycycline, etc.). The intensity of UVR

Table 16-1

Table 16-1 FITZPATRICK CLASSIFICATION OF SKIN TYPES

Skin Type	Reactivity to UVR	Phenotype Examples
I	Almost always sunburns, never tans	White skin, blond hair, blue or brown eyes, freckles
II	Usually sunburns, tans with difficulty	White skin; red, blond, or brown hair, blue, hazel or brown eyes
III	Sometimes sunburns, can tan gradually	White skin, any color hair, any color eyes
IV	Occasional sunburns, tans easily	White or brown skin, dark hair, dark eyes
V	Rarely sunburns, tans well	Brown skin, dark hair, dark eyes
VI	Almost never sunburns, tans well	Dark brown or black skin, dark hair, dark eyes

is augmented by reflective surfaces (snow, sand, water), altitude, and latitudes near the equator.

Genetics Skin phototypes are genetically determined.

PATHOPHYSIOLOGY

Sunburn induced erythema and edema are mediated by prostaglandin, histamine, and arachidonic acid. Systemic symptoms are mediated primarily by interleukins.

HISTORY

Mild reactions to sunlight begin 6 to 12 h after onset of exposure, peak at 24 h and fade at 3 to 5 days. Sunburns have a similar time course with blister formation on day 2 and desquamation on resolution.

Skin Symptoms The skin usually is pruritic, painful, and warm to touch. Severe sunburn over large surfaces creates fever, chills, malaise, and even prostration.

PHYSICAL EXAMINATION

Appearance of Patient In severe sunburn the patient is "toxic"—with fever, weakness, and lassitude.

Vital Signs In severe sunburn, tachycardia may be present.

Skin Findings

Type of Lesion Confluent erythema, edema, vesicles, and bullae confined to areas of exposure (Fig. 16-1).

Color Bright red.

Palpation Edematous areas are raised and tender.

Distribution of Lesions Typically confined to areas of exposure (in some instances sunburn can occur in areas covered with clothing, depending on the degree of exposure and the SPT of the person).

LABORATORY EXAMINATIONS

Dermatopathology Skin biopsy reveals damaged keratinocytes, "sunburn cells," in the epidermis with exocytosis of lymphocytes, vacuolization of melanocytes and Langerhans cells. In the dermis, there is vascular dilation, perivascular edema, and perivascular inflammation.

DIFFERENTIAL DIAGNOSIS

The distribution of the rash helps categorize the rash into a UVR mediated process. Sunburns are a normal reaction to overexposure of UVR, but other photoreactions such as lupus erythematosus or medication-induced photosensitivity should be considered.

COURSE AND PROGNOSIS

Sunburns self-resolve over 2 to 4 weeks and scarring rarely results. At most, there can be a permanent hypomelanosis, probably related to destruction of melanocytes.

MANAGEMENT

Treatment is symptomatic with:

1. Cold, wet compresses.
2. Baths with colloidal oatmeal (Aveeno).

3. Emollients such as:
   a. Hydrated petrolatum, Vaseline, mineral oil, Aquaphor, Lubriderm, Moisturel, and Eucerin creams.
4. Medicated ointments or creams (topical steroids/cortisones). Topical steroids are effective if used in appropriate strengths:
   a. Low potency steroids (Desowen, 1% hydrocortisone, 2.5% hydrocortisone) should be used on face or groin area, no more than bid × 2 weeks.
   b. Medium potency steroids (Elocon, Dermatop, Cutivate) should be used on the body or extremities no more than bid × 2 weeks.
   c. Strong steroids (Ultravate, Psorcon, Diprolene) are reserved for older children/adults on severely affected areas bid for no more than 2 weeks.

   Patients need to be cautioned about steroid side effects. (See page 48 for more details.)
5. Analgesics such as aspirin or ibuprofen may help alleviate the discomfort.

Severe cases may require:

1. Systemic steroids (prednisone 1 to 2 mg/kg per day divided QD to bid for 5 to 14 days).

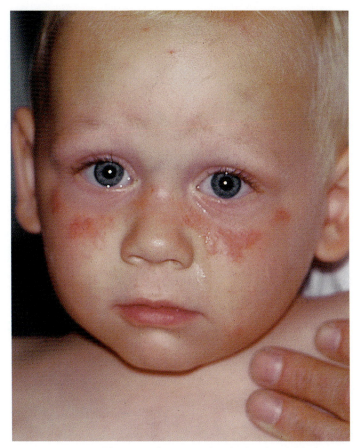

Figure 16-1   Acute sun damage   *Blistering plaques on the cheeks of a child after extended sunlight exposure.*

SOLAR URTICARIA

Solar urticaria is a distinctive reaction pattern of wheals that develop within minutes after exposure to sunlight or artificial ultraviolet radiation (UVR) and disappear within 1 h.

EPIDEMIOLOGY

Age Any age. More common in ages 30 to 40 years.

Gender F > M, 3:1.

Incidence Uncommon.

Etiology Possibly type 1, IgE-mediated hypersensitivity reaction.

PATHOPHYSIOLOGY

Solar urticaria may be induced by several different mechanisms. Some patients with solar urticaria have an inborn error of protoporphyrin metabolism. Others demonstrate passive transfer and reverse passive transfer tests supporting an allergic mechanism. For many, the mechanism is still unknown.

HISTORY

In solar urticaria, the patient experiences itching and burning that occurs within a few minutes of exposure to sunlight. Soon after, erythema appears, which develops into wheals, only in the sites of exposure. The wheals disappear within several hours. Some patients experience nausea and headache. Bronchospasm has been rarely reported. Sudden exposure of large surface areas can result in a generalized urticaria and an anaphylactic-like reaction.

PHYSICAL EXAMINATION

Skin Findings

Type Urticarial wheals, with a surrounding erythematous flare (Fig. 16-2).

Color Pink to red.

Distribution of Lesions The urticarial wheals occur less frequently on the habitually exposed areas (face and dorsa of the hands) than on the covered areas (arms, legs, and trunk).

LABORATORY EXAMINATIONS

Dermatopathology Skin biopsy shows the mild nonspecific changes of urticaria: vascular dilatation, dermal edema, and perivascular inflammation.

Phototesting is helpful in discovering the wavelengths involved, and can aid in the management of the disorder. Solar urticaria has been classified into several types depending on the action spectrum that elicits the eruption. Solar urticaria can be caused by UVB, UVA, and visible light, or a combination of them.

DIFFERENTIAL DIAGNOSIS

The diagnosis of solar urticaria is based on history and clinical induction of lesions by natural or artificial light under controlled conditions. Solar urticaria can be confused with polymorphic light eruption (PMLE), but in PMLE the lesions do not disappear in hours but last for days.

COURSE AND PROGNOSIS

Solar urticaria may undergo spontaneous remission, but it can take up to 5 to 8 years.

MANAGEMENT

Prevention

Sunblocks and sun avoidance.

Systemic Therapies

Antihistamines such as:
   a. Diphenhydramine (Benadryl, 5 mg/kg/day PO divided tid or qid).
   b. Hydroxyzine HCl (Atarax, 2 to 4 mg/kg/day divided tid or qid).
   c. Cetirizine HCl (Zyrtec 2.5 to 10 mg PO qd).
Other treatments:
   a. Antimalarials.
   b. Systemic steroids.
   c. Plasmapheresis.

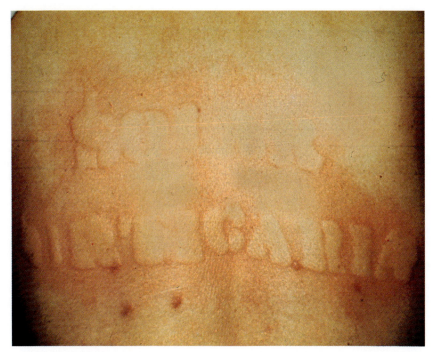

Figure 16-2   Solar urticaria   *Urticarial lesions on the back induced by solar irradiation 15 mins prior.* (Reproduced with permission from IM Freedberg et al., Dermatology in General Medicine, 5th edition. New York: McGraw-Hill, 1999).

Desensitization can be attempted with the specific wavelengths that elicit the eruption. This has been successful in maintaining a symptom-free life by using simple light treatments with or without psoralens in an attempt to slowly increase UVR tolerance.

POLYMORPHOUS LIGHT ERUPTION

Polymorphous light eruption (PMLE) is characterized by delayed abnormal skin reactions to UVR (290 to 480 nm). The various rash types include: erythematous macules, papules, plaques, and vesicles; however, in each patient the eruption is consistently monomorphous.

Synonyms Sun allergy, sun poisoning.

EPIDEMIOLOGY

Age Any age. Average age of onset: 23 years.

Gender M = F.

Incidence Most common child-onset photodermatitis.

Race All races.

Genetics In Native Americans (North and South America) there is a hereditary type of PMLE.

Etiology Unknown.

PATHOPHYSIOLOGY

The relation of the eruption to ultraviolet exposure is unknown. A delayed hypersensitivity reaction to an antigen induced by UVR is possible.

HISTORY

PMLE appears in spring or early summer, but will resolve by fall, suggesting a "hardening" response to UVR. The rash comes on suddenly, following minutes to days of sun exposure. PMLE most often appears in vacationing persons with an acute intense exposure to the sunlight. The rash appears within 18 to 24 hours after exposure and, once established, persists for 7 to 10 days, thereby limiting the vacationer's subsequent time outdoors.

PHYSICAL EXAMINATION

Skin Findings

Type Papules, macules, papulovesicles, rarely plaques (Fig. 16-3).

Color Pink to red.

Size 2 to 3 mm to > 1 cm.

Distribution The eruption often spares the face and areas habitually exposed to the sun. It is most frequently seen on the forearms and "V" area of the neck. The lesions may also occur on the trunk.

LABORATORY EXAMINATIONS

Dermatopathology Skin biopsy shows epidermal edema, spongiosis, vesicle formation, and mild liquefaction degeneration of the basal layer, but no atrophy or thickening of the basement membrane. A dense lymphocytic infiltrate is present in the dermis, with occasional neutrophils. There is edema of the papillary dermis and endothelial swelling.

DIFFERENTIAL DIAGNOSIS

PMLE is differentiated from other photodermatoses by its delayed onset of eruption, characteristic morphology, and histopathology. *Phototesting* can be done to confirm the diagnosis and help determine whether the action spectrum is UVB, UVA, or both. It is most important to rule out lupus erythematosus (LE) in the differential diagnosis. Skin biopsy, ANA, anti-Ro, and anti-La serologies will exclude LE. Photosensitivity eruptions caused by systemic drugs can be ruled out by history.

COURSE AND PROGNOSIS

The course is chronic and recurrent and may, in fact, become worse each season. Although some patients may develop "tolerance" by the end of the summer, the eruption usually recurs again the following spring, and/or when they travel to tropical areas in the winter. However, spontaneous improvement or even cessation of eruptions can occur after years.

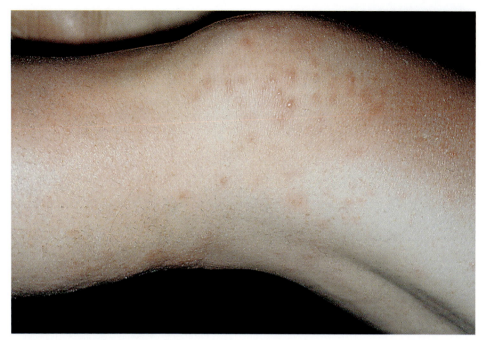

Figure 16-3 Polymorphous light eruption *Scattered erythematous papules on the legs of a child 24 hours after sun exposure.*

Prevention

Sunscreens and sun avoidance are recommended. Topical self-tanning products can help build-up a "tan" to prevent PMLE.

Systemic Therapy

Systemic beta carotene (solatene) can be helpful (dose 20 to 150 mg/d in children). Side effects include yellow skin, orange stools, and occasional GI upset. Antimalarials (hydroxychloroquine and chloroquine) are effective in some patients. Antimalarials (hydroxychloroquine and chloroquine) are effective in some patients.

Phototherapy

PUVA light treatments can also be attempted to help build "sun tolerance" for the following summer.

PHYTOPHOTODERMATITIS

Phytophotodermatitis is a streaky hyperpigmentation of the skin caused by contact with certain plants and concomitant exposure to sunlight. The inflammatory response is a phototoxic reaction usually due to psoralens found in plants such as limes, lemons, mangos, celery, parsnips, carrots, parsley, dill, figs, or meadow grass.

Synonyms Plant-induced photosensitivity, berloque dermatitis, Berlock dermatitis.

EPIDEMIOLOGY

Age Any age.

Gender M = F.

Incidence Common.

Etiology Furocoumarin compounds in the plants get onto (topically) or into (by ingestion) the skin. Subsequent sunlight exposure results in a photosensitive dermatitis.

HISTORY

The child usually gives a history of playing in grassy meadows or beach grass, making lemonade or lime-ade and the next day a streaky, erythematous (sometimes blistering) pattern appears, that leaves a residual hyperpigmentation.

PHYSICAL EXAMINATION

Skin Findings

Type Acutely: erythema, vesicles, and bullae. Chronically: residual dark hyperpigmentation (Fig. 16-4).

Shape of Individual Lesions Bizarre streaks, artificial patterns that indicate an "outside job."

Distribution and Arrangement of Multiple Lesions Scattered areas on the sites of contact, especially the arms, legs, and face.

Wood's Lamp Examination The sites of involvement can be detected by the enhancement of the erythema and pigmentation.

DIFFERENTIAL DIAGNOSIS

The diagnosis of phytophotodermatitis can be made if careful history elicits the exposure to furocoumarins and subsequent sunlight exposure. Phytophotodermatitis can sometimes be mistaken for child abuse with the linear hyperpigmented streaks of pigment being mistaken for resolving bruises.

COURSE AND PROGNOSIS

Most episodes of phytophotodermatitis fade spontaneously, but the pigmentation may last for weeks.

MANAGEMENT

Symptomatic Relief

- Baths with collodial oatmeal (Aveeno) on aluminum acetate (Domeboro soaks).
- Emollients such as hydrated petrolatum, Vaseline, mineral oil, Aquaphor, Lubriderm, Moisturel, and Eucerin creams.
- Medicated ointments or creams (topical steroids/cortisones). Topical steroids are effective if used in appropriate strengths. (See page 48 for more details.)

Systemic Therapy

- Analgesics such as aspirin or ibuprofen.
- Antihistamines such as Atarax (hydroxyzine, 2 to 4 mg/kg/day divided tid or qid) or Benadryl (diphenhydramine, 5 mg/kg/day divided tid or qid, not to exceed 300 mg a day).
- Systemic steroids (prednisone 1 to 2 mg/kg per day divided qd to bid for 5 to 14 days).

Post-inflammatory hyperpigmentation will gradually fade over a period of weeks to months.

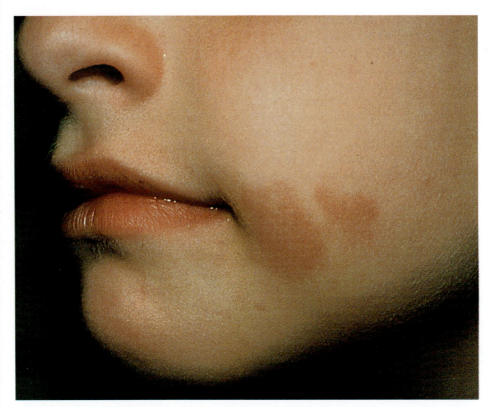

Figure 16-4 Phytophotodermatitis *Hyperpigmentation around the mouth after exposure to limes and sunlight.*

DRUG-INDUCED PHOTOSENSITIVITY

Drug-induced photosensitivity describes an adverse reaction of the skin that results from simultaneous exposure to certain drugs (via ingestion, injection, or topical application; see Table 16-2) and to ultraviolet radiation (UVR) or visible light. The chemicals may be therapeutic, cosmetic, industrial, or agricultural. There are two types of reaction: (1) phototoxic, which can occur in all individuals and is essentially an exaggerated sunburn response (erythema, edema, vesicles, etc.); and (2) photoallergic, which involves an immunologic response and the eruption is a rash.

Table 16-2 DRUGS THAT CAUSE PHOTOSENSITIVITY

Antibiotics
Amoxicillin
Ciprofloxacin
Clofazimine
Dapsone
Demeclocycline
Doxycycline
Enoxacin
Flucytosine
Griseofulvin
Lomefloxacin
Minocycline
Nalidixic acid
Norfloxacin
Ofloxacin
Oxyfloxacin
Oxytetracycline
Pyrazinamide
Sulfonamide
Tetracycline
Trimethoprim

Anticancer drugs
Dacarbazine (DTIC)
Fluorouracil
Flutamide
Methotrexate
Vinblastine

Antidepressants
Amitriptyline
Amoxapine
Clomipramine
Desipramine
Doxepin
Fluoxetine
Imipramine
Maprotiline
Nortriptyline
Phenelzine
Protriptyline
Trazodone
Trimipramine

Antihistamines
Astemizole
Cimetidine
Cyproheptadine
Diphenhydramine
Ranitidine
Terfenadine

Antihypertensives
β blockers
Captopril
Diltiazem
Methyldopa
Minoxidil
Nifedipine

Antiparasitics
Chloroquine
Quinine
Thiabendazole

Antipsychotic drugs
Chlorpromazine
Fluphenazine
Haloperidol
Perphenazine
Prochlorperazine
Thioridazine
Thiothixene
Trifluoperazine
Triflupromazine

Diuretics
Acetazolamide
Amiloride
Bendroflumethiazide
Benzthiazide
Chlorothiazide
Furosemide
Hydrochlorothiazide
Hydroflumethiazide
Methyclothiazide
Metolazone
Polythiazide
Triamterene
Trichlormethiazide

Hypoglycemics
Acetohexamide
Chlorpropamide
Glipizide
Glyburide
Tolazamide
Tolbutamide

**Nonsteroidal anti-
inflammatory drugs**
Benoxaprofen
Diclofenac

Diflunisal
Fenbufen
Ibuprofen
Indomethacin
Ketoprofen
Nabumetone
Naproxen
Phenylbutazone
Piroxicam
Sulindac

Sunscreens
Aminobenzoic acid
Avobenzone
Benzophenones
Cinnamates
Homosalate
Methyl anthranilate
PABA

**Miscellaneous
photosensitizing agents**
Alprazolam
Amantadine
Amiodarone
Benzocaine
Bergamot oil, oils of
citron, lavender, lime,
sandalwood, cedar
Carbamazepine
Chlordiazepoxide
Clofibrate
Contraceptives, oral
Desoximetasone
Disopyramide
Etretinate
Fluorescein
Gold salts
Griseofulvin
Hexachlorophene
Isotretinoin
6-Methylcoumarin
Musk ambrette
Promethazine
Quinine sulfate and
gluconate
Tretinoin
Trimeprazine

SOURCE: Reproduced with permission from TB Fitzpatrick et al., *Color Atlas and Synopsis of Clinical Dermatology*, 4th edition. New York: McGraw-Hill, 2001.

PHOTOTOXIC DRUG REACTION

Phototoxic drug reaction is an exaggerated sunburn response to UVR that can occur in all individuals exposed to sulfonamides, tetracyclines, doxycycline, amiodarone, thiazides, coal tar, furosemide, nalidixic acid, oxytetracycline, phenothiazines, piroxicam, and psoralens.

EPIDEMIOLOGY

Age   Can occur at any age, more common in older children and adults.

Gender   M = F.

Race   All types of skin color: black, white, and brown.

Incidence   Uncommon.

PATHOPHYSIOLOGY

Phototoxic reactions are caused by the formation of toxic photoproducts such as free radicals, or reactive oxygen species such as singlet oxygen. The principal sites of damage are nuclear DNA or cell membranes (plasma, lysosomal, mitochondrial, microsomal). The action spectrum is UVA. It is not known why some individuals show phototoxic reactions to a particular drug and others do not.

HISTORY

There are three patterns of phototoxic reaction: (1) immediate erythema and urticaria; (2) delayed sunburn type pattern developing within 16 to 24 h or later (48 to 72 h in psoralen phototoxic reactions); or (3) delayed (72 to 96 h) melanin hyperpigmentation.

PHYSICAL EXAMINATION

Skin Findings

Type   The skin lesions are those of an exaggerated sunburn (Fig. 16-5). In phototoxic drug reactions there is erythema, edema, and vesicle and bulla formation. An eczematous reaction pattern is not seen in phototoxic reactions. Marked brown epidermal melanin pigmentation can occur in the course of the erupton, and especially with certain drugs (chlorpromazine and

amiodarone) a gray dermal melanin pigmentation develops. After repeated exposure some scaling and lichenification can develop.

Distribution   Confined exclusively to areas exposed to light.

Nails   Photooncholysis can occur with certain drugs (e.g., psoralens, demethylchlortetracycline, and benoxaprofen).

LABORATORY EXAMINATIONS

Dermatopathology   Skin biopsy reveals inflammation, sunburn cells in the epidermis, epidermal necrobiosis, and intraepidermal and subepidermal vesiculation.

DIFFERENTIAL DIAGNOSIS

History of exposure to drug is most important as well as the type of morphologic changes in the skin characteristic of phototoxic drug eruptions: confluent erythema, edema, vesicles, and bullae. The differential diagnosis includes other photoreactions such as lupus erythematosus and the porphyrias.

COURSE AND PROGNOSIS

Phototoxic drug reactions disappear following cessation of drug. To implicate a specific drug, photopatch testing can be used. This test is especially helpful if the patient is on multiple potentially phototoxic drugs.

MANAGEMENT

Identification and elimination of the causative agent is required. Symptomatic treatment includes:

1.   Cold, wet compresses.
2.   Baths with colloidal oatmeal (Aveeno).

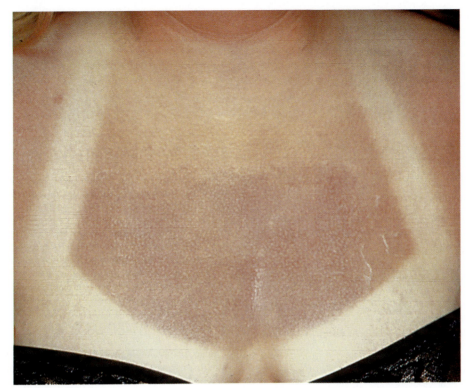

Figure 16-5 Phototoxic drug reaction *Intense sun sensitivity induced by tetracycline in a young girl who subsequently went to a tanning booth despite precautions.* (Slide courtesy of Lisa Cohen).

3. Emollients such as:
   a. Hydrated petrolatum (you must ask the pharmacist to get it), Vaseline, mineral oil, Aquaphor, Lubriderm, Moisturel, and Eucerin creams.
4. Medicated ointments or creams (topical steroids/cortisones). Topical steroids are effective if used in appropriate strengths (See page 48 for more details.)

5. Analgesics such as aspirin or ibuprofen may help alleviate the discomfort.

Severe cases may require:

1. Systemic steroids (Prednisone 1 to 2 mg/kg per day divided qd to bid for 5 to 14 days).

PHOTOALLERGIC DRUG REACTION

Photoallergic drug reactions are caused by photoproduct (the drug present in the skin absorbs light photons). This photoproduct then binds to a soluble or membrane-bound protein to form an antigen. Photoallergy depends upon individual immunologic reactivity and it develops in only a small percentage of persons exposed to these drugs.

EPIDEMIOLOGY

Age Any age, more common in adults.

Gender M = F.

Incidence Photoallergic drug reactions occur much less frequently than phototoxic drug sensitivity.

PATHOPHYSIOLOGY

Drug particles in the skin induce the formation of a photoproduct which conjugates with protein producing an antigen. The action spectrum involved is UVA.

HISTORY

The history may be more difficult in that initial sensitization induces a delayed hypersensitivity reaction and the eruption occurs on subsequent sensitization. Topically applied photosensitizers are the most frequent cause of photoallergic eruptions, e.g., halogenated salicylanilides (in soaps and other household products used to inhibit bacterial overgrowth) or musk ambrette. Systemic drugs can also cause a photoallergic reaction.

PHYSICAL EXAMINATION

Skin Findings

Type Eczematous plaques or flat-topped papular lichen planus-like eruptions.

Color Pink to red to purple.

Distribution of Lesions Areas exposed to light (Fig. 16-6), but there may be involvement of adjacent nonexposed skin.

LABORATORY EXAMINATIONS

Dermatopathology Skin biopsy shows epidermal spongiosis with lymphocytic infiltration.

DIFFERENTIAL DIAGNOSIS

History of exposure to drug is most important as well as the types of morphologic changes in the skin that are characteristic of photoallergic drug reactions (eczematous or lichenoid). Photoallergic drug reactions are difficult to diagnose and require the use of patch and photopatch tests done by a dermatologist. An eczematous reaction in the irradiated site but not in the nonirradiated site confirms photoallergy to the particular agent tested.

COURSE AND PROGNOSIS

Contact photoallergic dermatitis can persist for months to years. This is known as a persistent light reaction, originally caused by exposure to salicylanilides. In the persistent light reactor, an exposure to the originally offending agent does not occur and the action spectrum usually broadens to involve UVB but this is seen more in the adult rather than the childhood pop-ulation.

MANAGEMENT

Identification and elimination of the photoallergic agent is needed. Symptomatic treatment includes:

1. Cool, wet compresses.
2. Emollients such as hydrated petrolatum, Vaseline, mineral oil, Aquaphor, Lubriderm, Moisturel, and Eucerin creams.
3. Medicated ointments or creams (topical steroids/cortisones). Topical steroids are effective if used in appropriate strengths (see page 48 for more details).
4. Antihistamines such as Atarax (hydroxyzine, 2 to 4 mg/kg/day divided tid or qid) or Benadryl (diphenhydramine, 5 mg/kg per day divided tid or qid, not to exceed 300 mg a day).

Severe cases may require:

1. Systemic steroids (prednisone 1 to 2 mg/kg/day divided qd to bid for 5 to 14 days).

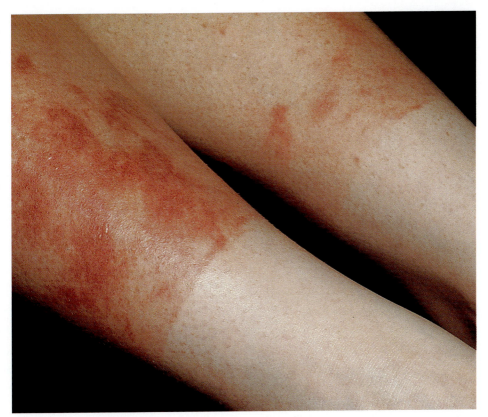

Figure 16-6 Photoallergic reaction *Erythema and edema with sunlight exposure in a patient sensitized to oral sulfonamides.*

ERYTHROPOIETIC PROTOPORPHYRIA

Erythropoietic protoporphyria (EPP) is the most common inherited metabolic disorder of porphyrin metabolism characterized by an acute sunburn like photosensitivity.

Synonym Erythrohepatic protoporphyria.

EPIDEMIOLOGY

Age Acute photosensitivity begins between ages 2–5 years old.

Gender M = F.

Race All ethnic groups.

Heredity Autosomal dominant.

Incidence Uncommon, cases reported from Europe, United Kingdom, and the United States.

Etiology An inherited deficiency of ferrochelatase.

PATHOPHYSIOLOGY

The specific enzyme defect occurs at the step in porphyrin metabolism in which protoporphyrin is converted to heme by the enzyme ferrochelatase. This leads to an accumulation of protoporphyrin, which is highly photosensitizing.

HISTORY

Duration of Onset of Lesions Stinging and itching may occur within a few minutes of sunlight exposure, erythema and edema appear after 1 to 8 h.

Seasonal Changes Photosensitivity is less common in the winter months in temperate areas.

Symptoms Burning or "stinging" sensation within minutes and may be the only abnormality. Children may choose to not go out in the direct sunlight after a few painful episodes. Symptoms occur when exposed to sunlight through window glass.

Systems Review Biliary colic, even in children.

PHYSICAL EXAMINATION

Skin Changes in Acute Reactions to Sunlight Exposure Bright red erythema, later edema with swelling of hands, urticaria, purpura on the nose and tips of ears. Vesicles or bullae rarely occur. These changes appear within 1 to 8 h and subside after several hours or days without obvious scarring.

Skin Changes Following Chronic Recurrent Exposures Shallow, often linear scars, especially on the nose and dorsa of the hands (aged knuckles). Diffuse wrinkling of the skin of the face (nose, around the lips, cheeks) with obvious thickening of the skin and a waxy color (Fig. 16-7). Crusted, erosive lesions may occur on the nose and lips. Absence of sclerodermoid changes, hirsutism, or hyperpigmentation.

General Medical Findings Hemolytic anemia with hypersplenism (rare). Cholelithiasis (12%), even in children. Stones contain large amounts of protoporphyrin. Liver disease may result from massive deposition of protoporphyrin in the hepatocytes; fatal hepatic cirrhosis is rare.

LABORATORY EXAMINATIONS

Porphyrin Studies Increased protoporphyrin in RBCs, plasma, and stools but no excretion in the urine. Decreased activity of the enzyme, ferrochelatase, in the bone marrow, liver, and in skin fibroblasts.

Liver Function Tests for liver function are indicated. Liver biopsy has demonstrated portal and periportal fibrosis and deposits of brown pigment in hepatocytes and Kupfer cells—with electron microscopy, needle-like crystals have been observed. About 20 patients have been reported with hepatic failure due to cirrhosis leading to portal hypertension.

Special Examination for Fluorescent Erythrocytes RBC in a blood smear exhibit a characteristic transient fluorescence when examined

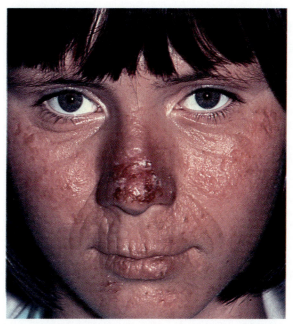

Figure 16-7 Erythropoietic protoporphyria *Fifteen-year-old with deep wrinkling and waxy thickening of the upper lip and cheeks.* (Reproduced with permission from TB Fitzpatrick et al., Color Atlas and Synopsis of Clinical Dermatology, 4th edition. New York: McGraw-Hill, 2001).

with a fluorescent microscope with a mercury or tungsten-iodide lamp that contains 400 nm radiation.

Dermatopathology

Skin Biopsy Marked eosinophilic homogenization and thickening of the blood vessels in the papillary dermis and an accumulation of an amorphous, hyaline-like basophilic substance in and around blood vessels.

Radiography Gall stones may be present.

DIFFERENTIAL DIAGNOSIS

In EPP there is photosensitivity but no rash, only an exaggerated sunburn response that appears much earlier than ordinary sunburn erythema. Also, the skin changes occur behind window glass. Finally, there are virtually no photosensitivity disorders in which the symptoms appear so rapidly (minutes) after exposure to sunlight. Porphyrin examination establishes the diagnosis with elevated free protoporphyrin levels in the RBCs and in the stool (but not urine, distinguishing it from the other more un-

common porphyrias). The fecal protoporphyrin is most consistently elevated.

COURSE AND PROGNOSIS

EPP persists throughout life but the photosensitivity may become less apparent in late adulthood.

MANAGEMENT

There is no treatment for the basic metabolic abnormality. Symptomatic relief includes:

1. Sunscreen and sun avoidance.
2. Betacarotene (180 mg PO qd). Therapeutic levels of carotenoids are achieved in 1 to 2 months. This treatment brings about an amelioration of the photosensitivity but does not completely eliminate the problem of photosensitivity. Patients on betacarotene can remain outdoors longer by a factor of 8 to 10, but still burn if exposures are too long. Nevertheless, many patients can participate in outdoor sports for the first time. There is no toxicity with prolonged treatment with betacarotene.

GENETIC DISORDERS ASSOCIATED WITH CUTANEOUS TUMORS

There are several inherited disorders with associated sensitivity or accelerated response to sun exposure. Most diseases are rare but need to be recognized at an early age so that preventative measures can be taken. These disorders can be divided into two groups:

1. Genetic disorders with prominent cutaneous malignancies:
   a. Xeroderma pigmentosum.
   b. Basal cell nevus syndrome.
2. Genetic disorders with prominent nonmalignant skin findings:
   a. Ataxia-telangiectasia.
   b. Bloom syndrome.
   c. Rothmund-Thomson syndrome.

XERODERMA PIGMENTOSUM

Xeroderma pigmentosum (XP) is a rare autosomal recessive genodermatosis, characterized by enhanced cellular photosensitivity to ultraviolet radiation and early onset of cutaneous malignancies. There are at least nine molecular forms of XP (complementation groups A through G plus a variant form).

EPIDEMIOLOGY

Age Infancy or early childhood.

Gender M = F.

Incidence 1:250,000 in the U.S. and Europe; 1:40,000 in Japan.

Etiology Defect in endonuclease, the enzyme that recognizes UV damaged regions of DNA.

Genetics Autosomal recessive; parents (obligate heterozygotes) are clinically normal.

PATHOPHYSIOLOGY

At this time there are nine known molecular defects as the basis for the clinical syndrome of XP. All the genes are integral for DNA repair, specifically the nucleotide excision repair. There are eight complementation groups (A through G, plus a variant form; see Table 16-3). The latter has a normal excision repair but has defective post-repair replication.

HISTORY

In about 50% of XP cases, there is a history of an acute sunburn reaction; the sunburn erythema may persist for days (in contrast to a normal sunburn, which disappears in a few days). The other patients appear to have normal sunburn reactivity. Freckle-like macules (lentigines) appear on the exposed areas by age 1 year in 50% of the patients, and in almost all patients by age 15. Solar keratoses develop at an early age, and the epithelial skin cancers (basal cell or squamous cell) appear by the eighth year of life. The skin becomes dry and leathery similar to a "farmer's skin" by the end of childhood. Most important are the series of malignancies that develop including melanoma, epithelial cancers, fibrosarcoma, and angiosarcoma. There is about a 2000-fold increase in the frequency of basal cell carcinoma, squamous cell carcinoma, and cutaneous malignant melanoma.

The eye is involved with equal frequency to the skin, and it is a prominent feature of the disease. Most striking is the photophobia with redness of the eyes due to conjunctival injection; later there is severe keratitis and vascularization leading to blindness. Ectropion is common and epithelial cancers and melanomas of the eyelids or anterior eye may develop.

A progressive neurologic degeneration occurs in 40% of the patients, either in infancy or by the second decade. There is a wide range of abnormalities: severe progressive mental retar-

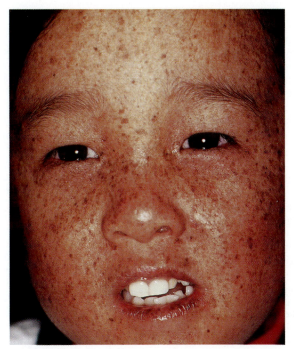

Figure 16-8 Xeroderma pigmentosum *Freckled hyperpigmented papules and keratoses on the face of a young child.*

dation, spasticity, seizures. The most common neurologic abnormalities are progressive sensorineural deafness and diminished to absent deep tendon reflexes.

PHYSICAL EXAMINATION

Skin Findings

Types Macules, telangiectasias, scaly keratoses (Fig. 16-8), basal cell carcinomas, and squamous cell carcinomas (Fig. 16-9).

Color Dark brown lentigines, guttate hypomelanotic macules, and red keratoses and carcinomas.

Distribution The skin changes occur on sunexposed areas (face, neck, forearms, and dorsa of arms, legs) but also in the areas covered with a single layer of clothing (i.e., shirt); the "double-covered" areas are spared (i.e., bathing trunk areas).

Mucous Membranes Telangiectasia can occur on the lips and the lingual mucous membrane: primary squamous cell carcinomas can occur on the tip of the tongue.

General Findings

Patients with XP have an increased risk of ocular cancers, brain sarcomas, leukemia, and lung and gastric carcinomas.

LABORATORY EXAMINATIONS

Dermatopathology

Skin biopsy shows findings consistent with lentigines, solar damage, actinic keratoses, and basal cell and squamous cell carcinomas.

Electron Microscopy Abnormal melanocytes with changes in melanosomes, melanin macroglobules (these are a special type of very large pigment particles resulting from the merging of autophagosomes with secondary lysosomes) are numerous.

SPECIAL EXAMINATIONS

Cultured cells from XP patients exhibit a striking inhibition of growth following exposure to UVR, and cellular recovery is considerably delayed. In one type of XP defect, present in 80% of XP patients, there is a deficiency of the initiation of excision repair acting on pyrimidine dimers. In the other group (called XP "variants"), which comprises about 20%, the fibroblasts exhibit a defect in "S" phase DNA replication following irradiation with UVR. Cell fusion studies permit a separation of the excision repair deficient types into eight groups: XPA through XPG and a variant form.

DIFFERENTIAL DIAGNOSIS

Some young patients with severe freckling or with multiple lentigines syndrome (LEOPARD syndrome) could be regarded as having XP, but at this age these patients do not have a history of acute photosensitivity, which is always present in XP, even in infancy. Also, there is no dermatoheliosis (telangiectasia, atrophy, or guttate hypomelanosis), which is present in XP, even in childhood. XP also has early skin cancers (squamous cell and basal cell carcinoma, malignant melanoma, fibrosarcoma, angiosarcoma).

COURSE AND PROGNOSIS

XP has a poor prognostic outcome. Metastatic melanoma or squamous cell carcinoma are the most frequent causes of death and over 60% of patients die by age 20. Some patients with mild involvement, however, may live beyond middle age. Early diagnosis and careful protection from sun exposure may prolong life substantially.

MANAGEMENT

XP is a very serious disease that requires constant attention from the first moment of diagnosis, not only to prevent exposure to UVR but to closely monitor the patient for the detection of skin malignancies, especially melanoma. Patients with XP need:

1. To be followed by a dermatologist every 3 months, not only to detect malignancies early but to constantly educate the patient (and the parents!) in effective sun protection and in the early recognition of skin cancers.
2. Strong UVA/UVB sunblocks worn daily, and sun avoidance between the hours of 10:00 and 15:00 is recommended.
3. Protective hats, clothing, and sunglasses with side shields are important.
4. Destruction of basal cell and squamous cell carcinomas can be achieved with:
   a. Topical 5-FU (Efudex cream).
   b. Surgical excision.
   c. Cryotherapy.
   d. Imiquimod (Aldara cream) is an immune-stimulating chemical currently approved for the treatment of genital warts. It can also be used off-label as a treatment for precancerous lesions. (Use qhs Monday, Wednesday and Friday until clinical clearing of the lesion. Sites should be monitored closely for recurrence.)
5. Ophthalmologic care with methylcellulose eyedrops and contact lenses are needed to protect the eyes from mechanical trauma in patients with deformed eyelids. Vision can be restored with corneal transplants.

Table 16-3   XERODERMA PIGMENTOSUM MOLECULAR DEFECTS

XP Group	Chromosome	Gene
XPA	9q22	XPA
XPB	2q21	XPB/ERCC3
XPC	3p25.1	XPC
XPD	19q13.2	XPD/ERCC2
XPE	11	XPE
XPF	16p13.3	XPF/ERCC4
XPG	13q32–33	XPG

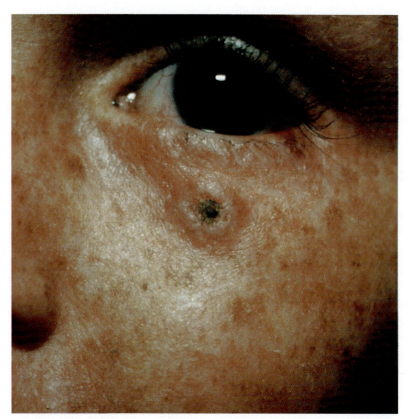

Figure 16-9 Xeroderma pigmentosum *Large nodular basal cell carcinoma on the cheek of a child with XP.*

6. Possible systemic therapies with oral 13-cis-retinoic acid. The limitation of this therapy is the dose-related irreversible calcification of ligaments and tendons. Additionally, the withdrawal of isotretinoin results in the reversal of its protective effect.

7. Genetic counseling and prenatal diagnosis by amniocentesis-measuring UV-induced unscheduled DNA synthesis in cultured amniotic fluid cells. There is as yet no laboratory test that can detect XP heterozygotes in the parents.

BASAL CELL NEVUS SYNDROME

Basal cell nevus syndrome is an autosomal dominant disorder characterized by the childhood onset of multiple basal cell epitheliomas and associated abnormalities or the bones, soft tissue, eyes, CNS, and endocrine organs.

Synonyms Nevoid basal cell carcinoma syndrome, multiple nevoid basal cell carcinoma syndrome, Gorlin syndrome.

EPIDEMIOLOGY

Age The basal cell epitheliomas may begin in ages 2 to 35 years, although several bony abnormalities are congenital.

Gender M = F.

Race Mostly white, but also occurs in blacks and Asians.

Incidence Rare.

Genetics Autosomal dominant with variable penetrance.

Precipitating Factors There appear to be more basal cell epitheliomas on the sun-exposed areas of the skin, but they can occur in covered areas also.

PATHOPHYSIOLOGY

The gene for basal cell nevus syndrome has been identified and located on chromosome 9q22-31. The PATCHED (PTC) gene encodes for a PTC protein, which binds and inhibits a transmembrane protein, SMOOTHENED (SMO). Inhibition of SMO signaling is critical for tumor suppression. Thus, loss of PTC results in cancer formation.

HISTORY

Patients with basal cell nevus syndrome have a characteristic facies, with frontal bossing, broad nasal root, and hypertelorism. The basal cell epitheliomas begin to appear singly in childhood or early adolescence and continue to appear throughout life; there may be thousands of skin cancers. Other congenital anomalies include undescended testes, hydrocephalus, blindness from coloboma, cataracts, and glaucoma.

PHYSICAL EXAMINATION

Skin Findings

Principal Lesions Basal cell carcinomas (translucent, 1- to 10-cm papules and nodules with and without ulcers) that are skin color or pigmented. Tumors on the eyelids, axillae, and neck tend to be pedunculated (Fig. 16-10A). Tumors can become invasive.

Arrangement Bilateral, symmetrical.

Distribution of Lesions Face, neck, trunk, axillae, usually sparing scalp and extremities.

Palmoplantar Lesions Palmar pits are present in 50% of patients and are pinpoint to several millimeters in size and 1.0 mm deep. There may be hundreds of lesions, especially on the lateral surfaces of the palms, soles, and fingers. The pits are the result of premature shedding of the horny layer. There may be a basal cell epithelioma and telangiectases at the bottom of the pit.

Bone Mandibular jaw cysts, which are multiple and may be unilateral or bilateral odontogenic keratocysts. Other bone lesions include defective dentition, bifid or splayed ribs, pectus excavatum, short fourth metacarpals, scoliosis, and kyphosis.

Eye Strabismus, hypertelorism, dystopia canthorum, and congenital blindness.

Central Nervous System Agenesis of the corpus callosum, medulloblastoma (Fig. 16-10B); mental retardation is rare.

Internal Neoplasms Fibrosarcoma of the jaw, ovarian fibromas, teratomas, and cystadenomas.

LABORATORY EXAMINATIONS

Dermatopathology Basal cell epitheliomas have identical histology to basal cell carcinomas: solid, adenoid, cystic, keratotic, superficial, and fibrosing types.

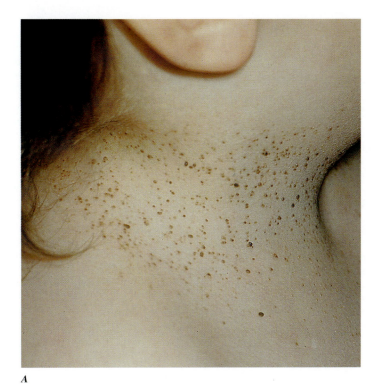

A

Figure 16-10   Basal cell nevus syndrome   *(A) Numerous basal cell epitheliomas on the neck of a child.*

Imaging Lamellar calcification of the falx is seen.

DIFFERENTIAL DIAGNOSIS

Basal cell nevus syndrome is often picked up by dentists or oral surgeons because of the mandibular bone cysts. Dermatologically, palmar pits and the early onset of multiple basal cell epitheliomas is diagnostic.

COURSE AND PROGNOSIS

The prognosis for individuals with basal cell nevus syndrome is good. Only the rare patients who develop medulloblastomas or aggressive deep epitheliomas are severely affected. The large number of skin cancers creates a lifetime problem of vigilance on the part of the patient and the physician. The multiple excisions can cause considerable scarring.

MANAGEMENT

Patients with basal cell nevus syndrome should be followed closely with regular skin examinations. The basal cell epitheliomas should be treated as they enlarge with:

1. Topical 5-FU (Efudex cream).
2. Surgical excision.
3. Cryotherapy.
4. Electrodesiccation.
5. Imiquimod (Aldara cream) an immune-stimulating compound currently approved for the treatment of genital warts, can also be used off-label as a treatment for precancerous lesions (qhs Monday, Wednesday, and Friday until clinical clearing of the lesion. Sites should be monitored closely for recurrence).
6. Radiation should be avoided and radiation therapy is NOT recommended.

Genetic counseling should be made available to the patient.

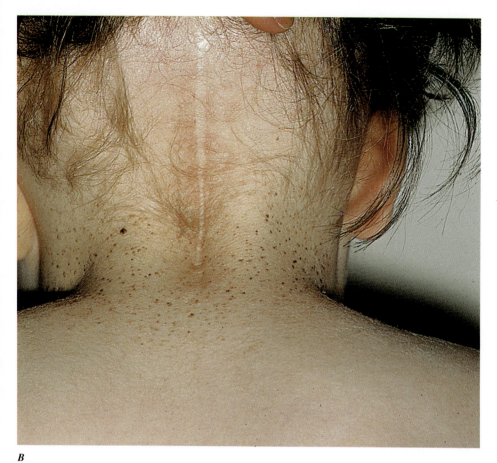

B

Figure 16-10 (continued)   Basal cell nevus syndrome   *(B) Scar from surgical removal of a medul-loblastoma on the same child.*

ATAXIA TELANGIECTASIA

Ataxia telangiectasia is a rare autosomal recessive syndrome characterized by progressive cerebellar ataxia, oculocutaneous telangiectasia, recurrent respiratory tract infections, and an increased susceptibility to lymphoreticular malignancies.

Synonym Louis-Bar syndrome.

EPIDEMIOLOGY

Age Telangiectasias typically appear between the ages of 3 to 5 years; ataxia may precede the skin findings.

Gender M = F.

Incidences Homozygotes > 1:40,000 births; gene frequency 1:100 (it is estimated that 1% of the unaffected population are heterozygous for this disorder and are trait carriers).

Genetics Autosomal recessive, mapped to chromosome 11q22–23.

PATHOPHYSIOLOGY

Ataxia telangiectasia is caused by a mutation in the ATM gene located on chromosome 11q22. Recent studies suggest that ATM functions to respond to chromosomal strand breakage. This would account for the observed chromosomal instability seen in the cells of patients with ataxia telangiectasia.

HISTORY

Ataxia telangiectasia initially presents with ataxia shortly after learning to walk. The skin findings appear from ages 3 to 5 years with fine symmetric telangiectases on the bulbar conjunctiva that subsequently involve the face, trunk, and extremities. With aging and continued sun exposure, the skin becomes sclerotic and acquires a mottled pattern of hypo- and hyperpigmentation.

PHYSICAL EXAMINATION

Skin Findings

Type Telangiectasias, sclerosis, atrophy, café au lait, follicular hyperkeratosis.

Color Red to dusky brown and mottled hypo- and hyperpigmentation.

Distribution Telangiectasia initially on the nasal and temporal areas of bulbar conjuctiva (Fig. 16-11), then involve eyelids, ears (Fig. 16-12), malar areas, neck, V of chest, antecubital and popliteal fossa, dorsal aspects of hands and feet. Sclerodermatous changes on the face (sad, mask-like facies), arms, and hands.

Hair Diffuse graying, hirsutism of arms/legs (Fig. 16-13).

Other Diffuse dry skin, eczematous and sebhorrheic dermatitis.

General Findings

Neurologic signs. Ataxia and clumsiness develop over the second year of life, intellectual deficit (30%), chroreoathetosis, drooling, peculiar ocular movements, sad mask-like facies, stooped posture with drooping shoulders and the head sunk forward and tilt to one side, peripheral neuropathy, spinal muscular atrophy. Recurrent sinopulmonary infections including acute rhinitis, chronic bronchitis, pneumonias, and bronchiectasis (75 to 80%). Immunologic deficits: impaired humoral responses (IgA and IgE deficiency) and cell-mediated immunity (lymphopenia, impaired lymphocyte transformation). Structural anomalies of thymus and lymph nodes. Neoplasms. Ten percent of individuals who survive to the late teens develop lymphoreticular malignancy (Hodgkin's, lymphosarcoma, reticular cell sarcoma, eukemia) or other neoplastic disorders (ovarian dysgerminoma, medulloblastoma, GI carcinoma).

DIFFERENTIAL DIAGNOSIS

Ataxia telangiectasia is a clinical diagnosis made from the finding of oculocutaneous telangiectasia in association with ataxia. Other conditions it may be confused with include: spider angiomas, angioma serpiginosum, hereditary hemorrhagic telangiectasia (Osler–Rendu–Weber disease), generalized essential telangiectasia, and telangiectasia macularis eruptiva perstans.

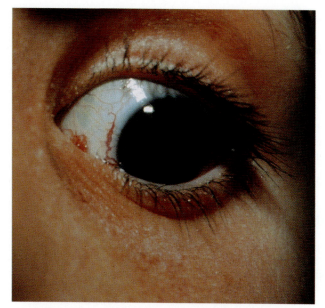

Figure 16-11   **Ataxia telangiectasia**   *Telangiectasia on the bulbar conjunctiva.*

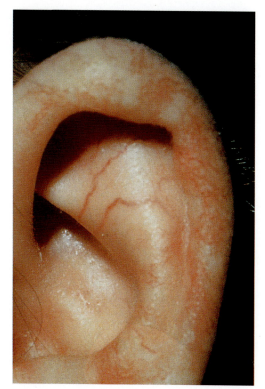

Figure 16-12   **Ataxia telangiectasia**   *Telangiectasia on the ear of a child.*

LABORATORY EXAMINATIONS

Dermatopathology Skin biopsy findings are nonspecific and reveal dilated blood vessels of the subpapillary plexus in telangiectatic areas.

Serology Elevated levels of serum α-fetoprotein.

Immunology Radiosensitivity assay of peripheral lymphocytes grown in culture with phytohematoglutin for 2 days.

Chemistry Glucose intolerance, elevated hepatic enzymes.

COURSE AND PROGNOSIS

Patients with ataxia telangiectasia have a poor prognosis. Death usually occurs at late childhood or early adolescence from bronchiectasis and respiratory failure secondary to recurrent sinopulmonary infections (lymphoreticular malignancies occur in 15% of patients). Individuals who survive beyond adolescence develop severe neurologic morbidity and are confined to a wheelchair and are unable to walk without assistance.

MANAGEMENT

Treatment for ataxia telangiectasia is supportive only:

1. Antibiotics are used for infection.
2. Respiratory therapy is used for bronchiectasis.
3. Physical therapy is used for contractures.
4. Sunscreens and sun avoidance will minimize actinic damage.
5. Genetic counseling is necessary and prenatal diagnosis is available (by measurement of α-fetoprotein in amniotic fluid and by increased spontaneous chromosomal breakages of amniocytes).

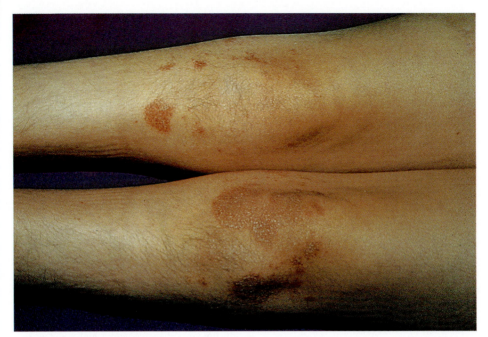

Figure 16-13   Ataxia telangiectasia   *Hirsutism on the lower legs and ecchymoses secondary to ataxia and numerous falls.*

BLOOM'S SYNDROME

Bloom's syndrome is a rare autosomal recessive disease characterized by photosensitivity, telangiectases, and severe intrauterine and postnatal growth retardation.

Synonym   Congenital telangiectatic erythema.

EPIDEMIOLOGY

Age   Skin findings apparent at 2 to 3 weeks of life.

Gender   Male predominance (80% of affected children).

Incidence   Most frequent among Ashkenazic Jews (carrier rate of 1:120); rare in the general population.

Genetics   Autosomal recessive.

PATHOPHYSIOLOGY

Bloom's syndrome has been mapped to chromosome 15q26.1. The gene has been designated BLM, which encodes for the BLM protein. In Bloom's syndrome, the BLM mutation impairs DNA helicase function. This results in an elevated frequency of chromosomal abnormalities and increased rate of sister chromatid exchanges (pathognomonic) and chromosomal breakage in cultured fibroblasts and leukocytes.

HISTORY

At birth, affected infants are born at term with reduced body weight and size. In infancy, a facial rash after exposure to light becomes prominent. The photosensitivity gradually resolves but erythema, telangiectases, mottled pigmentation, and scarring persist. Systemic symptoms include an abnormal facies and growth retardation.

PHYSICAL EXAMINATION

Skin Findings

Type   Facial erythema, bullae, bleeding, crusting of eyelids and lips upon light exposure (Fig. 16-14), telangiectasia, atrophy and scarring, scattered café au lait macules (50% of patients).

Color   Red to red-brown and mottled hyper- and hypopigmentation.

Distribution   Erythema and poikiloderma of malar areas, nose, around ears. Telangiectasia of ears and dorsa of hands, sparing trunk, buttocks, and lower extremities.

General Findings

Abnormal facies with narrow prominent nose, relatively hypoplastic malar area, receding chin, skeletal abnormalities (doliohocephaly, polydactyly, clubbed feet), cryptorchidism, severe infections of the respiratory and gastrointestinal tract secondary to cellular and humoral immune dysfunction, diabetes, and a high incidence of neoplastic disease (leukemia, Wilms' tumors, lymphosarcoma, lymphoma, carcinoma of oral cavity, and Gl tract). Normal intellectual and sexual development, although male infertility is common.

DIFFERENTIAL DIAGNOSIS

The diagnosis of Bloom's syndrome is suggested by history of low birth weight, presence of photosensitivity, and facial telangiectasia in a child of short stature (especially of Ashkenazic Jewish heritage). The diagnosis can be confirmed by chromosome analysis. The differential diagnosis for Bloom's syndrome includes: lupus erythematosus, Rothmund-Thomson syndrome, dyskeratosis congenita, hereditary acrokeratotic poikiloderma, Kindler's syndrome, Fanconi anemia, and xeroderma pigmentosum.

LABORATORY EXAMINATIONS

Dermatopathology   Skin biopsy reveals flattening of the epidermis, hydropic degeneration of the basal layer, and dilated capillaries in the upper dermis.

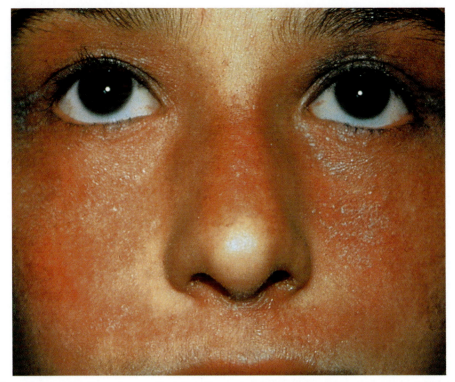

Figure 16-14 Bloom's syndrome *Facial erythema and desquamation after sun exposure with numerous telangiectases.*

Karyotype Increased chromatid exchange and chromosomal breakage.

Immunology Decreased immunoglobulins, reduced cellular proliferative response to mitogens, decreased proliferation in mixed lymphocyte reaction.

Sperm analysis Azoospermia.

Endocrinology High FSH response to LH-releasing hormone.

COURSE AND PROGNOSIS

Patients with Bloom's syndrome have a shortened life span because of fatal respiratory or GI tract infections and neoplastic disease. Approximately 20% of patients will develop neo-plasms; half of them before the age of 20 years. With increasing age, photosensitivity resolves and resistance to infection becomes more normal.

MANAGEMENT

There is no specific treatment for Bloom's syndrome. Management includes:

1. Sun avoidance, and regular use of sunscreens.
2. Antibiotics for the management of patients with respiratory or gastrointestinal infections.
3. Routine follow up and regular examinations.
4. Genetic counseling.

ROTHMUND-THOMSON SYNDROME

Rothmund-Thomson syndrome is a rare autosomal recessive disorder characterized by photosensitivity, skin atrophy, mottled pigmentation, and telangiectasia, in association with juvenile cataracts, short stature, ectoderm changes, and hypogonadism.

Synonyms Hereditary poikiloderma congenitale, poikiloderma atrophicans, and cataracts.

EPIDEMIOLOGY

Age Cutaneous poikiloderma changes may be present at birth, but usually make their appearance between 3 and 6 months of life.

Gender M > F, 2:1.

Incidence Rare.

Genetics Autosomal recessive inheritance.

PATHOPHYSIOLOGY

Rothmund-Thomson has been mapped to chromosome 8q24.3, the RECQL4 gene. This gene encodes for the protein RECQL4 helicase and mutations in the gene leads to dysfunctional DNA repair.

HISTORY

Skin changes are present at or soon after birth. One third of patients have photosensitivity and exhibit bullae formation after UVR exposure. However, the poikiloderma changes of the skin are diffuse on both sun-exposed and unexposed skin. Systemically, patients characteristically have short stature, abnormal facies, amenorrhea in females, undescended testes in males, and blindness.

PHYSICAL EXAMINATION

Skin Findings

Type Diffuse erythema followed by a reticulate pattern of telangiectasia (Fig. 16-15), scarring and atrophy, bullae and vesicles, verrucous hyperkeratoses.

Color Pink-red fading to reticulated hyper- and hypopigmentation, poikiloderma.

Distribution Erythema and poikiloderma on the cheeks (Fig. 16-16), chin, ears, forehead, extensor arms, legs, and buttocks. Verrucous hyperkeratoses on the hands, feet, knees, and elbows.

Hair Partial or total alopecia of scalp and eyebrows (50%). Sparse pubic and axillary hair. Occasional premature graying of hair.

Nails Rough, ridged, heaped-up, small or atrophic.

General Findings

Normal intelligence (except a few cases of mental retardation), short stature, triangular facial configuration (saddle nose, frontal bossing, wide forehead, narrow chin), cataracts (75%, usually before age of 7 years), bone defects (absence, hypoplasia, or dysplasia of long bones, absence or shortening of digits, cleft hand or foot, asymmetry in length of feet, osteoporosis), abnormal dentition (microdontia, failure of teeth to erupt).

DIFFERENTIAL DIAGNOSIS

The diagnosis of Rothmund-Thomson is suggested by the presence of photosensitivity and poikiloderma in a patient with short stature, skeletal abnormalities, cataracts, and normal intellectual ability. It must be differentiated from other photosensitive dermatoses such as Bloom's syndrome, dyskeratosis congenita, hereditary acrokeratotic poikiloderma, Kindler's syndrome, Fanconi anemia, and xeroderma pigmentosum.

LABORATORY EXAMINATIONS

Dermatopathology Skin biopsy shows flattening and thinning of the epidermis, with basal layer vacuolization, pigment incontinence with melanophages, and sclerotic collagen in the papillary dermis with loss of papillae.

Radiology X-ray of pelvic and long bones shows cystic spaces, osteoporosis, and sclerotic areas.

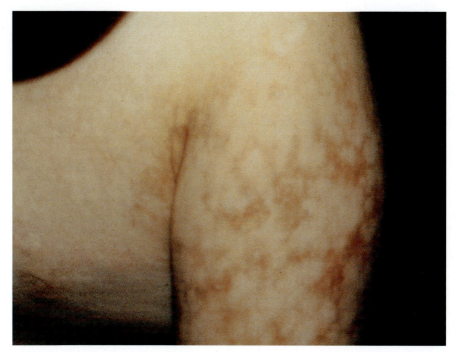

Figure 16-15 Rothmund-Thomson syndrome *Reticulated pattern of telangiectasia on the arm of a child.*

COURSE AND PROGNOSIS

Patients with Rothmund-Thomson syndrome have a normal life span and their photosensitivity decreases with age. Hyperkeratotic lesions of the extremities may transform into SCCs. There have also been case reports of osteosarcoma in Rothmund-Thomson patients.

MANAGEMENT

There is no specific treatment for Rothmund-Thomson syndrome. Preventive measures include:

1. Sunscreen use and sun avoidance.
2. Routine dermatologic exams are needed for appropriate treatment of precancerous keratoses and skin cancers.
3. Genetic counseling.

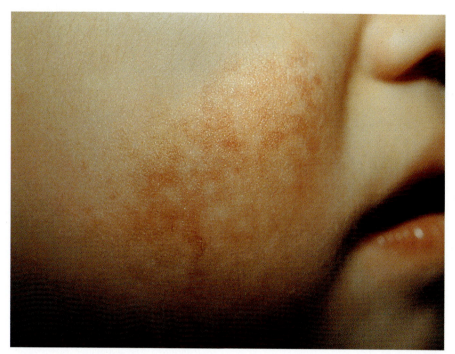

Figure 16-16   **Rothmund-Thomson syndrome**   *Erythema and poikiloderma on the cheek of a child.*

COLLAGEN VASCULAR DISORDERS

JUVENILE RHEUMATOID ARTHRITIS

Juvenile rheumatoid arthritis (JRA) is a generalized systemic disease of unknown etiology characterized by a transient macular, papular or urticarial rash and ensuing fever, adenopathy, splenomegaly, anemia, and arthralgia.

Synonym Still's disease.

EPIDEMIOLOGY

Age Biphasic-> first peak between 2 and 4 years of age, 2nd peak at adolescence.

Gender F > M, 2:1.

Prevalence Common.

Etiology Unknown.

HISTORY

The onset of JRA may be sudden or insidious depending on the age of the patient (the younger the more severe the systemic manifestations). Cutaneous eruptions occur in 25 to 50% of patients and may be the initial presentation. The rash of JRA is evanescent, and can be macular or urticarial. It tends to be precipitated by emotional, infectious, or surgical stress. Systemically, there may be associated fever, adenopathy, splenomegaly, anemia and arthralgias.

PHYSICAL EXAMINATION

Skin Findings

Type Macules and papules or edematous urticarial plaques (Fig. 17-1) with a slightly irregular or serpiginous border (seen in 25 to 50% of patients). Firm, nontender deep dermal or subcutaneous nodules (10% of patients). Periungal telangiectases (5% of patients).

Size Ranging from 2- to 6-mm papules to 8- to 9-cm larger plaques and nodules.

Color Salmon-pink to red papules; plaques surrounded by a zone of pallor (Fig. 17-2).

Distribution Maculopapular rash—areas of local trauma or heat nodules—most commonly on the olecranon process on the ulnar border of the forearm. Can also occur on dorsal aspect of the hands, knees, ears, and over pressure areas such as scapulae, sacrum, buttocks, and heels.

Other Palms and soles: thenar and hypothenar eminences may be erythematous.

General Findings

Skin over joints can become atrophic, smooth, and glossy. High fevers, lymphadenopathy, splenomegaly, single joint involvement (50% of patients) or symmetric polyarthritis with painful, warm, slightly erythematous joints and motion limitation (knee involvement: 90%, finger joints: 75%, wrists and ankles: 66% of patients), spindling of fingers (spindle-shaped deformity of fingers because of involvement of proximal > distal interphalangeal joints, seen in 50% of patients).

DIFFERENTIAL DIAGNOSIS

The diagnosis of JRA is made based on clinical characteristics and history of arthritis lasting for more than 6 weeks, with appropriate studies to exclude other causes such as other autoimmune diseases, urticaria, rheumatic fever,

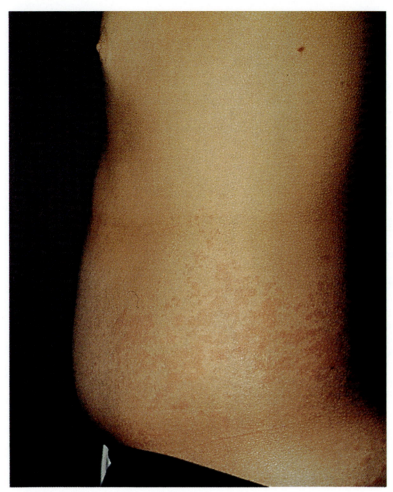

Figure 17-1 **Juvenile rheumatoid arthritis** *Transient macular rash on the body characteristic of JRA.*

hypersensitivity reactions, granuloma annulare, sarcoid, and other granulomatous diseases. Up to 80% of patients with JRA will have a positive rheumatoid factor.

LABORATORY EXAMINATIONS

Dermatopathology   Skin biopsy shows edematous collagen fibers and perivascular cell infiltrate with neutrophils, plasma cells and histiocytes.

Hematology   Leukocytosis, anemia, elevated sedimentation rate, hypoalbuminemia, and hyperglobulinemia.

Serology   Positive Rh factor by latex fixation in 80% of patients.

Radiology   Joint destruction in late disease.

COURSE AND PROGNOSIS

The course and prognosis of JRA is variable. The younger the age of onset, the more prominent the systemic manifestations. The rash typically precedes the systemic symptoms by up to 3 years. The disease may end after a few months and never recur, or it may recur after months or years of remission. The disease typically improves by puberty and 80 to 85% of patients achieve remission. Only 10% have residual severe crippling arthritis.

MANAGEMENT

For active disease:

1. Aspirin (70-100 mg/day for children up to 25 kg of weight, maintain serum levels of 20 to 30 mg/dL).
2. Nonsteroidals such as:
   a. Indomethacin.
   b. Naprosyn.

For severe cases that are resistant to other therapies, have crippling deformities, iridocyclitis, or vasculitis:

1. Systemic corticosteroids.
2. Immunosuppressives.
   a. MTX.
   b. Azathioprine.
   c. Chlorambucil.
   d. Cyclophosphamide.
3. For nonresponsive polyarthritis:
   a. Gold (1 mg/kg of the salt for a total of 500 mg once a week).
4. For structural correction of severe deformities, surgery is a last resort.

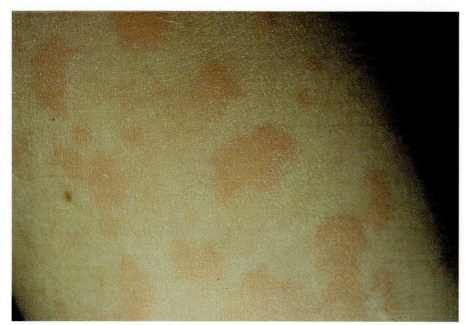

Figure 17-2   Juvenile rheumatoid arthritis   *Faint erythematous, urticarial plaques on the torso of a child.*

SYSTEMIC LUPUS ERYTHEMATOSUS

Systemic lupus erythematosus (SLE) is a serious multisystem disease involving connective tissue and blood vessels; the clinical manifestations include fever (90%); skin lesions (85%); arthritis; and renal, cardiac, and pulmonary disease.

EPIDEMIOLOGY

Age All ages; 15 to 25% of cases occur in patients < 20 years old. Peak childhood incidence at age 11 to 13. Peak adult incidence at age 30 (females), or at age 40 (males).

Gender Prepubertal: M = F. Adults: F > M, 8:1.

Genetics Family history (< 5%) suggests a hereditary component.

PATHOPHYSIOLOGY

The tissue injury in the epidermis results from the deposition of immune complexes at the dermoepidermal junction. Immune complexes selectively generate the assembly of the membrane-attack complex, which mediates membrane injury.

HISTORY

Up to 80% of patients with SLE have cutaneous disease (malar rash, discoid lesions, photosensitivity, or atrophy) and in 25% of patients, the skin is the first presenting symptom.

PHYSICAL EXAMINATION

Skin Findings

Type Erythematous, confluent, macular malar butterfly eruption (Fig. 17-3) with fine scaling; erosions and crusts (seen in 30 to 60% of patients). Lifting of scale reveals follicular projections, "carpet-tacks." Erythematous, discrete, papular or urticarial lesions (face and arms). Discoid papules as in chronic DLE (face and arms). Rarely, "palpable" purpura (vasculitis). Rarely, urticarial lesions with purpura (urticarial vasculitis), (seen in 7 to 22% of patients). Rarely, bullae, often hemorrhagic (acute flares). See Table 17-1.

Color Bright red.

Shape Round or oval.

Arrangement Diffuse involvement of the face in light-exposed areas. Scattered discrete lesions (face, forearms, and dorsa of hands).

Distribution Localized or generalized.

Sites of Predilection Face (80%); scalp (discoid lesions); presternal, shoulders; dorsa of the forearms, hands, fingers, fingertips (vasculitis).

Hair Discoid lesions associated with patchy alopecia. Diffuse alopecia.

Mucous Membrane Ulcers arising in purpuric necrotic lesions on palate (80%), buccal mucosa, or gums (Fig. 17-4).

Other Periungual telangiectases and palmar erythema are also seen.

General Findings

Arthralgia or arthritis (15%), renal disease (50%), pericarditis (20%), pneumonitis (20%), gastrointestinal (due to arteritis and sterile peritonitis), hepatomegaly (30%), splenomegaly (20%), lymphadenopathy (50%), peripheral neuropathy (14%), CNS disease (10%), seizures, or organic brain disease (14%).

LABORATORY EXAMINATIONS

Dermatopathology Skin biopsy shows epidermal atrophy, liquefaction degeneration of the dermoepidermal junction, edema of the dermis, dermal inflammatory infiltrate (lymphocytes), and fibrinoid degeneration of the connective tissue and walls of the blood vessels

Other Organs The fundamental lesion is fibrinoid degeneration of connective tissue and walls of the blood vessels that is associated with an inflammatory infiltrate of plasma cells and lymphocytes.

Immunofluorescence The lupus band test (direct immunofluorescence demonstrating IgG, IgM, and C1q) shows granular or globular deposits of immune reactants in a bandlike pattern along the dermoepidermal junction. This is positive in lesional skin in 90% and in clinically

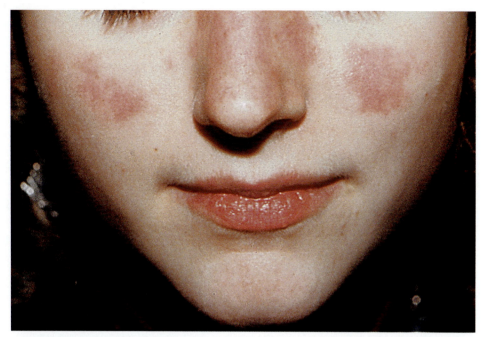

Figure 17-3 Systemic lupus erythematosus *Erythematous, edematous plaques in a "butterfly distribution" on the face.*

normal skin (sun-exposed, 70% to 80%; non-sun-exposed, 50%); in the latter case, indicative of renal disease and hypocomplementemia.

Serologic ANA positive (> 95%); peripheral pattern of nuclear fluorescence and antidouble-stranded DNA antibodies are specific for SLE; low levels of complement (especially with renal involvement). SS-A (Ro) autoantibodies are present in a subset of subacute cutaneous lupus erythematosus (SCLE) in which there is extensive skin involvement and photosensitivity. SS-B(La) antibodies also coexist in 50% of the cases.

Hematologic Anemia [normocytic, normochromic, or rarely hemolytic Coombs' positive, leukopenia (< 4000/mm^3)], elevated ESR (a good guide to activity of the disease).

DIAGNOSIS

The diagnosis of SLE can be made if four of the following criteria are present.

1. Malar rash (butterfly appearance).
2. Discoid rash.
3. Photosensitivity.
4. Oral ulcers.
5. Arthritis.
6. Serositis (pleuritis or pericarditis).
7. Renal complications (proteinuria or cellular casts).
8. Neurologic disorder (seizures or psychosis).
9. Hematologic disorder (anemia, leukopenia, thrombocytopenia).
10. Immunologic disorder (+ LE prep, anti-DNA, anti-Sm, false + FPR).
11. ANA (90% of patients have a titer of 1:32 or greater).

COURSE AND PROGNOSIS

SLE is a lifelong controllable disease with a survival rate of > 90%. Mortality is secondary to renal failure, CNS lupus, cardiac failure, or infection.

MANAGEMENT

1. Sun protection and avoidance and rest.
2. NSAIDs and salicylates are useful for mild disease (arthritis).

SYSTEMIC LUPUS ERYTHEMATOSUS

Table 17-1 ABBREVIATED GILLIAM CLASSIFICATION OF SKIN LESIONS ASSOCIATED WITH LE

I. LE-specific skin disease (cutaneous LE[a] [CLE])
    A. Acute cutaneous LE [ACLE]
        1. Localized ACLE (malar rash; butterfly rash)
        2. Generalized ACLE (macolupapular lupus rash, malar rash, photosensitive lupus dermatitis)
    B. Subacute cutaneous LE [SCLE]
        1. Annular SCLE
        2. Papulosquamous SCLE (disseminated DLE, subacute disseminated LE, maculopapular photosensitive LE)
    C. Chronic cutaneous LE (CCLE)
        1. Classic discoid LE (DLE)
            a. Localized DLE
            b. Generalized DLE
        2. Hypertrophic/verrucous DLE
        3. Lupus profundus
        4. Mucosal DLE
            a. Oral DLE
            b. Conjunctival DLE
        5. Lupus tumidus (urticarial plaque of LE)
        6. Chilblains LE (chilblains lupus)
        7. Lichenoid DLE (LE/lichen planus overlap)
II. LE-nonspecific skin disease
    These range from necrotizing and urticarial vasculitis to livedo reticularis, Raynaud's phenomenon, dermal mucinosis, and bullous lesions in LE

[a]Alternative or synonymous terms are listed in parentheses; abbreviations are indicated in brackets.
SOURCE: Reproduced with permission from TB Fitzpatrick et al., Color Atlas and Synopsis of Clinical Dermatology, 4th edition. New York: McGraw-Hill, 2001.

3. Topical steroids are useful to treat cutaneous lesions. (See page 48 for more details.)

Systemic therapies include:

1. Antimalarials.
2. Systemic corticosteroids. The indications for prednisone (1 to 2 mg/kg per d po divided bid) include CNS involvement, renal involvement, severely ill patients without CNS involvement, and hemolytic crisis.
3. Immunosuppressive drugs may be necessary if renal disease is severe.
    a. Azathioprine.
    b. Cyclophosphamide.

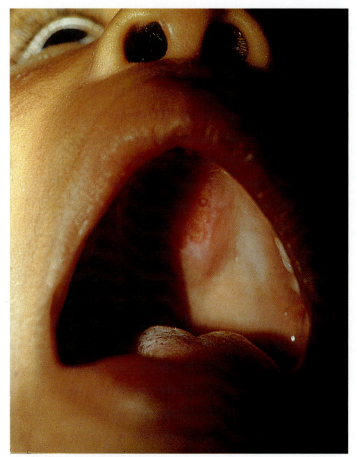

Figure 17-4 Systemic lupus erythematosus *Ulcers on the hard palate in a child with systemic lupus erythematosus.*

DERMATOMYOSITIS

Dermatomyositis (DM) is a systemic disease characterized by violaceous (heliotrope) inflammatory changes of the eyelids and periorbital area; erythema of the face, neck, and upper trunk; and flat-topped violaceous papules over the knuckles associated systemically with a polymyositis.

EPIDEMIOLOGY

Clinical Spectrum Ranges from DM with only cutaneous inflammation to polymyositis with only muscle inflammation.

Age Onset in childhood 25% (peak 5 to 12 years old). With adult DM, (> 50 years), 20% have an associated malignancy.

Gender F > M, 2:1.

Etiology Unknown. Often preceded by a viral illness.

Genetics Increased frequency of HLA-B8/HLA-DR3 in children and HLA-B14 in adults suggests a genetic predisposition exists.

PATHOPHYSIOLOGY

Acute and chronic inflammation of striated muscle accompanied by segmental necrosis of myofibers resulting in progressive muscle weakness.

HISTORY

In childhood DM, frequently there is a history of a preceding viral illness followed by fever, muscle weakness, fatigue, and a rash. Unlike adult DM, juvenile DM has decreased rate of malignancies and the mortality is low.

PHYSICAL EXAMINATION

Skin Findings

Types Periorbital heliotrope (reddish-purple) flush usually associated with some degree of edema. Dermatitis with varying degrees of erythema and scaling; may evolve to erosions and ulcers which heal with stellate, bizarre scarring. Flat-topped, violaceous papules (Gottron's papule/sign) with varying degrees of atrophy. Periungual erythema, telangiectasia, thrombosis of capillary loops, infarctions. Calcification in subcutaneous tissues and fascia common later in course of juvenile DM; may evolve to calcinosis universalis. Palmar erythema, skin atrophy, poikiloderma, calcinosis.

Color Reddish purple heliotrope color.

Distribution Photodistributed dermatitis—forehead, malar area (Fig. 17-5), neck, upper chest. Gottron's papules—dorsa of knuckles (sparing interarticular areas; Fig. 17-6) and nape of neck. ± Periungal telangectasia.

Mucous Membranes Vivid red hue on gumline, ulceration, white plaques on tongue and mucosa.

General Examination

Progressive muscle weakness affecting proximal/limb girdle muscles. Difficulty or inability to rise from sitting or supine position without using arms. Occasional involvement of facial/bulbar, pharyngeal, and esophageal muscles. Muscle tenderness and atrophy.

DIFFERENTIAL DIAGNOSIS

The diagnostic criteria for DM are a characteristic rash and two of the following.

1. Proximal muscle weakness.
2. Elevated serum "muscle enzyme" levels.
3. Diagnostic muscle biopsy.
4. Characteristic electromyographic (EMG) changes.

The differential diagnosis for DM includes lupus erythematosus, mixed connective tissue disease, steroid myopathy, trichinosis, and toxoplasmosis.

LABORATORY EXAMINATIONS

Dermatopathology Skin biopsy shows a flattening of epidermis, hydropic degeneration of basal cell layer, edema of upper dermis, scattered inflammatory infiltrate, PAS+ fibrinoid deposits at dermoepidermal junction and around

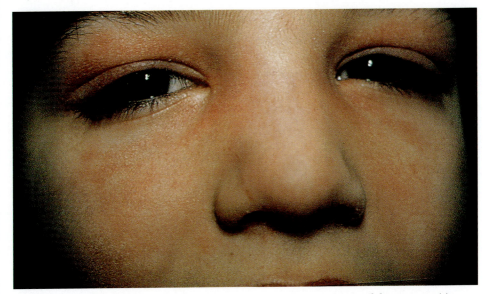

Figure 17-5 Dermatomyositis *Violaceous periorbital rash characteristic of dermatomyositis.*

upper dermal capillaries, and an accumulation of acid mucopolysaccharides in dermis. A muscle biopsy of a weak or tender muscle (i.e., deltoid, supraspinatus, gluteus, quadriceps) will show segmental necrosis within muscle fibers with loss of cross-striations; waxy/coagulative type of eosinophilic staining; ± regenerating fibers; inflammatory cells, histiocytes, macrophages, lymphocytes, plasma cells. Vasculitis may also be seen.

Chemistry During acute active phase elevation of creatine phosphokinase most specific for muscle disease; also aldolase, glutamic oxaloacetic transaminase, lactic dehydrogenase.

Urine Elevated 24-h creatinine excretion (> 200 mg/24 h).

Electromyography Increased irritability on insertion of electrodes, spontaneous fibrillations, pseudomyotonic discharges, positive sharp waves; excludes neuromyopathy. With evidence of denervation, suspect coexisting tumor.

ECG Evidence of myocarditis; atrial, ventricular irritability, atrioventricular block.

X-Ray of Chest ± Interstitial fibrosis.

COURSE AND PROGNOSIS

Dermatitis and polymyositis usually are detected at the same time; however, skin or muscle involvment can occur initially, followed at some time by the other. Juvenile DM, unlike adult DM, is rarely associated with Raynaud's phenomenon, malignancies, or mortality. In children, morbidity is higher with less functional recovery; 33% of patients will have spontaneous remission in 1 to 2 years; 33% of patients will have 1 to 2 relapses; and 33% of patients will have persistent symptoms > 2 years.

MANAGEMENT

1. Sun protection and avoidance.
2. NSAIDs and salicylates.
3. Topical steroids are useful to treat cutaneous lesions. (See page 48 for more details.)

Most childhood cases of DM require systemic steroids.

1. Systemic corticosteroids:
   a. Prednisone (1 to 3 mg/kg per d po divided bid until muscle enzymes have normalized).

In severe cases, immunosuppressive drugs may be necessary.

1. Azathioprine (Imuran, 1 to 3 mg/kg per d not to exceed 200 mg/d).
2. Methotrexate (1 mg/kg per week not to exceed 25 mg/week).
3. Cyclosporin (2.5 to 5 mg/kg per d).

Other possible therapies include:

1. Plasmapheresis.
2. Antimalarials.
3. Hydroxychloroquine.

In the acute stages, children may need hospitalization to monitor for palatorespiratory muscle involvement with myositis. In such cases, adequate respiration and prevention of aspiration is needed.

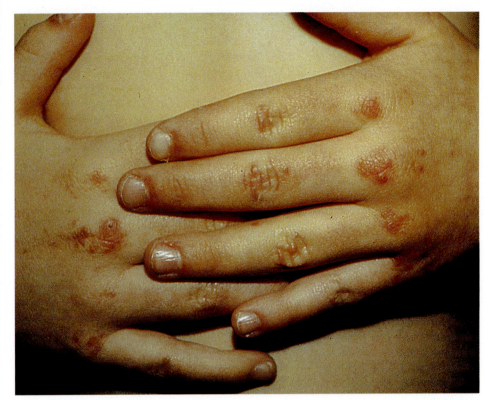

Figure 17-6   Dermatomyositis   *Gottron papules on the dorsa of the knuckles.*

MORPHEA

Morphea is a localized cutaneous sclerosis characterized by early violaceous-colored plaques later evolving to ivory-colored sclerotic areas, which may be solitary, linear, or generalized.

Synonyms Localized scleroderma, circumscribed scleroderma.

EPIDEMIOLOGY

Age Onset in childhood, young adults. Average age of onset is 5 years old.

Etiology Unknown. Possibly infection-related from *Borrelia* in western Europe. Lichen sclerosis may be somehow related.

HISTORY

The onset of morphea is insidious with erythematous violaceous plaques that evolve into firm, waxy, ivory-colored sclerotic areas.

PHYSICAL EXAMINATION

Skin Findings

Classification by pattern of involvement
Circumscribed or localized: plaques or bands.
Linear: extremity.
Frontoparietal: En coup de sabre; linear morphea occurring on the head with or without hemiatrophy of face.
Pansclerotic: generalized involvement (trunk, extremities, face, scalp with sparing of fingertips and toes) with deep atrophy of the underlying dermis, fat, fascia, muscle, and bone.

Type *Plaques:* initially, indurated but poorly defined areas. In time, surface become smooth and shiny; hair follicles and sweat duct orifices disappear. *Vesicles, bullae, purpura, telangiectasia:* may be seen later in course. Deep involvement of tissue may be associated with atrophy of muscle and bone, with resultant growth disturbance in children and flexion contracture; pseudoainhum-like lesion may occur circumferentially on limb with subsequent distal edema. Scalp involvement results in scarring alopecia.

Size Few mm to several cm.

Color Initially, purplish; after months to years becomes ivory colored (Fig. 17-7). With generalized morphea, may have generalized hyperpigmentation in involved areas.

Shape Round or oval.

Palpation Indurated, hard. May be hypoesthetic.

Arrangement Usually multiple, bilateral, asymmetric. May be linear on extremity or scalp.

Distribution *Localized:* trunk, limbs, face, genitalia. Less commonly, axillae, perineum, areola.
Linear: usually on extremity.
Frontoparietal: scalp and face.
Generalized: initially on trunk (upper, breasts, abdomen), thighs.

Hair and Nails Scarring alopecia with scalp involvement of plaque, generalized, or frontoparietal morphea. Nail dystrophy in linear lesions of extremity or pansclerotic morphea.

Mucous Membranes With linear morphea of head, may have associated hemiatrophy of tongue.

General Examination

Involvement around joints may lead to flexion contractures, especially of hands and feet. Deeper involvement of tissue associated with atrophy and fibrosis of muscle. Extensive involvement may result in restricted respiration. With linear morphea of head, may have associated atrophy of ocular structures and atrophy of bone.

DIFFERENTIAL DIAGNOSIS

The diagnosis of morphea is made by clinical history, physical findings, and at times, confirmed by skin biopsy. The differential diagnosis includes: progressive systemic sclerosis, lichen sclerosis et atrophicus, eosinophilic fasciitis, eosinophilia-myalgia syndrome as-

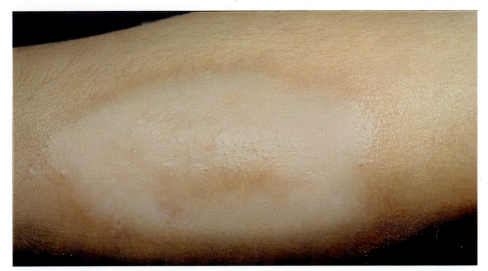

Figure 17-7 Morphea *Sclerotic depigmented plaque on the shin of a young child.*

sociated with L-tryptophan ingestion, acro-dermatitis chronica atrophicans, and sclero-derma.

LABORATORY EXAMINATIONS

Dermatopathology Skin biopsy shows swelling and degeneration of collagen fibrils; with later lesions these become homogeneous and eosinophilic. Slight infiltrate, perivascular or diffuse; lymphocytes, plasma cells, macrophages. Later, dermis thickened with few fibroblasts and dense collagen; inflammatory infiltrate at dermal-subcutis junction; dermal appendages progressively disappear. Pansclerotic lesions show fibrosis and disappearance of subcutaneous tissue, fibrosis broadening as well as sclerosis of fascia. Silver stains can be performed to rule out *B. burgdorferi* infection.

Serology Serologic testing can be performed to rule out *B. burgdorferi* infection.

COURSE AND PROGNOSIS

Guttate and plaque-like lesions of morphea in children tend to improve in 3 to 5 years, but can persist for life.

MANAGEMENT

1. Physical therapy is warranted for lesions overlying joints, which may impede mobility.
2. Topical steroids are of limited use.
   a. Low potency steroids (Desowen, 1% hydrocortisone, 2.5% hydrocortisone) should be used on face or groin area, no more than bid × 2 weeks.
   b. Medium potency steroids (Elocon, Dermatop, Cutivate) should be used on the body or extremities no more than bid × 2 weeks.
   c. Strong steroids (Ultravate, Psorcon, Diprolene) are reserved for older children and adults on severely affected areas bid for no more than 2 weeks. (See page 48 for more details.)
3. Intralesional steroids are also of limited use.
4. Topical vitamin D (Dovonex applied bid to lesions) has also been tried with mixed results.

Severe cases may require systemic therapies, such as systemic steroids, antimalarials, phenytoin, methotrexate, penicillamine, salazoprine, cyclosporine, colchicine, calcipitriol, but many are of limited benefit.

SCLERODERMA

Scleroderma is a rare but severe multisystem disorder characterized by sclerotic changes of the skin, lungs, heart, GI tract, joints, and kidneys.

Synonyms Progressive systemic sclerosis, systemic sclerosis, systemic scleroderma.

EPIDEMIOLOGY

Age All ages. Uncommon in children. Average age of onset 30 to 50 years old.

Gender F > M, 4:1.

Etiology Unknown.

Clinical Variant CREST syndrome, i.e., Calcinosis cutis + Raynaud's phenomenon + Esophageal dysfunction + Sclerodactyly + Telangiectasia.

Genetics Familial cases reported.

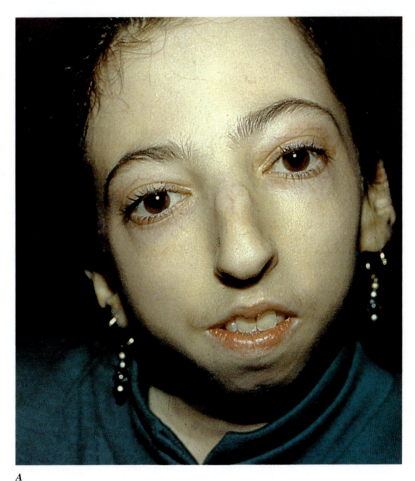

A

Figure 17-8 **Scleroderma** *(A) Mask-like facies in a patient with scleroderma.*

PATHOPHYSIOLOGY

The pathogenesis of systemic sclerosis is unknown. The primary event might be endothelial cell injury in blood vessels. Early in the course of the disease, target organ edema occurs followed by fibrosis; the cutaneous capillaries are reduced in number and the remaining vessels dilate and proliferate, becoming visible telangiectasias. Fibrosis is also present due to overproduction of collagen by fibroblasts.

HISTORY

Raynaud's phenomenon with digital pain, coldness, rubor, with pain and tingling of the fingertips and toes is usually the first sign of scleroderma. Patients with scleroderma have a characteristic tightening of the facial features producing a pinched-nose, pursed-lip appearance (Fig. 17-8A). Systemic involvement leads to migratory polyarthritis, heartburn, dysphagia, constipation, diarrhea, abdominal bloating, malabsorption, weight loss, exertional dyspnea, and dry cough.

PHYSICAL EXAMINATION

Skin Findings

Types of Lesions
Hands and feet: Early in course, Raynaud's phenomenon with triphasic color changes (i.e., pallor, cyanosis, rubor). Nonpitting edema of hands and feet. Painful ulcerations at fingertips, knuckles; heal with pitted scars. Later, sclerodactyly with tapering fingers, waxy shiny atrophic skin; flexion contractures (Fig. 17-8B); bony resorption results in loss of distal phalanges. Cutaneous calcification over bony prominences and end of fingers associated with white exudate from ulcerations (Fig. 17-8C). Matlike telangiectasia especially on face, neck, upper trunk, hands; also lips, oral mucous membranes, GI tract.
Face: Early, periorbital edema; later, edema and fibrosis result in loss of normal facial lines, masklike, thinning of lips, small mouth, radial perioral furrowing, small sharp nose.

Color Hyperpigmentation, generalized. In areas of sclerosis, postinflammatory hyper- and hypopigmentation.

Palpation Early, skin feels indurated, stiff; later, tense, smooth, hardened, bound down. Leathery crepitation over joints, especially knees.

Distribution Fingers, hands, upper extremities, trunk, face, lower extremities.

Hair and Nails Thinning/complete loss of hair on distal extremities. Loss of sweat glands with anhidrosis. Periungual telangiectasia with giant sausage-shaped capillary loops. Nails grow clawlike over shortened distal phalanges.

Mucous Membranes Sclerosis of sublingual ligament; uncommonly, painful induration of gums, tongue.

General Examination

Lung Restricted movement of chest wall due to pulmonary fibrosis.

Musculoskeletal System Carpal tunnel syndrome. Muscle weakness.

DIFFERENTIAL DIAGNOSIS

Systemic sclerosis is diagnosed when the characteristic sclerosis of the face and hands is recognized. Other sclerotic entities that need to be considered in the differential diagnosis include mixed connective tissue disease, eosinophilic fasciitis, lupus erythematosus, dermatomyositis, morphea, chronic graft-versus-host disease, lichen sclerosis et atrophicus, polyvinyl chloride exposure, and adverse drug reaction (pentazocine, bleomycin).

LABORATORY EXAMINATIONS

Dermatopathology On skin biopsy, a mild cellular infiltrate around dermal blood vessels, eccrine coils, subcutaneous tissue will be evident. Later lesions show effacement of the rete ridges; paucity of blood vessels, thickening and hyalinization of vessel walls, narrowing of lumen; atrophied dermal appendages; calcium deposits and homogenized collagen.

Serology Immunofluorescence staining shows speckled antinuclear antibodies.

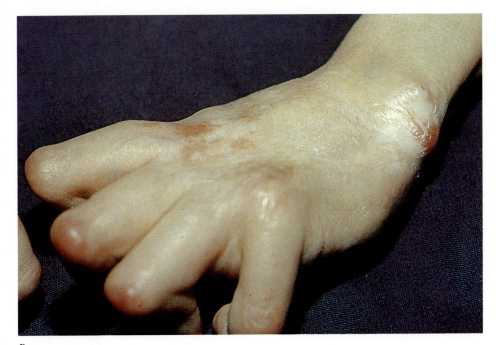

B

Figure 17-8 (continued)   Scleroderma   (B) *Debilitating joint contractures of the hands.*

COURSE AND PROGNOSIS

The course of systemic sclerosis is characterized by slow relentless progression of skin and/or visceral sclerosis; 80% of patients die within 10 years after the onset of symptoms. The leading cause of death is renal failure followed by cardiac and pulmonary dysfunction. Spontaneous remissions do occur. CREST syndrome progresses more slowly and has a more favorable prognosis.

MANAGEMENT

The treatment of scleroderma is primarily symptomatic.

1. Avoidance of vasospastic agents is recommended (cold, stress, fatigue).
2. Minimizing trauma to the extremities.
3. For polyarthritis, salicylates and NSAIDs are helpful.
4. For Raynaud's phenomenon the following are helpful, but their use in children is strictly off-label.
   a. Nifedipine (Procardia).
   b. Pentoxifylline (Trental).
5. For GI involvement and reflux, the patient should try to eat small frequent meals, to elevate the head of the bed, and antacids.

For severe cases, systemic theraputic modalities such as corticosteroids, extracorporeal photophoresis, calcipotriol, D-penicillamine, colchicine, and potassium p-aminobenzoate have been tried and are of limited benefit.

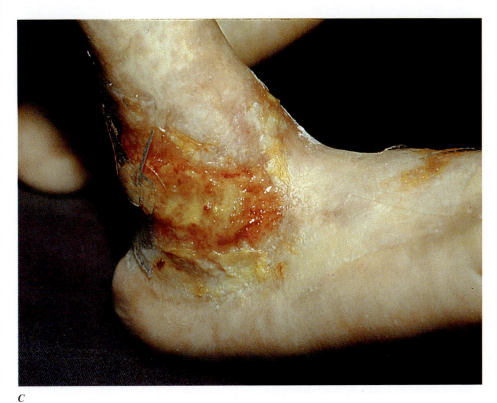

C

Figure 17-8 (continued) **Scleroderma** *(C)* *Ulceration of sclerotic ankle with extruding white calcified material.*

ENDOCRINE AUTOIMMUNE DISORDERS AND THE SKIN

ACANTHOSIS NIGRICANS

Acanthosis nigricans (AN) is a diffuse velvety thickening and hyperpigmentation of the skin, chiefly in axillae and other body folds, the etiology of which may be related to factors of hereditary, associated endocrine disorders, obesity, drug administration, and, in one rare form, malignancy.

EPIDEMIOLOGY

Classification
Type 1—hereditary benign AN: no associated endocrine disorder.

Type 2—benign AN: various endocrine disorders associated with insulin resistance: insulin-resistant diabetes mellitus, hyperandrogenic states, acromegaly and gigantism, Cushing's disease, glucocorticoid therapy, diethylstilbestrol and oral contraceptives, growth hormone therapy, hypogonadal syndromes with insulin resistance, Addison's disease, hypothyroidism.

Type 3—pseudo AN: complication of obesity; more commonly seen in patients with darker pigmentation. Obesity produces insulin resistance.

Type 4—drug-induced AN: nicotinic acid in high dosage, stilbestrol in young males, oral contraceptives.

Type 5—malignant AN: paraneoplastic, usually adenocarcinoma; less commonly, lymphoma.

Age *Type 1:* onset during childhood or puberty.

PATHOPHYSIOLOGY

Epidermal changes may be caused by hypersecretion of pituitary peptide, or nonspecific growth-promoting effect of hyperinsulinemia.

HISTORY

Usually insidious onset, first visible change is darkening of pigmentation.

PHYSICAL EXAMINATION

Skin Findings

Type of Lesion Darkening of pigmentation, skin appears dirty. As skin thickens, appears velvety; skin lines further accentuated; surface becomes rugose, mammillated (Fig. 18-1).

Type 3 AN: velvety patch on inner, upper thigh at site of chafing; often has many skin tags in body folds, especially axillae, groins.

Type 5 AN: hyperkeratosis and hyperpigmentation more pronounced. Hyperkeratosis of palms and soles, involvement of oral mucosa and vermilion border of lips.

Color Dark brown to black.

Palpation Velvety texture.

Distribution of Lesions Most commonly, axillae, neck (back, sides); also groin, anogenitalia, antecubital fossa, knuckles, submammary, umbilicus.

Mucous Membranes Oral mucosa, velvety texture with delicate furrows.

Type 5: mucous membranes and mucocutaneous junctions commonly involved; warty papillomatous thickenings periorbitally, periorally.

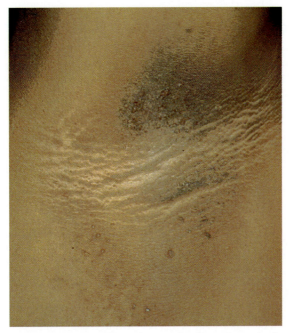

Figure 18-1   Acanthosis nigricans   *Hyperpigmented velvety plaque in the axillary area.*

General Examination

Examine for underlying endocrine disorder in benign AN and search for malignancy in malignant AN.

DIFFERENTIAL DIAGNOSIS

History and physical examination differentiate this entity from confluent and reticulated papillomatosis (Gougerot–Carteaud syndrome). The finding of abundant *Pityrosporum orbiculare* and response to minocycline therapy may support the latter diagnosis.

LABORATORY EXAMINATIONS

Dermatopathology   Papillomatosis, hyperkeratosis; epidermis thrown into irregular folds, showing varying degrees of acanthosis.

COURSE AND PROGNOSIS

Type 1: accentuated at puberty, and, at times, regresses when older.
Type 2: may regress subsequent to significant weight loss.

Type 3: resolves when causative drug discontinued.
Type 4: AN may precede other symptoms of malignancy by 5 years; removal of malignancy may be followed by regression of AN.

MANAGEMENT

Treatment of acanthosis nigricans should include a careful work-up to exclude any underlying endocrine disorder. In children, acanthosis nigricans is rarely a sign of an underlying malignancy. Correction of any underlying disorder (obesity, endocrine disease) improves the skin condition. Cosmetically, acanthosis nigricans is difficult to treat, but some improvement may be gained with:

1. Topical retinoic acid.
    a.   Tretinoin (Retin A, Renova).
    b.   Adapelene (Differin).
2. Topical hydroxy acids.
    a.   Lactic acid (Lac-Hydrin, Epilyt).
    b.   Glycolic acid (Aquaglycolic).
    c.   10 to 20% urea (Carmol).
3. Gentle loofah or "Buf-Puf."

NECROBIOSIS LIPOIDICA DIABETICORUM

Necrobiosis lipoidica diabeticorum (NLD) is a cutaneous disorder often associated with diabetes mellitus (DM). The lesions are distinctive, sharply circumscribed, multicolored (red, yellow, brown), atrophic macules occurring on the anterior and lateral surfaces of the lower legs.

EPIDEMIOLOGY

Age Adolescents, young adults, can also be seen in juvenile diabetic patients.

Gender F > M, 3:1, in both diabetic and non-diabetic forms.

Incidence Less than 1% of diabetics, > two thirds of patients with NLD have overt diabetes mellitus, and 90% of the remainder can be shown to develop an abnormal glucose tolerance.

Precipitating Factor A history of preceding trauma to the site can be a factor in the initial development of the lesions, and for this reason, NLD is often present on the shins and over the bony areas of the feet.

PATHOPHYSIOLOGY

The granulomatous inflammatory reaction is believed to be due to alterations in the collagen. The arteriolar changes in the areas of necrobiosis of the collagen have been thought by some to be precipitated by aggregation of platelets.

HISTORY

NLD skin lesions evolve slowly and enlarge over months. The skin lesions are typically asymptomatic, but ulcerated lesions are painful.

Systems Review Diabetes may or may not be present at the time of onset of lesions; diabetes mellitus, however, develops in the majority of patients.

PHYSICAL EXAMINATION

Skin Findings

Types of Lesions
Characteristic lesions: early lesions are small and dusky red, and as the lesions enlarge, the center becomes atrophic and there is usually a raised brownish-red border; there are waxy yellow atrophic areas, in which many well-marked telangiectases are seen throughout the center of the lesion where the atrophy is most prominent (Fig. 18-2).
Less common lesions: nodules the color of the skin, and rarely on the elbows small annular lesions without epidermal atrophy appear and these closely mimic granuloma annulare or sarcoidosis.
Ulcers: (shallow, painful, and slow-healing) not infrequently develop.

Shape Serpiginous, irregularly irregular.

Arrangement Often symmetrical.

Distribution More than 80% occur on the legs and feet (shins, bony areas of the feet, heels); other areas include arms, trunk, or the face and scalp.

LABORATORY EXAMINATIONS

Dermatopathology On skin biopsy, the lower dermis shows sclerotic collagen and obliteration of the bundle pattern, necrobiosis of connective tissue, and concomitant granulomatous infiltration. Fat-containing foam cells are often present, imparting the yellow color to the clinical lesion. There is a "microangiopathy," with thickening of the capillary walls with endothelial thickening and focal deposits of PAS-positive material.

Immunofluorescence Presence of immunoglobulins and complement (C3). Immune complexes may occur in the walls of the small blood vessels.

Special Techniques *Special stains:* fat stains.

Chemistry Evidence of frank diabetes, or an abnormal glucose tolerance.

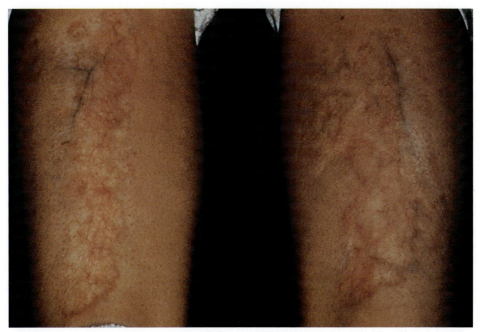

Figure 18-2 Necrobiosis lipoidica diabeticorum *Well-demarcated yellow-orange plaques on the bilateral shins of a young female diabetic patient.*

DIFFERENTIAL DIAGNOSIS

The diagnosis is usually made with clinical history and physical examination. It can be confirmed by skin biopsy. The differential diagnosis includes xanthomas, sarcoidosis, and granuloma annulare.

COURSE AND PROGNOSIS

The lesions are indolent and can enlarge to involve large areas of the skin surface unless treated. Up to 30% of the patients have clinical DM, 30% have an abnormal glucose tolerance test, and 30% have a normal glucose tolerance.

The severity of NLD is not related to the severity of the diabetes mellitus. Furthermore, control of the diabetes has no effect on the course of NLD.

MANAGEMENT

Most patients are most upset by the clinical appearance of the lesions rather than the symptoms. Lesions can be improved with:

Corticosteroids Topical steroids, with or without occlusion, are of slight benefit. Cordran tape is a flurandrenolide-impregnated adhesive tape that is useful for this condition. Intralesional steroids can be used in more resistant cases.

GRANULOMA ANNULARE

Granuloma annulare (GA) is a common self-limited dermatosis of unclear etiology, clinically characterized by dermal papules arranged in an annular configuration commonly on the dorsa of the hands, feet, elbows, and knees.

EPIDEMIOLOGY

Age Usually children, but can be any age.

Gender F:M 2:1.

Etiology Unknown. Reported to follow insect bites, trauma, viral infections (EBV, VZV, HIV), sun exposure, PUVA therapy, tuberculin skin test. Generalized GA may be associated with diabetes mellitus.

Genetics Familial cases have been reported.

PATHOPHYSIOLOGY

Unclear. It is thought that GA probably represents an immune-mediated necrobiotic inflammation of collagen and elastin fibers.

HISTORY

The solitary skin lesions appear sporadically and are asymptomatic. Most self-resolve in a few months to years. More generalized GA can persist for years and have a more recalcitrant course.

PHYSICAL EXAMINATION

Skin Lesions

Type Firm, smooth, shiny, dermal papules and plaques. Some nodules or subcutaneous swellings.

Size 1 to 5 cm.

Color Color of the skin to erythematous to violaceous.

Shape Papules are dome-shaped.

Arrangement Annular (Fig. 18-3) or arciform.

Distribution Isolated lesion can occur anywhere on the body. Generalized GA can affect a localized region or entire body.

Sites of Predilection

Solitary annular lesions: dorsa of hands and feet, extensor surfaces of arms and legs, and trunk.
Subcutaneous nodules: palms, legs, buttocks, scalp.

DIFFERENTIAL DIAGNOSIS

The diagnosis of GA is usually made from the history and clinical examination. A skin biopsy can be confirmatory. The differential diagnosis includes lichen planus, tinea, psoriasis, papular sarcoid, annular erythema, SCLE, erythema multiforme, erythema chronicum migrans.

LABORATORY EXAMINATIONS

Dermatopathology Skin biopsy reveals palisading granulomas in the upper/mid reticular dermis with a central zone of necrobiotic collagen surrounded by histiocytes, lymphocytes, and a few giant cells.

COURSE AND PROGNOSIS

Solitary lesions of GA have a good prognosis. More than 50% of lesions resolve in 2 years, but there is a 40% recurrence rate. Disseminated GA has a persistent and more recalcitrant course, but is uncommonly seen in children. Up to 21% of patients with generalized GA have diabetes mellitus.

MANAGEMENT

The skin lesions are typically asymptomatic and will eventually self-resolve, thus treatment is unnecessary. Symptomatic or extensive lesions can be treated with:

1. Topical steroids with or without occlusion.
   a. Low potency steroids (Desowen, 1% hydrocortisone, 2.5% hydrocortisone)

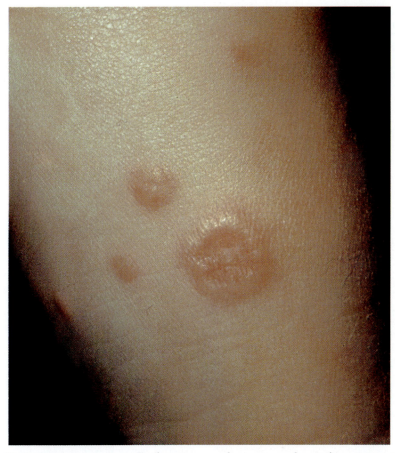

Figure 18-3 Granuloma annulare *Erythematous papules in an annular configuration on the leg.*

should be used on face or groin area, no more than bid × 2 weeks.

b. Medium potency steroids (Elocon, Dermatop, Cutivate) should be used on the body or extremities no more than bid × 2 weeks.

c. Strong steroids (Ultravate, Psorcon, Diprolene) are reserved for older children and adults on severely affected areas bid for no more than 2 weeks. Cordran tape is a flurandrenolide-impregnated adhesive tape that is useful for this condition.

2. Intralesional steroids can be used in more resistant cases. Other treatment modalities include cryotherapy, PUVA.

ALOPECIA AREATA

Alopecia areata (AA) is a localized loss of hair in round or oval areas without any visible inflammation, typically on the scalp. Alopecia totalis is the loss of all the scalp hair and alopecia universalis is the loss of the scalp and all body hair.

EPIDEMIOLOGY

Age   Children are frequently affected; 60% of patients present before age 20 years.

Gender   M = F.

Incidence   Up to 2% of dermatology visits in the U.S. and UK.

Family   History of AA seen in 10 to 42% of cases.

Etiology   Thought to be an autoimmune disease of T lymphocytes directed against the hair follicles. May be associated with other autoimmune disorders such as vitiligo, familial multiendocrine syndrome, and thyroid disease (Hashimoto's disease). Emotional problems, especially life crises, could reportedly precipitate some cases of AA.

HISTORY

Patients usually report abrupt hair loss and will present with an asymptomatic bald spot on the scalp. More spots may appear and in severe cases, can lead to loss of all the scalp and/or body hair. Most cases of localized areas in the scalp slowly regrow hair over a period of weeks to months.

PHYSICAL EXAMINATION

Skin Lesions

Hair

Type   Well-circumscribed area of non-scarring alopecia (Fig. 18-4) with diagnostic proximally-tapered short hairs called "exclamation point hairs" (Fig. 18-5).

Shape   Round to oval.

Size   1 cm to several cm.

Distribution   Localized (to scalp or body) or regional with total loss of scalp hair (alopecia totalis) or generalized with total loss of scalp and body hair (alopecia universalis).

Sites of Predilection   Scalp, eyebrows, eyelashes, pubic hair, beard.

Nails

Dystrophic changes (20%): fine stippling like "hammered brass" (Fig. 18-6).

DIFFERENTIAL DIAGNOSIS

Alopecia areata can usually be diagnosed clinically especially with the presence of exclamation point hairs. The differential diagnosis includes telogen effluvium, trichotillomania, androgenetic alopecia, secondary syphilis ("moth-eaten" appearance in beard or scalp), or tinea capitis.

LABORATORY EXAMINATIONS

Dermatopathology   Peribulbar lymphocytic infiltrate, miniaturized hairs with fibrous tracts, and pigment incontinence. There is also a decreased anagen-to-telogen ratio.

COURSE AND PROGNOSIS

In the majority of patients, hair will regrow in less than 1 year without treatment. Total alopecia is rare. Recurrences of alopecia, however, are frequent and 7 to 10% of cases can have a chronic form of the condition. Repeated attacks, nail changes, and total alopecia before puberty are poor prognostic signs.

MANAGEMENT

No treatment changes the course of the disease, but some palliative options include:

1. Topical steroids are of limited benefit.
    a. Clobetasol propionate ointment (qd–bid × 6 weeks only, as skin atrophy can occur).

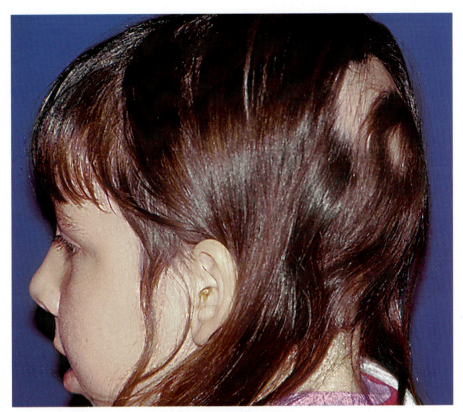

Figure 18-4 Alopecia areata, scalp *Sudden onset of well-circumscribed areas of non-scarring alopecia in an otherwise healthy child.*

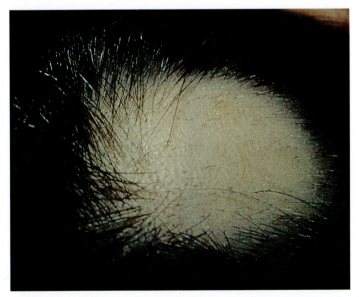

Figure 18-5 Alopecia areata, scalp *Oval area of non-scarring alopecia on the scalp with evidence of "exclamation point hairs" (short hairs that taper proximally).*

ALOPECIA AREATA

2. Intralesional steroids (for children > 10 years) is most useful.
   a. Triamcinolone acetonide (diluted 2.5 to 5 mg/mL, 0.1 mL injected intradermally per site, not to exceed 3 mL total q4 to 6 weeks).
3. Minoxidil (Rogaine 5% solution applied bid).
4. Anthralin (0.25 to 1% cream applied qd).
5. Topical immunotherapy with sensitizers include squaric acid dibutyl ester (SADBE) and diphenylcyclopropenone (DPCP).

For more severe or refractory cases, systemic approaches, such as corticosteroids, photochemotherapy, and immunotherapy can be used, but relapses are common and thus these approaches are not highly recommended.

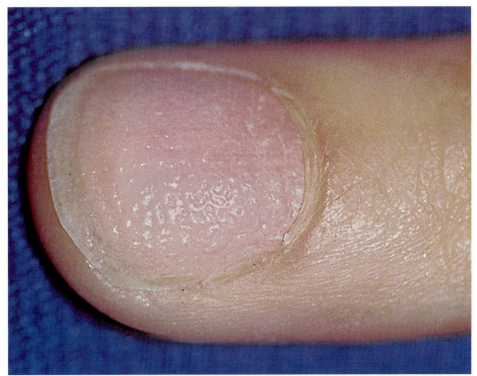

Figure 18-6   Alopecia areata, nails   *Pitting in organized transverse rows giving the nail a "hammered brass" appearance.*

SKIN SIGNS OF RETICULOENDOTHELIAL DISEASE

HISTIOCYTOSIS

LANGERHANS CELL HISTIOCYTOSIS (HISTIOCYTOSIS X)

Langerhans cell histiocytosis (LCH) is an idiopathic group of disorders characterized histologically by proliferation and infiltration of tissue by Langerhans cell-type histiocytes. These fuse into multinucleated giant cells and form granulomas with eosinophils. Clinically, LCH is characterized by lytic bony lesions and cutaneous findings that range from soft tissue swelling to eczema- and seborrheic dermatitis-like changes and ulceration.

Synonyms Type II histiocytosis, nonlipid reticuloendotheliosis, eosinophilic granulomatosis.

CLASSIFICATION

The disorders of xanthohistiocytic proliferation involving histiocytes, foam cells, and mixed inflammatory cells are divided into Langerhans cell (histiocytic X) (LCH) and non-Langerhans cell (non-histiocytic X) histiocytoses. LCH is classified as follows:

1. Localized LCH:
    a. Bone (for two adjacent lesions).
    b. Lymph node.
    c. Skin.
2. Disseminated LCH:
    a. Bone, multifocal.
    b. Bone and soft tissue or soft tissues alone (except skin and isolated lymph node).
    c. Organ dysfunction (liver, lungs, hemopoietic system).

Benign Unifocal LCH: most benign form. Typically manifested by a single osteolytic bony lesion. Skin and soft tissue lesions may or may not also be present (known as eosinophilic granuloma).

Benign Multifocal LCH: similar to unifocal LCH; however, bony lesions are multiple and interfere with function of neighboring structures. Multifocal LCH involves bones, skin (30% of patients, second most frequently involved organ), soft tissue, lymph nodes, lungs, and pituitary. Triad of lytic skull lesions, exophthalmos, and diabetes insipidus (known as Hand–Schüller–Christian disease).

Malignant Letterer–Siwe syndrome (LSS): the most aggressive of multifocal LCH forms, with skin involvement (in 30% of patients) and infiltration of various organs causing organomegaly and thrombocytopenia guarded prognosis.

PATHOPHYSIOLOGY

The proliferating Langerhans cell appears to be primarily responsible for the clinical manifestation. The stimulus for the proliferation is unknown. It may be secondary to a disturbance of intracellular lipid metabolism, a reactive response to infection, or a neoplastic process.

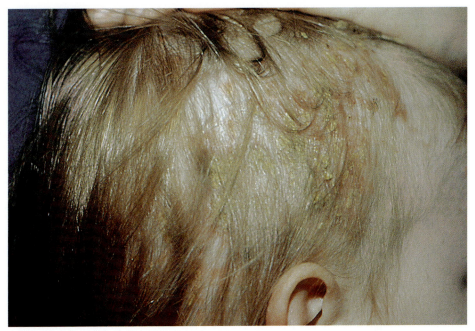

Figure 19-1 Histiocytosis X *Erythematous plaques with seborrhea-like scale on the scalp of an infant.*

EPIDEMIOLOGY

Age
Unifocal LCH: Children > 6 years old and adults.
Multifocal LCH: Children ages 2 to 6 years old.
LSS: Children < 3 years old.

Gender M > F.

Incidence Rare. 0.5 per 100,000 children in U.S.

HISTORY

Unifocal LCH: patient presents with pain and/or swelling over underlying bony lesion, a spontaneous fracture, disruption of teeth with mandibular disease, otitis media due to mastoid involvement, or a recalcitrant ulcer on oral or genital mucosa. Often, lesions are asymptomatic and diagnosed on radiographs for unrelated disorders. Systemic symptoms are uncommon.
Multifocal LCH: patient usually presents with erosive lesions that are exudative, pruritic, or painful, with poor response to local treatments.

Associated disorders include otitis media caused by destruction of temporal and mastoid bones, proptosis due to orbital masses, loose teeth with infiltration of maxilla or mandible, anterior and/or pituitary dysfunction with involvement of sella turcica. Diabetes insipidus occurs secondary to hypothalamic or pituitary involvement. Lung involvement can lead to a chronic cough or pneumothorax. Hand–Schüller–Christian disease: triad of lytic skull lesions, exophthalmos, and diabetes insipidus.
LSS: infant appears systemically ill with a course that resembles a systemic infection or malignancy. A generalized skin eruption with sebborrhea, petechiae, and purpura is followed by fever, anemia, thrombocytopenia, adenopathy, hepatosplenomegaly, and/or skeletal lesions.

PHYSICAL EXAMINATION

Skin Findings

Type

Unifocal LCG:

1. Swelling over bony lesion, over long or flat bone, tender.

2. Cutaneous/subcutaneous nodule, yellowish, may be tender and break down, occurring anywhere.
3. Sharply marginated ulcer with a necrotic base usually in genital and perigenital region or oral mucous membrane (gingiva, hard palate).

Multifocal LCH: As in unifocal LCH; in addition, regionally localized (head) or generalized eruptions. Papulosquamous, seborrheic dermatitis-like, eczematous dermatitis-like lesions; sometimes vesicular; lesions may be purpuric, necrotic; areas may coalesce with loss of epidermis; may become heavily crusted. Intertriginous lesions may be exudative and become secondarily infected and ulcerate. Mandibular and maxillary bone involvement may result in loss of teeth.

Palpation   Area overlying bony lesions may be tender; papulosquamous eruption usually rough due to crusting; removal of crusts occurs easily and leaves erosions and punched-out, flat ulcers.

Distribution   Tumorous swelling: calvarium, sphenoid bone, sella turcica, mandible, long bones of upper extremities. Papulosquamous eruptions on scalp (Fig. 19-1), face, and trunk, particularly abdomen and buttocks (Fig. 19-2). Skin lesions can be discrete and localized or disseminated and generalized. Ulcers: vulva, gingiva. Eczema- and seborrhea-like changes seen on scalp and in intertriginous areas; erosions occur in groin, axillae, retroauricular, neck.

General Findings

Unifocal LCH: pain and swelling over affected bony lesion, painful ulcer.
Multifocal LCH: bony lesions occur in calvarium, sphenoid bone, sella turcica, mandible, long bones of upper extremities, and vertebrae.
LSS: fever, hepatosplenomegaly, lymphadenopathy, involvement of lungs, bone marrow; thrombocytopenia.

DIFFERENTIAL DIAGNOSIS

All forms of LCH require confirmation of diagnosis by biopsy (skin, bone, or soft tissue/internal organs). Because skin is the organ most frequently involved after the bone, skin biopsies have great diagnostic significance (see below). Histiocytosis X is generally diagnosed by history, physical examination, and skin or organ biopsy. Often, bony lesions are detected as the first presenting symptom. The differential diagnosis includes seborrheic dermatitis, systemic infections (viral, bacterial, fungal), or a neoplastic disorder.

LABORATORY EXAMINATIONS

Histopathology   Constant histologic feature of LCH is proliferation of Langerhans cells that have abundant pale eosinophilic cytoplasm with indistinct cell borders; a folded, indented, kidney-shaped nucleus with finely dispersed chromatin; and small inconspicuous nucleoli. For diagnostic purposes, Langerhans cells in LCH have to be recognized by morphologic, ultrastructural (Birbeck granules on electron microscopy), histochemical, and immune histochemical markers (CD1a+, ATPase+, S-100+, alpha-D mannosidase+, peanut agglutinin+).

Radiographic Findings
Unifocal LCH: single osteolytic lesion in a long or flat bone (in children, calvarium, femur; in adults, rib).
Multifocal LCH: osteolytic lesions in calvarium, sphenoid bone, sella turcica, mandible, and/or long bones of upper extremities. Chest: diffuse micronodular and interstitial infiltrate in midzones and bases of lungs with sparing of costophrenic angles; later, honeycomb appearance, pneumothorax. Extent of osseous involvement established by bone scanning.
LSS: scans show organomegaly.

COURSE AND PROGNOSIS

Unifocal LCH: benign course with excellent prognosis for spontaneous resolution. Only 10% go on to multifocal LCH.
Multifocal LCH: spontaneous remissions possible. Prognosis worse with pulmonary involvement (seen in 30% of patients).
LSS: commonly fulminant and fatal. Spontaneous remissions uncommon. Current staging on scoring systems for evaluation of prognosis are based on number of organs involved, presence or absence of organ dysfunction, and age. The worst prognosis is in children < 6 months old with multifocal LCH and organ dysfunction. Death is caused by pulmonary, hepatic, or splenic involvement.

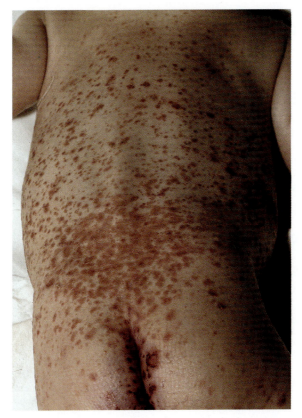

Figure 19-2 Langerhans cell histiocytosis *Erythematous papules and nodules with purpura on the back and buttocks on a child.* (Reproduced with permission from TB Fitzpatrick et al., Color Atlas and Synopsis of Clinical Dermatology, 4th edition. New York: McGraw-Hill, 2001).

MANAGEMENT

Unifocal LCG:

1. Bony lesions.
   a. Curettage removal of the lesion with or without bony chip packing.
   b. Low-dose (300 to 600 rads) radiotherapy.
2. Extraosseous soft tissue lesions.
   a. Surgical excision.
   b. Low-dose radiotherapy.

Multifocal LCG:

1. Diabetes insipidus and growth retardation treated with.
   a. Vasopressin.
   b. Human growth hormone.

2. Bony lesions treated with.
   a. Low-dose radiotherapy.
3. Aggressive disease can be systemically treated with.
   a. Corticosteroids.
   b. Vinblastine.
   c. Methotrexate.
   d. Epipodophyllotoxin (Etoposide).
4. For discrete cutaneous lesions.
   a. Topical corticosteroids.
   b. PUVA.
   c. Topical nitrogen mustard.

LSS: immunosuppressive drugs offer the most hope. They include prednisone, nitrogen mustard, vinblastine, vincristine, methotrexate, cyclophosphamide, and chlorambucil.

NON-HISTIOCYTOSIS DISORDERS

JUVENILE XANTHOGRANULOMA

Juvenile xanthogranulomas (JXG) are a benign, self-healing disease of infancy and childhood characterized by one or several red to yellow papules and nodules on the skin and rarely in other organs. The absence of Langerhans cells (no Birbeck granules on electron microscopy) differentiates JXG from the histiocytosis disorders.

Synonym Nevoxanthoendothelioma (a misnomer).

EPIDEMIOLOGY

Age Birth to 9 months of age.

Gender M = F.

Incidence Most common form of the non-histiocytosis X disorders.

Etiology Unclear. Possibly reactive granuloma to unknown cause.

HISTORY

Asymptomatic cutaneous JXGs are present at or soon after birth, may proliferate in number and size for 1 to 2 years and then both cutaneous and visceral lesions involute spontaneously within 3 to 6 years.

PHYSICAL EXAMINATION

Skin Findings

Type Papules to nodules

Color Initially red-brown (Fig. 19-3), transitioning to yellow quickly.

Size 2 to 20 mm in diameter.

Number Solitary or multiple (can be hundreds; Fig. 19-4).

Palpation Firm or rubbery.

Distribution Face, scalp, neck, proximal aspects of extremities or trunk, mucous membranes or mucocutaneous junctions.

Other Features Up to 20% have café au lait macules of neurofibromatosis. Ocular involvement is the most common extracutaneous manifestation. Mucous membrane involvement occasionally seen. Occasionally, systemic lesions affecting lungs, bones, kidneys, pericardium, colon, ovaries, and testes may be noted.

DIFFERENTIAL DIAGNOSIS

JXG is diagnosed by history, clinical presentation, and sometimes confirmed by skin biopsy. The differential for JXG includes nodular urticaria pigmentosa, benign cephalic histiocytosis, generalized eruptive histiocytoma, self-healing reticulohistiocytoma, tuberous xanthoma, papular xanthoma, nodular forms of histiocytosis X, and nevi.

LABORATORY EXAMINATIONS

Dermatopathology Skin biopsy of an early lesion shows a monomorphous, non-lipid-containing histiocytic infiltrate occupying the upper half and, sometimes, the entire thickness, of the dermis. Later, lesions show foamy cells, foreign body giant cells, and Touton giant cells in the superficial dermis and periphery of the infiltrate. Fat stains are positive.

Electron Microscopy EM shows histiocytes with pleomorphic nuclei, pseudopods, and elongated irregular dense bodies.

COURSE AND PROGNOSIS

JXG skin lesions are often present at birth or present during the first 9 months of life, run a benign course, often increasing in number until 1 to 1½ years of life and then spontaneously in-

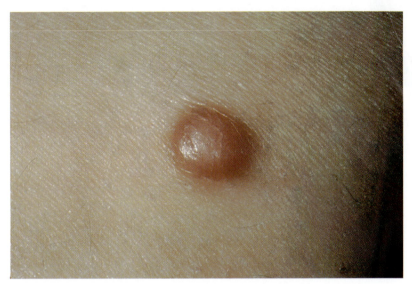

Figure 19-3 Juvenile xanthogranuloma *Solitary red-brown nodule on the arm of a small child.*

volute. Rarely, systemic lesions involving the eyes, lung, pericardium, meninges, liver, spleen, and testes also occur. The patient's general health is not affected and development progresses normally.

Ocular tumors are the most worrisome due to complications such as glaucoma, hemorrhage, and blindness. In rare instances, JXG may be seen in conjunction with neurofibromatosis and these patients have an increased risk of leukemia.

MANAGEMENT

No treatment is necessary for the cutaneous lesions. Ocular lesions require radiation and/or topical or systemic steroids to avert complications of glaucoma, hemorrhage, or blindness.

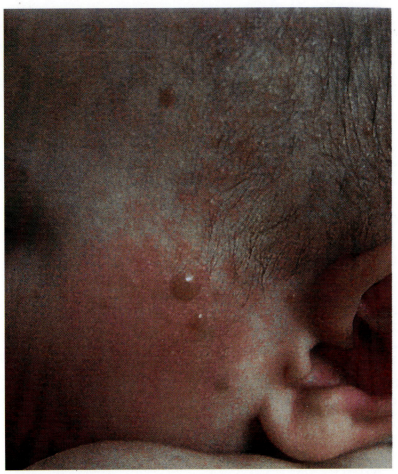

Figure 19-4   Juvenile xanthogranuloma   *Scattered 3–7 mm yellow-red papules on the face of a child with generalized lesions.*

MASTOCYTOSIS SYNDROMES

Mastocytosis is associated with an abnormal accumulation of mast cells within the skin and, rarely, other organs (the liver, spleen, and lymph nodes). In childhood, mastocytosis appears in three forms.

1. Individual lesions (solitary mastocytoma).
2. Generalized (urticaria pigmentosa).
3. Diffuse cutaneous mastocytosis.

In very rare instances, there is a malignant form of mast cell leukemia.

Synonyms Bullous mastocytoma, bullous urticaria pigmentosa, bullous mastocytosis.

EPIDEMIOLOGY

Age Birth to 2 years old; 50% of patients present with lesions in childhood, 50% present after age 15.

Gender M = F.

Incidence Uncommon. Estimated to occur in 1/8000 patients.

Prevalence 20,000 cases estimated in the United States.

Etiology Unknown.

Genetics Reported familial cases, but majority are sporadic.

PATHOPHYSIOLOGY

Mast cells contain vasoactive substances such as histamine (leads to urticaria and GI symptoms), prostaglandin D_2 (leads to flushing and cardiac and GI symptoms), heparin, and neutral protease/acid hydrolases.

HISTORY

In children, mastocytosis typically begins before age 2 with one to many scattered cutaneous lesions. The lesions may be flat or slightly raised but have a tendency to become red and form an urticarial wheal or bullae with gentle mechanical irritation, exercise, hot baths, or histamine releasing drugs (alcohol, dextran, polymyxin B, morphine, codeine). With extensive cutaneous involvement, the flushing episode may be accompanied by headache, diarrhea, wheezing, or syncope. Diffuse cutaneous mastocytosis presents as a diffusely erythrodermic infant with a boggy or doughy appearance.

PHYSICAL EXAMINATION

Skin Findings

Type Macule/papule that can become urticarial wheals/plaques or bullae when gently stroked (Darier's sign; Fig. 19-5).

Color Reddish-brown hyperpigmented color.

Size 1 mm to several cm.

Number Solitary lesions or multiple (hundreds; Fig. 19-6).

Distribution Any site. Multiple lesions are typically symmetric on trunk, extremities, and neck. Reported rare cases involving scalp, face, palms, soles, or mucous membranes.

General Findings

Rarely, hepatosplenomegaly.

DIFFERENTIAL DIAGNOSIS

Diagnosis of any mastocytosis disorder is made by history and physical examination; 90% of cutaneous lesions will demonstrate a positive Darier's sign (urticaria after gentle rubbing). Skin biopsy can confirm clinical suspicion. The differential diagnosis includes lentigines, juvenile xanthogranuloma, nevi, histiocytosis X, secondary syphilis, papular sarcoid, and generalized eruptive histiocytoma.

LABORATORY EXAMINATIONS

Dermatopathology Skin biopsy shows an abnormal accumulation of mast cells in the dermis. Mast cell infiltrates may be sparse (spindle-shaped mast cells) or dense (cube-shaped mast

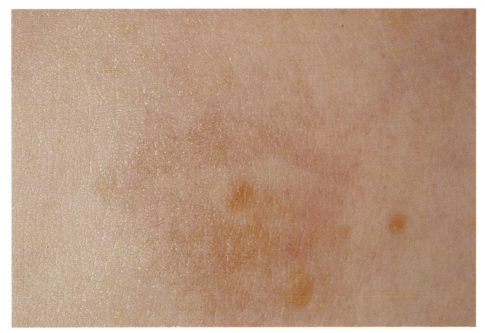

Figure 19-5 Mastocytosis, Darier's sign *Reddish-brown macules that urticate with mild trauma indicative of mastocytosis.*

cells). They can have metachromatic staining with Giemsa's or toluidine blue dyes.

Urine Patients with extensive cutaneous involvement may have increased 24-hour urinary histamine excretion (2 to 3 times normal, which is 36 ± 15 μg).

Bone Marrow Biopsy In bone marrow biopsies of children with urticaria pigmentosa, up to 18% can have mast cell infiltration.

COURSE AND PROGNOSIS

When seen in children <10 years old, all forms of mastocytosis have a good prognosis. Most childhood disease has limited cutaneous involvement; 50% of cases spontaneously remit by adolescence and another 25% of cases resolve by adulthood. Systemic involvement appears to affect < 5% of children with mastocytosis. This percentage is much higher in adults with mastocytosis and the prognosis is much worse. When systemic involvement occurs, mast cells infiltrate the bones, liver, spleen, and lymph nodes. The presence of mast cells in the peripheral blood of patients with mastocytosis is a grave prognostic sign.

MANAGEMENT

Solitary mastocytosis and urticaria pigmentosa cutaneous lesions self-resolve and need no treatment. Moderate sunlight exposure can help diffuse skin lesions resolve. Patients with numerous lesions or diffuse cutaneous mastocytosis should be counseled to avoid potential mast-cell degranulating drugs such as: aspirin, NSAIDs, codeine, opiates, procaine, alcohol, polymyxin B, radiographic dyes, ketorolac, toradol, scopolamine, D-tubocurarrine, gallamine, decamethonium, pancuronium, hot baths, vigorous rubbing after baths or showers, tight clothing, and extremes of temperature.

Antihistamines may be helpful and concomitant use of H_1- and H_2-blockers is suggested.

1. H_1-blockers
   a. Diphenhydramine (Benadryl, 5 mg/kg per d PO divided tid or qid).
   b. Hydroxyzine HCl (Atarax, 2 to 4 mg/kg per d divided tid or qid).
2. To avoid the sedation effects, a nonsedating H_1-blocker may be preferred.
   a. Cetirizine HCl (Zyrtec 2.5 to 10 mg PO qd).

3. In resistant cases, H_2-blockers can used in combination with H_1-blockers.
   a. Cimetidine (Tagamet, 10 to 40 mg/kg per d PO divided qid).
   b. Ranitidine hydrochloride (Zantac, 2 to 4 mg/dose PO bid).
4. A combination H_1- and H_2-blocker antidepressant used in low doses may be helpful, but pediatric use is strictly off-label.
   a. Doxepin (Sinequan or Adapin, 5 to 10 mg PO qd).

Other medications that have been helpful for diffuse cutaneous involvement include:

1. Oral cromolyn sodium (disodium cromoglycate 20 to 40 μg/kg per d divided qid).

2. PUVA can help but relapses after discontinuation are frequently seen.

Patients with mastocytosis should carry an epinephrine pen (Epi-pen) because severe allergic reactions can occur. Additional diagnostic evaluation should be performed in patients with evidence of further organ system involvement such as GI bleeding, abdominal pain, enlarged liver or spleen, bone pain, or blood abnormalities. Those tests might include liver/spleen imaging and/or bone imaging (x-ray or bone scan).

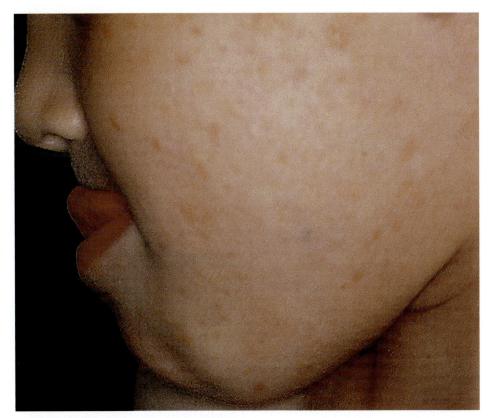

Figure 19-6   Mastocytosis, urticaria pigmentosa   *Numerous scattered red-brown macules on the body of the same child.*

LYMPHOMATOID PAPULOSIS

Lymphomatoid papulosis (LyP) is a recurrent self-healing papulovesicular dermatosis of trunk and extremities with histologic features suggestive of lymphocytic atypia and a low, but real, risk of malignant transformation.

EPIDEMIOLOGY

Age Ranges from very young to very old; average age of about 40 years.

Gender M = F.

Incidence Rare.

Etiology Unclear.

PATHOPHYSIOLOGY

The pathophysiology of LyP is unknown. The presence of antigens associated with Hodgkin's lymphoma as well as the detection of antibodies to HTLV-I in some patients suggests that the disease is a low-grade lymphoma contained by the host immune response.

HISTORY

LyP begins as asymptomatic or mildly pruritic macules and papules that appear in crops within 1 to 4 weeks. Lesions may resolve within 3 to 6 weeks or persist for longer periods. If present, it should be followed and if constitutional symptoms (low grade fever, malaise, night sweats) occur, a work-up for progression to lymphoma may be indicated.

PHYSICAL EXAMINATION

Skin Findings

Type Papules and vesiculopapules with a smooth, scaly, crusty, or ulcerative surface. Active lesions have hemorrhagic centers and resolve with variliform scars. Occasionally, large ulcerating nodules or plaques may occur.

Color Reddish-brown to hyperpigmented (Fig. 19-7).

Size 2 to 30 mm in diameter.

Arrangement Lesions appear in crops, limited to one or two areas of the body or widespread.

Distribution Trunk and proximal extremities, occasionally on hands, feet, scalp.

Mucous Membranes Oral and genital mucosa rarely can be affected.

General Findings

Regional or generalized lymphadenopathy may be present.

DIFFERENTIAL DIAGNOSIS

The diagnosis of LyP is made on history and physical examination and can be confirmed by skin biopsy. The differential for LyP includes pityriasis lichenoides et varioliformis acuta (PLEVA), cutaneous Hodgkin's lymphoma, or cutaneous T-cell lymphoma (CTCL).

LABORATORY EXAMINATIONS

Dermatopathology Skin biopsy shows a moderately dense mixed cell infiltrate with a wedge or band-like distribution on the upper dermis. The infiltrate is composed of histiocytes, eosinophils, plasma cells, and strikingly atypical lymphocytes with convoluted nuclei. According to the principal morphologic type, LyP is classified into type A, which consists of large atypical lymphocytes with multinucleated variants and cells resembling Sternberg–Reed cells, and type B, composed of cerebriform lymphocytes similar to cells in CTCL.

Immunohistology Dominant cells in LyP express Ki-1 antigen (Ber-H2) previously associated with Hodgkin's disease and Sternberg–Reed cells.

COURSE AND PROGNOSIS

Up to 10 to 20% of adult cases of LyP evolve into malignant lymphoma (CTCL, Hodgkin's disease, non-Hodgkin's lymphoma), malignancy is rare in childhood. In 90% of childhood cases, the lesions usually resolve after

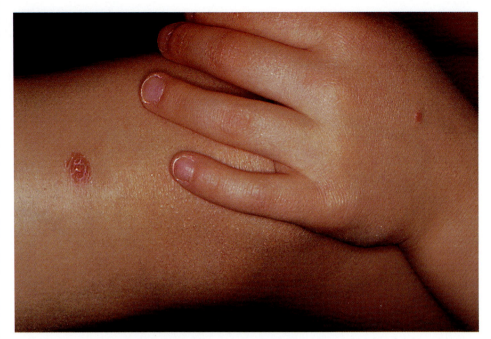

Figure 19-7 Lymphomatoid papulosis *Few scattered red-brown papules and nodules on the extremities of a young otherwise healthy child.*

3 to 8 weeks or may have a slightly prolonged course. Development of nodules or tumors may be a useful clinical sign for malignant transformation of the disease and patients with such lesions should have a systemic work-up.

MANAGEMENT

No treatments have been proven to be consistently effective. Many childhood cases resolve spontaneously or with sunlight exposure. Pruritic symptoms and lesions can be treated topically with steroids. (See page 48 for more details.)

Because of the risk of malignant transformation, especially in adults, careful long-term follow-up is recommended.

For more severe or refractory and extensive disease in adults, reported systemic treatments such as steroids, antibiotics (tetracycline, erythromycin), sulfones, PUVA, electron beam therapy, low dose methotrexate, acyclovir, retinoids, chlorambucil, cyclophosphamide, cyclosporin, or interferon alpha-2b have been tried.

CUTANEOUS T-CELL LYMPHOMA

Cutaneous T-cell lymphoma (CTCL) applies to T-cell lymphoma that first manifests in the skin and slowly progresses to lymph nodes and internal organs, terminating as a malignant lymphoma.

Synonym Mycosis fungoides.

EPIDEMIOLOGY

Age Any age. Usually seen in adults ages 50 to 70 years.

Gender M > F, 2:1.

Incidence Two per 1,000,000 population. Accounts for 1% of deaths from lymphoma (about 200 deaths per year in the United States).

Etiology Unknown. Possible antigenic stimulation to human T lymphotrophic virus (HTLV) in some patients.

HISTORY

Skin symptoms are the presenting symptom of CTCL and last for months to years, often preceded by nonspecific or false-negative diagnoses such as psoriasis, nummular dermatitis, or parapsoriasis. The skin lesions may wax and wane and are asymptomatic or mildly pruritic. Systemically, the patient feels well until the visceral organs become involved.

PHYSICAL FINDINGS

Skin Findings

Type Plaques, scaling or not scaling, at first superficial, much like "eczema" or psoriasis, and later becoming thicker or "infiltrated" (Fig. 19-8). Nodules and tumors are seen in later stage CTCL, with or without ulcers.

Color Red to pink or violaceous in color.

Shape Round, oval, arciform, annular, concentric or bizarre configurations.

Size > 3.0 cm.

Arrangement Randomly distributed discrete plaques, nodules, and tumors, or diffuse involvement with erythroderma (Sézary's syndrome) and palmoplantar keratoderma.

Distribution Often spares exposed areas (in early stages). No typical distribution pattern, random localization.

Sézary's Syndrome

This is a leukemic form of CTCL consisting of (1) erythroderma, (2) lymphadenopathy, (3) elevated WBC (> 20,000) with a high proportion of so-called Sézary cells, (4) hair loss, and (5) pruritus.

General Examination

In late disease, lymphadenopathy and/or splenomegaly may be present.

DIFFERENTIAL DIAGNOSIS

In the early stages, the diagnosis of CTCL is difficult to recognize. Clinical lesions may be typical but histologic confirmation may not be possible for years despite repeated biopsies. Fresh tissue can be sent for analysis of cellular makeup by the use of monoclonal antibodies. A high index of suspicion is needed in patients with atypical or refractory psoriasis, eczema, and poikiloderma atrophicans vasculare. Repeated biopsies may be necessary.

LABORATORY EXAMINATIONS

Repeated and multiple (three) biopsies are often necessary.

Dermatopathology Skin biopsy will show T cells with hyperchromatic, irregularly shaped nuclei. Mitoses may be present. In the epidermis, there are scattered microabscesses. In the dermis, there is a bandlike and patchy infiltrate of atypical lymphocytes extending to skin appendages. Monoclonal antibody techniques identify most atypical cells as helper/inducer T cells.

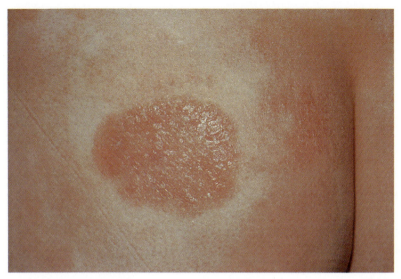

Figure 19-8   Cutaneous T-cell lymphoma   *An isolated plaque on the buttock of a child.* (Slide courtesy of Chi Rosenberg, MD.)

COURSE AND PROGNOSIS

Children typically live for 10 to 15 years before CTCL ever progresses to any worrisome degree.

MANAGEMENT

Children with CTCL need routine follow-up and conservative symptomatic treatment such as:

1. Sunlight exposure.
2. Anti-pruritic creams.
    a. Pramoxine (Prax, Pramasone).
    b. Menthol/camphor (Sarna).
3. Topical steroids. (See page 48 for more details.)

For histologically proven plaque-stage CTCL, treatment possibilities include PUVA, topical nitrogen mustard, total electron beam therapy, interferon, or extracorporeal PUVA photochemotherapy.

CUTANEOUS BACTERIAL INFECTIONS

IMPETIGO

Impetigo is a superficial infection of the skin characterized by honey-colored crusts and due to *Streptococcus pyogenes, Staphylococcus aureus*, or both.

Synonyms   Bullous impetigo, blistering distal dactylitis.

EPIDEMIOLOGY

Age   Preschool children and young adults.

Gender   M = F.

Incidence   Common. Accounts for up to 10% of dermatology visits.

Etiology   Bullous impetigo is caused by phage group II streptococcus. Vesiculopustular impetigo is caused by beta-hemolytic streptococcus.

Predisposing Factors   Colonization of the skin and/or nares of the patient or patient's family members.

HISTORY

The skin lesions begin as erythematous areas progressing to superficial vesicles and bullae, which rupture and form honey-colored crusts. Systemic symptoms are rare but can include fever and lymphadenopathy.

PHYSICAL EXAMINATION

Skin Findings

Type   Erythematous macules → transient thin-roofed vesicles of bullae → crusts and erosions.

Color   Golden-yellow "stuck on" crusts (hallmark of impetigo; Fig. 20-1).

Size and Shape   1.0 to 3.0 cm; round or oval; central healing.

Arrangement   Scattered discrete lesions, some large confluent lesions; satellite lesions occur by autoinoculation.

Distribution   Face, arms, legs, buttocks, distal fingers (Fig. 20-2), toes.

DIFFERENTIAL DIAGNOSIS

The honey-colored crusts of impetigo are diagnostic and Gram's stain or nasal culture will help to demonstrate causative organism. In the early vesicular stage impetigo may simulate *varicella* and *herpes simplex*.

LABORATORY EXAMINATIONS

Dermatopathology   Skin biopsy (usually not performed) would show an acantholytic cleft in the stratum granulosum with leukocytes and cocci.

Gram's Stain   Gram-positive cocci, in chains or clusters, may be present.

Culture   Group A streptococci and sometimes a mixed culture of streptococci and *S. aureus* can be cultured from lesions or nasopharynx. Use of a moistened culture swab to dissolve crusts may be necessary to isolate the pathogens.

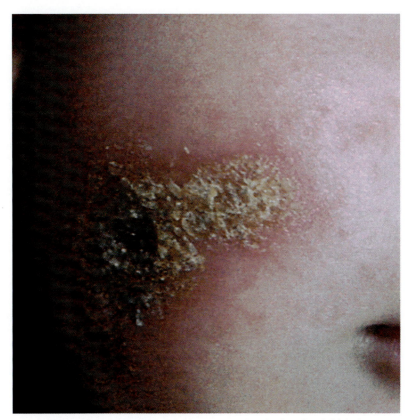

Figure 20-1 Impetigo, bullous *Honey-colored crusts on the cheeks of a child with impetiginized eczema. Skin cultures grew* S. aureus.

COURSE AND PROGNOSIS

Impetigo is a benign but recurrent and contagious condition. Untreated it can persist for weeks and continue to spread. Once treatment is initiated, the clinical response is swift and effective. In rare cases of beta-hemolytic streptococcal impetigo, acute glomerulonephritis or scarlet fever can ensue.

MANAGEMENT

Preventive measures include:

1. Antibacterial soaps and washes.
   a. Dial antibacterial soap.
   b. Lever 200 antibacterial soap.
   c. Benzoyl peroxide (Panoxyl bar or Benzac wash).
2. All close household and/or family members should be treated at the same time because asymptomatic nasal carriage of the pathogenic bacteria can occur.
3. For uncomplicated cases of impetigo, topical treatment is effective. Topical mupirocin antibiotic ointment (Bactroban applied tid to skin lesion and nasal passages for 7 to 10 d) is highly effective in eliminating both group A streptococci as well as *S. aureus* and is an effective treatment of impetigo.

Systemic antibiotic therapy may be considered for moderate to severe or refractory (i.e., mupirocin-resistant) cases.

1. If staphylococci are present.
   a. Dicloxacillin (25 to 50 mg/kg per d PO divided qid for 10 d).
   b. Cephalexin (25 to 50 mg/kg per d divided PO qid for 10 d, not to exceed 4 g/d).
   c. Amoxicillin plus clavulanic acid (20 to 40 mg/kg per d PO divided tid × 10 d).
2. If caused by group A streptococci alone.
   a. Benzathine penicillin (600,000 U IM qd in children < 7 years, 1.2 million U if > 7 years for 10 d).
   b. Penicillin V (25 mg/kg per d PO divided tid–qid, not to exceed 3 g/day for 10 d).
   c. Cephalexin (25 to 50 mg/kg per d divided PO qid for 10 d, not to exceed 4 g/d).
3. If the patient is allergic to penicillin.
   a. Erythromycin (30 to 50 mg/kg per d PO divided qid × 10 d, not to exceed 2 g/d).
   b. Clarithromycin (50 to 250 mg PO qd × 10 d).
   c. Azithromycin (50 to 250 mg PO qd × 5 to 7 d).
   d. Clindamycin (15 mg/kg per d PO divided qid for 10 d).

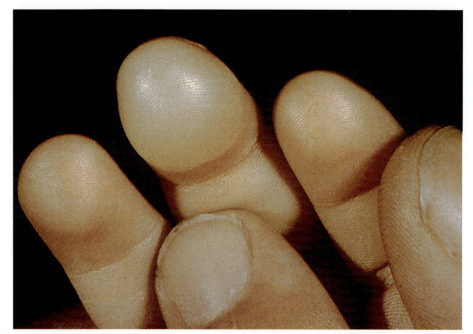

Figure 20-2 Blistering distal dactylitis *Tense fluid-filled blister on the fingertip of a young boy with* S. aureus *nasal carriage.* (Slide courtesy of Lisa M. Cohen).

ECTHYMA

Ecthyma is a deep or ulcerative bacterial infection of the skin characterized by ulcers on the buttocks or legs of children.

Synonyms Ecthyma minor, ecthyma major.

EPIDEMIOLOGY

Age Children, adolescents, elderly.

Gender M = F.

Incidence Common.

Etiology Skin bacterial organisms (group A streptococci or *S. aureus,* or both) grow in excoriations, insect bites, and sites of trauma.

HISTORY

Lesions begin as excoriations or insect bites with superinfection leading to saucer-shaped ulcer with a raised margin. The lesions are pruritic and tender and heal slowly, usually with scar formation. Systemic symptoms are rare but can include fever and lymphadenopathy.

PHYSICAL EXAMINATION

Skin Findings

Type Vesicle or pustule progressing to an ulcer with subsequent scar formation (Fig. 20-3).

Color Violaceous to dirty yellowish-gray crust.

Shape and Size Round or oval, 0.5 to 3.0 cm.

Palpation Indurated, tender.

Arrangement Scattered, discrete.

Sites of Predilection Ankles, dorsa of feet, thighs, buttocks.

DIFFERENTIAL DIAGNOSIS

The diagnosis of ecthyma is made by history and clinical examination and can be confirmed by Gram's stain and bacterial culture.

LABORATORY EXAMINATIONS

Culture Group A streptococci, staphylococci.

COURSE AND PROGNOSIS

Lesions persist for weeks and are slow to heal. They often heal with a resultant scar.

MANAGEMENT

Ecthyma should be treated with warm soaks to remove crusts. Topical and systemic therapy may be indicated. (See page 456 for more details.)

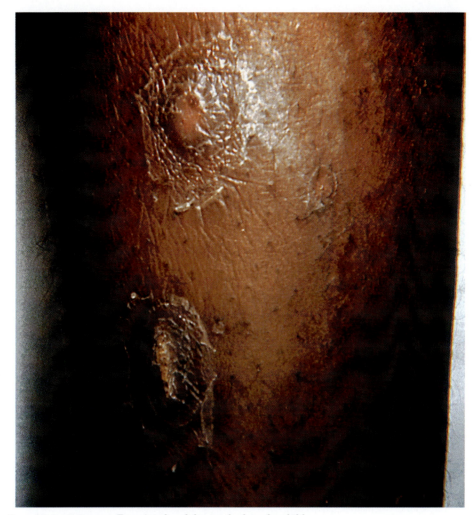

Figure 20-3   Ecthyma   *Excoriated nodules on the leg of a child.*

FURUNCLES AND CARBUNCLES

A furuncle is an acute, deep-seated, red, hot, very tender, inflammatory nodule that evolves from a staphylococcal folliculitis. A carbuncle is a large lesion of coalescing furuncles.

Synonyms Boils, abscesses.

EPIDEMIOLOGY

Age Children, adolescents, and young adults.

Gender M > F.

Incidence Common.

Predisposing Factors Chronic staphylococcal carrier state in nares or perineum, friction of collars or belts, obesity, bactericidal defects (e.g., in chronic granulomatosis), defects in chemotaxis and in hyper-IgE syndrome, diabetes mellitus.

HISTORY

Furuncles begin as a folliculitis that becomes deeper and larger from friction or maceration. Systemic symptoms are rare but can include low-grade fever and malaise.

PHYSICAL EXAMINATION

Skin Findings

Type Hard nodule, fluctuant, pustule on top covering central necrotic plug → ruptures into an ulcer, with erythematous halo.

Color Bright red.

Palpation Indurated, firm, tender.

Distribution Isolated single lesions or a few multiple lesions (Fig. 20-4).

Arrangement Scattered, discrete.

Sites of Predilection Occur only where there are hair follicles and in areas subject to friction and sweating: neck, scalp, face, axillae, buttocks, thigh, and perineum.

LABORATORY EXAMINATION

Blood culture in cases with fever and/or constitutional symptoms before beginning treatment; if blood culture is positive, IV antibiotics are necessary.

Skin Culture Incision and drainage of lesions for Gram's stain, culture and antibiotic sensitivity studies.

DIFFERENTIAL DIAGNOSIS

Furuncles and carbuncles are a clinical diagnosis and the diagnosis of hidradenitis suppurativa (cystic lesions in axillae, groin, vulva; presence of double comedones) should be ruled out clinically.

COURSE AND PROGNOSIS

Furuncles and carbuncles resolve with incision and drainage, and systemic antibiotic treatment. At times, however, furunculosis is complicated by bacteremia and possible hematogenous seeding of heart valves, joints, spine, long bones, and viscera (especially kidneys). Some patients are subject to recurrent furunculosis and these patients and their family members need to be treated simultaneously and aggressively.

MANAGEMENT

Simple furunculosis is treated by local application of heat. Incision and drainage is commonly required, particularly for carbuncles. No systemic antibiotics are needed except in patients with systemic symptoms.

Furunculosis with surrounding cellulitis or with fever should be treated with systemic antibiotics.

1. Dicloxacillin (25 to 50 mg/kg per d PO divided qid for 1 to 2 weeks).
2. Cephalexin (25 to 50 mg/kg per d divided PO qid for 1 to 2 weeks, not to exceed 4 g/d).
3. Amoxicillin plus clavulanic acid (20 to 40 mg/kg per d PO divided tid for 1 to 2 weeks).

If the patient is allergic to penicillin:

1. Erythromycin (30 to 50 mg/kg per d PO divided qid × 1 to 2 weeks, not to exceed 2 g/d).

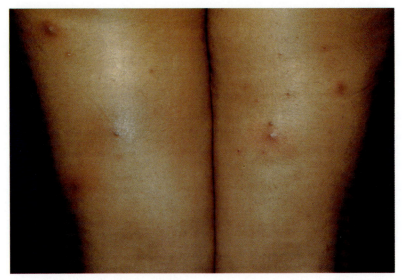

Figure 20-4   Furuncle   *Scattered inflammatory papules, pustules, and nodules on the posterior thighs.*

2. Clarithromycin (50 to 250 mg PO qd × 1 to 2 weeks).
3. Azithromycin (50 to 250 mg PO qd × 5 to 7 d).
4. Clindamycin (15 mg/kg per d PO divided qid for 1 to 2 weeks).

Recurrent furunculosis may be difficult to control. This may be related to persistent staphylococci in the nares, perineum, and body folds. Effective control can sometimes be obtained with:

1. Frequent showers (not baths).
2. Antibacterial soaps and washes.
    a. Povidone-iodine soap.
    b. Dial antibacterial soap.
    c. Lever 2000 anti-bacterial soap.
    d. Benzoyl peroxide (Panoxyl bar or Benzac wash).
3. Topical mupirocin antibiotic ointment (Bactroban applied tid to skin lesion and nasal passages for 7 to 10 d) is highly effective in eliminating both group A streptococci as well as *S. aureus*. All close household and/or family members should be treated at the same time because asymptomatic nasal carriage of the pathogenic bacteria can occur.
4. Systemic antibiotics at lower doses on a daily basis prophylactically may be needed to avoid relapses.

FOLLICULITIS

A folliculitis is a superficial or deep inflammation (often bacterial) of hair follicles. Different types occur on different regions of the body (Table 20-1).

Table 20-1 SPECIFIC TYPES OF FOLLICULITIS

Location	Synonym	Etiology
Neck	Acne keloidalis, folliculitis keloidalis nuchae	*S. aureus*, ingrown, curly hair
Back	Periporititis suppurtiva	*Candida albicans*
Buttocks, body	Hot tub folliculitis, whirlpool folliculitis, pseudomonas folliculitis	*Pseudomonas aeruginosa* in hot tubs
Face (beard region in adolescents)	Folliculitis barbae, sycosis barbae, pseudofolliculitis barbae	*Staphylococcus aureus*, ingrown hair

EPIDEMIOLOGY

Age   Any age.

Incidence   Common.

Etiology   Often bacterial: *Staphylococcus aureus* most common. Can also be caused by occlusive dressings, tar, or mineral oils.

HISTORY

Folliculitis begins with inflammation of the follicular ostium that may be symptomatic or pruritic. The lesions self-resolve with gentle cleansing and no systemic symptoms are noted.

PHYSICAL EXAMINATION

Skin Findings

Type   Papules or pustules confined to the ostium of the hair follicles.

Color   Yellow or gray with surrounding erythema.

Size   1 to 5 mm.

Arrangement   Scattered discrete or more frequently grouped (Fig. 20-5).

Distribution   Scalp, face, buttocks, extremities.

LABORATORY EXAMINATIONS

Gram's Stain   Look for gram-positive cocci.

Culture   *Staphylococcus aureus, Candida albicans, Pseudomonas aeruginosa,* less likely *Streptococcus, Proteus,* or *S. epidermidis.*

DIFFERENTIAL DIAGNOSIS

The diagnosis of folliculitis is made by history and the physical finding of a folliculocentric dermatitis. The differential diagnosis includes: acne, flat warts, molluscum contagiosum, tinea barbae, tinea corporis, and pustular niiliaria.

MANAGEMENT

In the treatment of folliculitis, occlusive agents (clothes, etc.) should be removed.

For uncomplicated cases, folliculitis can be managed with:

1. Antibacterial soaps and washes:
   a. Dial antibacterial soap.
   b. Lever 2000 antibacterial soap.
   c. Benzoyl peroxide (Panoxyl bar or Benzac wash).
2. Topical mupirocin antibiotic ointment (Bactroban applied tid to skin lesions and nasal passages for 7 to 10 d) is highly effective in eliminating both group A streptococci as well as *S. aureus*. All close household and/or family members should be treated at the same time because asymptomatic nasal carriage of the pathogenic bacteria can occur.
3. Systemic antibiotic therapy may be considered for moderate to severe or refractory cases. (See page 456 for more details.)

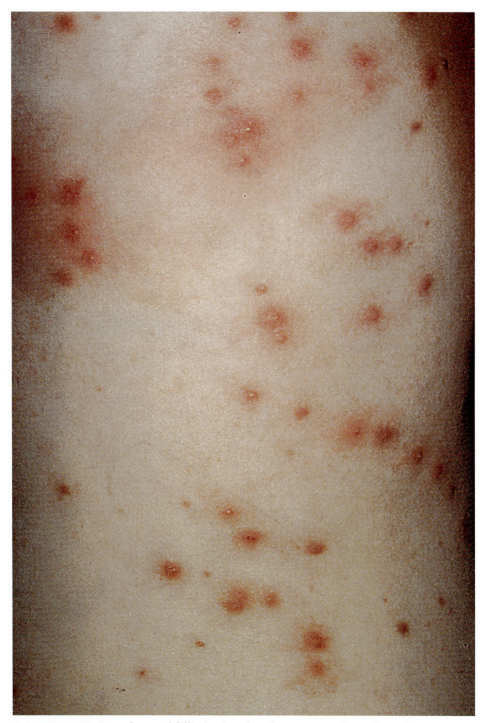

Figure 20-5   Folliculitis   *Scattered follicular-based erythematous papules and pustules.*

CELLULITIS

Cellulitis is an acute, spreading infection of dermal and subcutaneous tissues, characterized by a red, hot, tender area of skin, often at the site of bacterial entry.

EPIDEMIOLOGY

Age   Children < 3 years.

Gender   M = F.

Incidence   Common.

Etiology   Bacterial, usually *Haemophilus influenzae,* group A streptococci, or *Staphylococcus aureus.* Less commonly, pneumococci or *Neisseria meningitidis.*

Transmission   Entry via break in the skin (puncture, laceration, abrasion, surgical site), underlying dermatosis (tinea pedis, atopic dermatitis). In children *H. influenzae* enters through middle ear or nasal mucosa.

PATHOPHYSIOLOGY

A break in the skin allows bacterial entry and proliferation in the soft tissues with a marked inflammatory response.

HISTORY

Cellulitis occurs 1 to 3 days after a break in the skin (wound, trauma) as a red, tender, hot swelling of the skin and underlying tissues. Systemic symptoms such as malaise, anorexia, fever, chills can occur and an associated bacteremia may be present.

PHYSICAL EXAMINATION

Skin Findings

Type   Breaks in the skin, wounds, chronic dermatosis with edematous sharply defined, irregular, and slightly elevated plaques.

Size   Few to several cm.

Color   Red to purple *(H. influenzae).*

Palpation   Firm, hot, tender.

Distribution   Cheek, periorbital area (Fig. 20-6), head, neck, extremities.

Lymph Nodes   Can be enlarged and tender, regionally.

DIFFERENTIAL DIAGNOSIS

The diagnosis of cellulitis is suspected for any large, red, hot, tender, spreading, erythematous plaques, especially if systemic fever, malaise, chills, and sweats are present. Positive bacterial cultures are obtained in only 25% of cases. Facial, orbital, and periorbital cellulitls require special attention, early recognition, and systemic treatment because of the risk of serous visual impairment in untreated cases. The differential diagnosis includes contact dermatitis, urticaria, annular erythemas, and drug eruptions.

LABORATORY EXAMINATIONS

Dermatopathology   Skin biopsy will show edema and inflammation. Special stains for organisms can be performed.

Laboratory Examination of Blood   White cell count and sedimentation rate may be elevated.

Cultures   Cultures of the skin can be aspirated or biopsied at the leading edge of inflammation. Blood cultures are positive in only one quarter of cases.

COURSE AND PROGNOSIS

The prognosis for cellulitis is good if early detection and treatment is initiated. Late recognition increases risk of hematogenous or lymphatic involvement and more systemic disease (i.e., seeding of the heart valve, CNS, etc.). Periorbital cellulitis warrants hospitalization, identification of causative organism, and prompt systemic therapy to avoid permanent sequelae such as blindness.

MANAGEMENT

Identifying the organism that is causing the cellulitis can aid in choosing the correct antibiotic coverage.

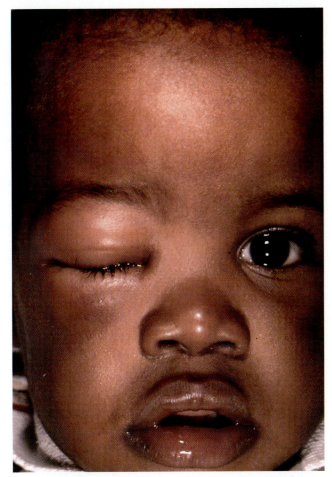

Figure 20-6 **Cellulitis, *Haemophilus influenzae*** *Two-year-old with a right periorbital cellulitis.* (Reproduced with permission from TB Fitzpatrick et al., Color Atlas and Synopsis of Clinical Dermatology, 4th edition. New York: McGraw-Hill, 2001).

H. influenzae cellulitis can be treated with:

1. Cefotaxime (100 to 200 mg/kg per d PO divided tid × 7 to 14 d).
2. Ceftriaxone (50 to 100 mg/kg per d IM/IV qd × 7 to 14 d).
3. Chloramphenicol (75 to 100 mg/kg per d PO divided qid × 7 to 14 d).

Ampicillin-resistant organisms can be treated with:

1. Cefixime (8 mg/kg per d PO qd × 7 to 14 d).

Staphylococcal and streptococcal cellulitis can be treated with systemic antibiotics. (See page 456–457 for more details.)

For cellulitis in which an organism cannot be identified:

1. Cefazolin (50 to 100 mg/kg per d divided tid × 10 d not to exceed 6 g/d).

For severe refractory cases, facial and/or periorbital cellulitis usually requires hospitalization and IV antibiotics until clinical improvement is noted.

ERYSIPELAS

Erysipelas is a superficial infection of the skin caused by group A beta-hemolytic streptococci (GAS).

EPIDEMIOLOGY

Age   Young children.

Gender   M = F.

Incidence   Uncommon.

Etiology   GAS from an external break in the skin or pharynx, or less likely, internal hematogenous spread.

HISTORY

Two to 5 days after a break in the skin, a red, hot, tender, well-demarcated erythematous plaque begins to form and enlarge around the inoculation site. Systemic symptoms are rare.

PHYSICAL EXAMINATION

Skin Findings

Type   Well-demarcated infiltrated plaque usually surrounding a wound (excoriation, laceration).

Color   Bright red (Fig. 20-7).

Palpation   Firm, hot, tender.

Distribution   Any site.

Sites of Predilection   Bridge of nose, cheeks, face, scalp.

General Findings

Usually none. May have fever and malaise.

DIFFERENTIAL DIAGNOSIS

Erysipelas is diagnosed by its characteristic distribution on the bridge of nose and cheek(s) and confirmed by group A beta-hemolytic streptococcal identification. The facial rash can be confused with lupus, sunburn, contact dermatitis, urticaria, or dermatomyositis.

LABORATORY EXAMINATIONS

Gram's Stain   Gram's stain of tissue or wound swab may show gram-positive cocci.

Culture   Blood tissue or wound swab cultures may grow beta-hemolytic streptococcus.

COURSE AND PROGNOSIS

Once identified and treated, erysipelas has a good prognosis.

MANAGEMENT

The treatment for erysipelas is:

1.   Benzathine penicillin (600,000 U IM qd in children < 7 years, 1.2 million U if > 7 years for 10 d).
2.   Penicillin V (25 mg/kg per d PO divided tid–qid for 10 d, not to exceed 3 g/d).
3.   Cephalexin (25 to 50 mg/kg per d divided PO qid for 10 d, not to exceed 4 g/d).

Penicillin-allergic individuals can be treated with:

1.   Erythromycin (30 to 50 mg/kg per d PO divided qid × 10 d, not to exceed 2 g/d).
2.   Clarithromycin (50 to 250 mg PO qd × 10 d).
3.   Azithromycin (50 to 250 mg PO qd × 5 to 7 d).
4.   Clindamycin (15 mg/kg per d PO divided qid for 10 d).

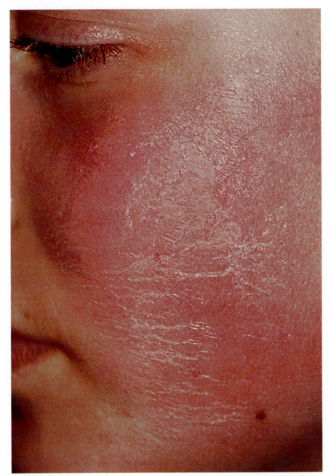

Figure 20-7 **Erysipelas, group A streptococcus** *Erythematous warm, tender plaque on the cheek.*

PERIANAL STREPTOCOCCAL INFECTION

Perianal streptococcal infection is characterized by a bright, red perianal dermatitis that leads to pruritus, pain, fissures, and resultant behavioral defecation disorders.

Synonyms Perianal streptococcal cellulitis, streptococcal perianal disease.

EPIDEMIOLOGY

Age Childhood.

Gender M = F.

Incidence Uncommon.

Etiology GAS.

HISTORY

Perianal streptococcal infection typically presents as a perianal itching or pain. No systemic symptoms are usually present. Perianal streptococcal dermatitis may also first present as guttate or recurrent psoriasis acting as the infectious precipitant.

PHYSICAL EXAMINATION

Skin Findings

Type Well-demarcated plaque

Color Bright red

Size Few to several cm.

Distribution Perianal area (Fig. 20-8).

DIFFERENTIAL DIAGNOSIS

Perianal streptococcal infection is diagnosed by its characteristic distribution and a positive skin culture. It can be clinically confused with psoriasis, candidiasis, contact dermatitis, atopic dermatitis, pinworm infection, or sexual abuse.

LABORATORY EXAMINATIONS

Skin cultures of the area will grow beta-hemolytic streptococcus.

COURSE AND PROGNOSIS

Treated perianal streptococcal infection has a very good prognosis but relapses (seen in up to 40% of cases) occur requiring retreatment. Untreated cases can lead to perianal fissures, streaks of blood on the stool, and behavioral defecating disabilities.

MANAGEMENT

The treatment for perianal streptococcal infection is:

1. Benzathine penicillin (600,000 U IM qd in children < 7 years, 1.2 million U if > 7 years for 10 to 14 d).
2. Penicillin V (25 to 50 mg/kg per d PO divided tid–qid, not to exceed 3 g/d for 10 to 14 d).
3. Cephalexin (25 to 50 mg/kg per d divided PO qid for 10 to 14 d, not to exceed 4 g/d).

If the patient is allergic to penicillin.

1. Erythromycin (30 to 50 mg/kg per d PO divided qid × 10 to 14 d, not to exceed 2 g/d).
2. Clarithromycin (250 mg PO qd × 10 to 14 d).
3. Azithromycin (250 mg PO qd × 10 to 14 d).
4. Clindamycin (15 mg/kg per d PO divided qid for 10 to 14 d).

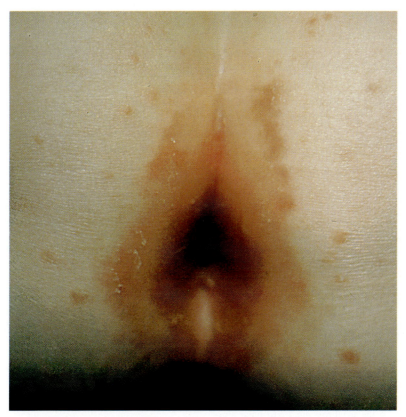

Figure 20-8 **Perianal streptococcal infection** *Perianal erythema and fissures. A skin culture revealed beta-hemolytic streptococcus.*

SCARLET FEVER

Scarlet fever is a group A streptococcal infection of the tonsils, pharynx or skin, associated with a characteristic diffuse erythematous exanthem.

Synonyms Scarletina, surgical scarlet.

EPIDEMIOLOGY

Age All ages, between ages 1 to 10 years.

Incidence Uncommon.

Etiology Group A beta-hemolytic *Streptococcus pyogenes* (GAS). Uncommonly, exotoxin-producing *Staphylococcus aureus*.

Season Seen more commonly in late fall, winter, and early spring.

Other Household member(s) may be a streptococcal carrier.

PATHOPHYSIOLOGY

Group A streptococcal erythrogenic toxin production produces the clinical findings of scarlet fever and depends on the presence of a temperate bacteriophage. Patients with prior exposure to the erythrogenic toxin have anti-toxin immunity and neutralize the toxin. The scarlet fever syndrome therefore does not develop in these patients. Since several erythrogenic strains of beta-hemolytic streptococcus cause infection, it is theoretically possible to have a second episode of scarlet fever. Additionally, several strains of *Staphylococcus aureus* can produce an exotoxin and simulate a scarlitiniform exanthem.

HISTORY

The rash of scarlet fever appears within 2 to 3 days after onset of streptococcal infection (of nose, throat, ears, or skin). Systemic symptoms can include fever, malaise, and/or a sore throat.

PHYSICAL EXAMINATION

Skin Findings

Type of Lesion Finely punctate erythema is first noted on the upper part of the trunk. Exanthem fades within 4 to 5 days and is followed by brawny desquamation on the body and ex-tremities (Fig. 20-9) and by sheet-like exfoliation on the palms and soles (Fig. 20-10).

Color Exanthem is pink to scarlet at the onset. Face becomes flushed but with a perioral pallor. Initial punctate lesions become confluently erythematous (i.e., scarlatiniform). Linear petechiae (Pastia's sign) occur in body folds. Intensity of the exanthem varies from mild to moderate erythema confined to the trunk to an extensive purpuric eruption.

Palpation Sandpaper texture to skin.

Distribution Erythema starts on the chest and then spreads to the extremities. Erythema accentuated at pressure points and in body folds. Linear petechiae (Pastia's sign) noted in antecubital and axillary folds.

Mucous Membranes Pharynx and/or tonsils beefy red. Tongue initially is white with scattered red swollen papillae (white strawberry tongue). By the fourth or fifth day, the hyperkeratotic membrane is sloughed and the lingular mucosa appears bright red (red strawberry tongue; Fig. 20-11). Punctate erythema and petechiae may occur on the soft palate.

General Examination

Fever, malaise, headache, sore throat, vomiting, and anterior cervical lymphadenitis.

DIFFERENTIAL DIAGNOSIS

The diagnosis is made by recognizing the characteristic exanthem. It can be confirmed by detecting strep antigen in a rapid test, culturing group A beta-hemolytic *S. pyogenes* from the throat or wound, and/or documenting rise in the antistreptolysin-O titer. Scarlet fever can be confused with staphylococcal infection, viral exanthems, and drug eruptions.

LABORATORY EXAMINATIONS

Dermatopathology Skin biopsy shows perivascular neutrophilic inflammation with dilated small blood vessels.

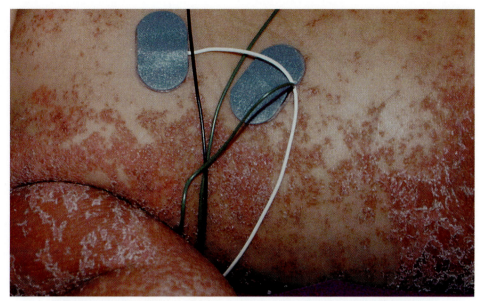

Figure 20-9 Scarlet fever, exanthem *Brawny desquamation on the torso and extremities of a child.*

Gram's Stain Reveals gram-positive cocci.

Bacterial Culture Throat or wound culture will grow beta-hemolytic streptococcus.

Serology Will demonstrate a fourfold rise in antistreptolysin-O titer.

COURSE AND PROGNOSIS

Uncomplicated scarlet fever has a good prognosis. As with all streptococcal disease, the possibility of worrisome sequelae needs to be assessed (i.e., acute rheumatic fever, acute glomerulonephritis).

MANAGEMENT

The treatment for scarlet fever can be with:

1. Benzathine penicillin (600,000 U IM qd in children < 7 years, 1.2 million U if > 7 years for 10 to 14 d).

2. Penicillin V (25 mg/kg per d PO divided tid–qid for 10–14 d, not to exceed 3 g/d.

3. Cephalexin (25 to 50 mg/kg per d divided PO qid for 10 to 14 d, not to exceed 4 g/d).

If the patient is allergic to penicillin, the possible systemic therapies include:

1. Erythromycin (30 to 50 mg/kg per d PO divided qid × 10 to 14 d, not to exceed 2 g/d).

2. Clarithromycin (50 to 250 mg PO qd × 10 to 14 d).

3. Azithromycin (50 to 250 mg PO qd × 5 to 7 d).

4. Clindamycin (15 mg/kg per d PO divided qid for 10 d).

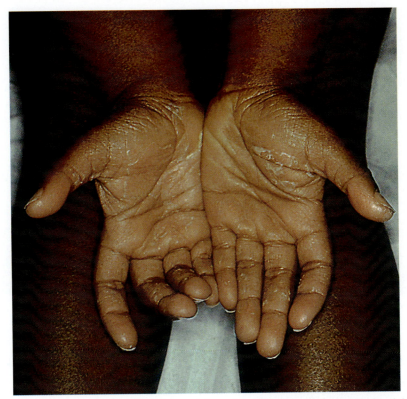

Figure 20-10   Scarlet fever, late desquamation   *Palmar desquamation on the hands of a child.*

CUTANEOUS BACTERIAL INFECTIONS

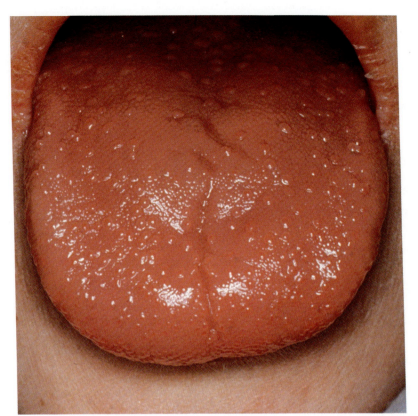

Figure 20-11   Scarlet fever, early exanthem   *Bright red tongue with prominent papillae on the fifth day after onset of group A streptococcal pharyngitis.* (Reproduced with permission from TB Fitzpatrick et al., Color Atlas and Synopsis of Clinical Dermatology, 3rd edition. New York: McGraw-Hill, 1997).

STAPHYLOCOCCAL SCALDED-SKIN SYNDROME

Staphylococcal scalded-skin syndrome (SSSS) is a toxin-mediated epidermolytic disease characterized by erythema and widespread detachment of the superficial layers of the epidermis. It is caused by certain strains of staphylococci.

Synonyms   Pemphigus neonatorum, Ritter's disease.

EPIDEMIOLOGY

Age   Newborns and infants < 5 years old.

Etiology   *Staphylococcus aureus* of phage group II (types 3A, 3B, 5S or 71).

PATHOPHYSIOLOGY

SSSS is predominantly a disease of newborns and infants because after age 10, the majority of people are thought to have staphylococcus antibodies, or a greater ability to localize and metabolize the staphylococcal exotoxin, thus limiting widespread dissemination of the toxin. In newborns and infants, *Staphylococcus aureus* colonizes the nose, conjunctivae, or umbilical stump without causing a clinically apparent infection. Certain strains can produce an exotoxin (exfoliation, epidermolysin) that is transported hematogenously to the skin. The exfoliative toxin causes acantholysis and intraepidermal cleavage within the stratum granulosum. This leads to generalized sloughing of the superficial epidermis.

HISTORY

SSSS begins as fever, malaise, and generalized erythema that progresses to a scarlitiniform eruption. The child appears irritable and inconsolable. The skin then develops fluid bullae and exfoliates (giving the child a "scalded" appearance). Eventually, if properly treated, the skin will heal without scarring.

PHYSICAL EXAMINATION

Skin Findings

Type   Tender, ill-defined macular erythema progresses to a diffuse papular eruption followed by a flaccid bullae and desquamation (Fig. 20-12).

Color   Pink to red.

Palpation   Gentle lateral pressure causes shearing off of superficial epidermis (Nikolsky's sign).

Distribution of Lesions   Begins periorifically on face, neck, axillae, groins; becoming more widespread in 24 to 48 hours.

Mucous Membranes   Usually uninvolved.

General Examination

Fever, malaise, irritability, inconsolability, crying when held secondary to painful skin.

DIFFERENTIAL DIAGNOSIS

The diagnosis of SSSS can be made by clinical presentation and confirmatory laboratory examinations (see below). The differential diagnosis for SSSS includes toxic epidermal necrolysis, erythema multiforme, or other bullous diseases.

LABORATORY EXAMINATIONS

Dermatopathology   A skin biopsy or simply a "jelly roll" (taken by rolling the sloughed skin on the wooden end of a cotton tipped swab) of the sloughed skin will demonstrate cleavage of the skin at the level of the stratum granulosum.

Tzanck Smear   Scraping the base of a blistering lesion will demonstrate a skin split at the granular layer.

Gram's Stain   Do not Gram's stain sloughing skin (recall sloughing is due to the exotoxin, no organisms are in the skin). Gram's stain of infected source (i.e., umbilical stump, nose, pharynx, conjunctiva, etc.) will show gram-positive cocci.

Bacterial Culture   Sloughing skin will not yield and bacteria culture results since it is toxin-mediated. Bacterial culture of the primary infection site (nose, umbilical stump, pharynx,

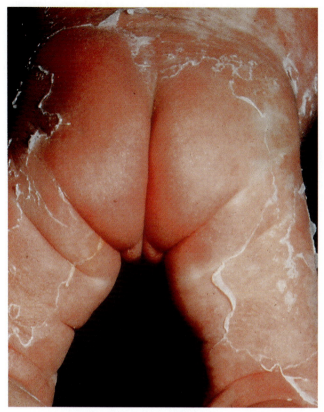

Figure 20-12   Staphylococcal scalded skin-syndrome   *Diffuse sheet-like desquamation of the entire body.*

conjunctiva, etc.) will grow *Staphylococcus aureus*.

COURSE AND PROGNOSIS

Following adequate antibiotic treatment, the superficially denuded areas of SSSS heal in 3 to 5 days following full-body desquamation of the superficial epidermis.

MANAGEMENT

Treatment for SSSS is dependent on early recognition and prompt identification of the primary infectious source. Once the infectious source of *Staphylococcus aureus* is cleared, the production of exotoxin is stopped.

The treatment of choice is a penicillinase-resistant agent such as dicloxicillin (25 to 50 mg/kg per day PO divided qid for 10 to 14 d).

In seriously affected newborns, hospitalization and treatment with oxacillin (200 mg/kg per day IV divided q6h) may be needed.

Topical care includes:

1. Gentle cleansing baths and compresses.
2. Topical mupirocin antibiotic ointment (Bactroban applied tid to skin lesion and nasal passages for 7 to 10 d) is highly effective in eliminating *S. aureus*. All close household and/or family members should be treated at the same time because asymptomatic nasal carriage of the pathogenic bacteria can occur.
3. Topical silver sulfadiazine (Silvadene) can also help protect denuded areas.

TOXIC SHOCK SYNDROME

Toxic shock syndrome (TSS) is an acute toxin-mediated illness caused by *Staphylococcus aureus* and characterized by rapid onset of fever, generalized skin and mucosal erythema, hypotension, and multisystem failure, sometimes leading to shock.

Synonym   Staphylococcal scarlet fever.

EPIDEMIOLOGY

Age   Predominantly adolescence and young. Can less often be seen in children or older adults.

Gender   F >> M.

Race   White > Black.

Incidence   Uncommon.

Etiology   *Staphylococcus aureus* producing TSS toxin-1 (TSST-1).

Risk Factors   Up to 95% of TSS cases in women using highly absorptive vaginal tampon during menses. The other 15% are seen with surgical wounds, vaginal contraceptive devices, nasal packings postop, etc.

PATHOPHYSIOLOGY

TSS is caused by *Staphylococcus aureus* colonization and the subsequent production of TSST-1 leading to a decrease in vasomotor tone, leakage of intravascular fluid, hypotension, and end-organ failure.

HISTORY

TSS starts with high fever and systemic symptoms, which may include myalgias, muscle tenderness, hypotension, headache, confusion, disorientation, seizures, diarrhea, or dyspnea. The skin is diffusely red and painful and the patient appears severely ill.

PHYSICAL EXAMINATION

Skin Findings

Mucous Membranes   Intense injection of the bulbar conjunctivae and possible subconjunctival hemorrhages (Fig. 20-13A). Tongue may be strawberry red in appearance. Ulcerations may be present.

Type   Generalized erythroderma is followed by a maculopapular eruption and edema. Petechiae and bullae may be present but are uncommon. Later, there is desquamation of the skin, especially on the palms and soles (Fig. 20-13B, C).

Color   Bright red.

Distribution   Generalized.

Sites of Predilection   Edema is most marked on face, hands, feet.

Hair and Nails

May be shed. Telogen effluvium (loss of the hair) may be seen 2 to 6 months later.

General Findings

Fever, malaise, myalgia, vomiting, diarrhea, hypotension, and shock.

DIFFERENTIAL DIAGNOSIS

TSS is suspected in menstruating, tampon-using females seen with diffuse erythema, edema, and fever. The differential diagnosis of TSS includes staphylococcal scalded-skin syndrome, scarlet fever, erythema multiforme, toxic epidermal necrolysis, drug reaction, viral infection, Kawasaki's disease, other bacterial infections, urticaria, or juvenile rheumatoid arthritis.

The Centers for Disease Control and Prevention has set a list of criteria for the diagnosis of TSS. Four of the following criteria plus desquamation or five of the criteria without desquamation must be present.

1. Fever > 38.9°C (102°F).
2. Rash (diffuse erythema and edema).
3. Desquamation 1 to 2 weeks after acute episode.
4. Hypotension.
5. Involvement of three or more organ systems: GI, muscles, mucous membranes, kidney, liver, hematologic, or CNS.

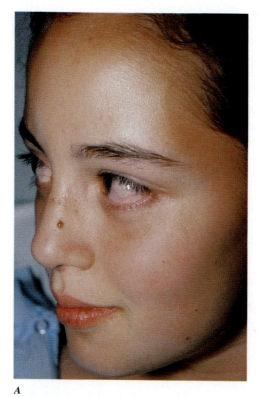

A

Figure 20-13 Toxic shock syndrome *(A) Facial edema and conjunctival injection in a young woman with toxic shock syndrome.*

6. Negative blood and CSF cultures, negative serologic tests for Rocky Mountain spotted fever, leptospirosis, and measles.

LABORATORY EXAMINATIONS

Dermatopathology Skin biopsy shows confluent epidermal necrolysis, vacuolar changes at the dermal-epidermal junction and a superficial and interstitial inflammatory infiltrate.

Gram's Stain Vaginal exudates will show many leukocytes and gram-positive cocci in clusters.

Bacterial Cultures The possibly affected sites (vagina, throat, nose, conjuncitiva, blood, or stool) will grow *S. aureus*.

COURSE AND PROGNOSIS

Untreated TSS has a high morbidity and mortality rate. Treating TSS reduces the mortality rate from 15% to 3% and deaths are secondary to refractory hypotension, respiratory distress, cardiac arrhythmias, cardiomyopathy, encephalopathy, metabolic acidosis, liver necrosis, or disseminated intravascular coagulation.

MANAGEMENT

Cases usually require hospitalization in an intensive care unit to optimize fluid, electrolytes, metabolic, and nutritional support. If a tampon is present, it should be removed and the area should be irrigated to reduce bacterial overgrowth. The patient should be started on an intravenous penicillinase-resistant penicillin.

1. Oxacillin (150 to 200 mg/kg per d IV divided q6h).
2. Cefazolin (50 to 100 mg/kg per d IV divided tid, not to exceed 6 g/d).

Future tampon use should be discouraged.

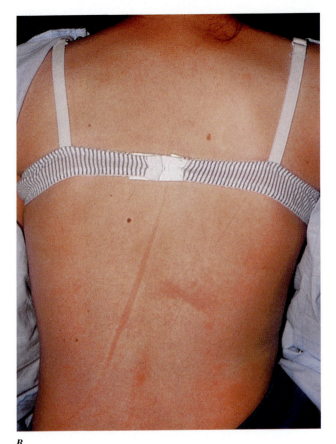

B

Figure 20-13 (continued)   Toxic shock syndrome   *(B) Diffuse erythema and a maculopapular eruption on the back of the same woman.*

CUTANEOUS BACTERIAL INFECTIONS

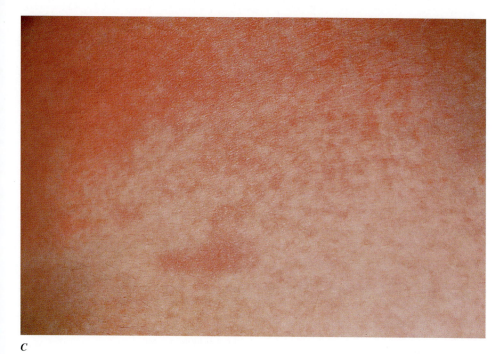

C

Figure 20-13 (continued)   Toxic shock syndrome   *(C) Close up of the bright red papular rash coalescing into a confluent plaque.*

ERYTHRASMA

Erythrasma (Greek, "red spot") is a superficial bacterial infection caused by *Corynebacterium minutissimum* affecting the intertriginous areas of the toes, groin, or axillae.

EPIDEMIOLOGY

Age   Seen in children ages 5 to 14 years, but much more common in adults.

Gender   M = F.

Incidence   Uncommon.

Predisposing Factors   May coexisit with tinea cruris or tinea pedis.

Etiology   *Corynebacterium minutissimum.*

HISTORY

Erythrasma begins in body folds such as the web spaces between the toes, the groin, or the axillac. It tends to be chronic for months or years with symptoms of pruritus or pain from maceration. Systemic symptoms are not present.

PHYSICAL EXAMINATION

Skin Findings

Type   Scaling (fine) macules, sharply marginated patches and plaques.

Color   Red or brownish red.

Arrangement   Scattered discrete lesions coalescing into confluent patches.

Sites of Predilection   Toe web spaces (Fig. 20-14), groin, axilla, intergluteal fold.

DIFFERENTIAL DIAGNOSIS

Erythrasma is often confused with a dermatophyte infection (i.e., tinea pedis, tinea cruris), seborrheic dermatitis, candidal infection, or intertrigo.

LABORATORY EXAMINATIONS

KOH   Examination reveals rods and filaments as opposed to hyphae or spores of tinea.

Wood's Lamp   Fluoresces; erythrasma a characteristic coral-red color due to the production of porphyrins by the corynebacterial organisms.

COURSE AND PROGNOSIS

Erythrasma tends to be a chronic condition persisting for months to years if untreated. There are only minor skin symptoms of pruritus or maceration and no systemic symptoms. Relapses after treatment are common, typically about 6 months later.

MANAGEMENT

Erythrasma can be controlled and prevented with:

1. Antibacterial soaps and washes.
    a. Dial antibacterial soap.
    b. Lever 2000 antibacterial soap.
    c. Benzoyl peroxide (Panoxyl bar or Benzac wash).
    d. Povidone-iodine soap.
2. Topical erythromycin or clindamycin solutions applied bid can improve the condition.
3. Less restrictive clothing.
4. Topical imidazoles can also improve the condition.
    a. Clotrimazole (Lotrimin, Mycelex).
    b. Econazole (Spectazole).
    c. Miconazole (Micatin).
    d. Ketoconazole (Nizoral).
    e. Oxiconizole (Oxistat).

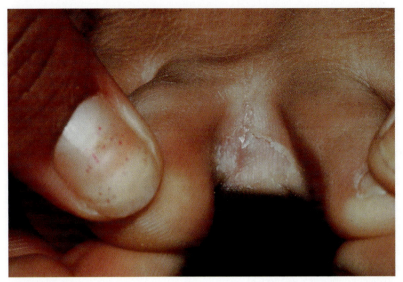

Figure 20-14 Erythrasma *Scale and maceration in the toe-web spaces that fluoresces with a Wood's lamp.*

MENINGOCOCCEMIA

Meningococcemia is a severe bacterial septicemia characterized by fever, petechial or purpuric lesions, hypotension, and signs of meningitis associated with high morbidity and mortality.

Synonym Waterhouse–Friderichsen syndrome.

EPIDEMIOLOGY

Age Highest incidence in children aged 6 months to 1 year; lowest in persons over 20 years.

Gender M = F.

Incidence Uncommon.

Risk Groups Asplenic patients or persons with complement deficiency (C5 to C8).

Etiology *Neisseria meningitidis*, a gram-negative organism that seeds the blood from the nasopharynx (carrier rate: 5% to 15%).

Transmission Person-to-person through inhalation of droplets of infected nasopharyngeal secretions.

Season Highest incidence, midwinter, early spring; lowest in midsummer.

Geography Worldwide. Occurs in epidemics or sporadically.

PATHOPHYSIOLOGY

The primary focus of *N. meningitidis* is usually a subclinical nasopharynx infection. Hematogenous dissemination of the diplococcus seeds the skin and meninges. An endotoxin is thought to be involved in causing hypotension and vascular collapse. Meningococci are found within endothelial and PMN cells leading to local endothelial damage, thrombosis, and necrosis of the vessel walls. Edema and the infarction of overlying skin, with extravasation of RBCs is responsible for the characteristic macular, papular, petechial, hemorrhagic, and bullous lesions. Similar vascular lesions occur in the meninges and in other tissues. The frequency of hemorrhagic cutaneous manifestations in meningococcal infections, compared to infections with other gram-negative organisms, may be due to increased potency and/or unique properties of meningococcal endotoxins for the dermal reac-

tion. Chronic meningococcemia is rarely seen in children but during perodic fevers, rash, and joint manifestations, meningococci can be isolated from the blood. It is thought that an unusual host–parasite relationship is central to this persistent infection. In fulminant meningococcemia, disseminated intravascular coagulation can be seen.

HISTORY

Acute meningococcemia may present as a flu-like illness with spiking fevers, chills, arthralgias, and myalgias. Hemorrhagic skin lesions and profound hypotension may be evident within a few hours of onset. Chronic meningococcemia manifests as intermittent fevers, rashes, myalgias, arthralgias, headaches, and anorexia.

PHYSICAL EXAMINATION

Skin Findings

Type At outset, few macular and papular petechiae with smudged appearance and transient urticarial, macular and papular lesions. In fulminant disease, purpura, ecchymosis, and confluent, often bizarre-shaped grayish to black necrotic areas are associated with disseminated intravascular coagulation (Fig. 20-15).

Color Pink to red with pale grayish center.

Distribution Trunk, extremities, but can be anywhere, including face, palms, and soles.

Mucous Membranes Petechiae on conjunctiva and other mucous membranes.

General Examination

Patient appears acutely ill with marked prostration, high fevers, tachypnea, tachycardia, and hypotension. Up to 50% to 88% of patients with meningococcemia develop meningitis and show signs of meningeal irritation and altered consciousness. Rarely, septic arthritis, purulent pericarditis, and bacterial endocarditis can oc-

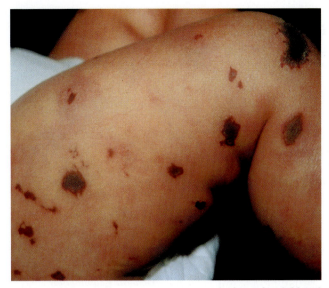

Figure 20-15 **Meningococcemia** *Stellate necrotic areas on the legs of a child with meningococcemia.*

cur. Fulminant meningococcemia can sometimes lead to adrenal hemorrhage (Waterhouse–Friderichsen syndrome).

DIFFERENTIAL DIAGNOSIS

The diagnosis of meningococcus is made by clinical impression confirmed by cultures. If suspected, meningococcal disease is so severe that treatment should be initiated before final culture results are grown (can take 24 to 48 hours). Meningococcemia can mimic other acute bacteremias and endocarditis, acute "hypersensitivity" vasculitis, enteroviral infections, Rocky Mountain spotted fever, toxic shock syndrome, Henoch-Schönlein purpura, typhoid fever, erythema multiforme, or gonococcemia

LABORATORY EXAMINATIONS

Dermatopathology Skin biopsy will show swollen endothelial cells with vascular lumina occluded by thrombi. Blood vessel walls may also show necrosis. Meningococcal organisms may be demonstrated in the lumina of vessels, within thrombi in perivascular spaces or in the cytoplasm of endothelial cells.

Cultures Blood culture and CSF cultures and Gram's stain will reveal gram-negative diplo-

cocci. A culture of a skin biopsy will be positive in up to 85% of cases.

Latex Agglutination The most rapid diagnostic test for meningeal meningococcus is with latex agglutination performed on the CSF fluid looking for the presence of *N. meningitidis*.

COURSE AND PROGNOSIS

Meningococcemia, if undiagnosed and untreated, ends fatally. Adequately treated, recovery rate for meningitis or meningococcemia is > 90%. Mortality for severe disease or Waterhouse–Friderichsen syndrome remains very high. Prognosis is poor when late symptoms or purpura and ecchymosis are present at time of diagnosis.

MANAGEMENT

Prompt recognition and treatment of meningococcemia is critical.

Treatment includes penicillin G (100,000 to 400,000 U/kg per day IV divided q4h).

For penicillin-allergic individuals IV chloramphenicol (100 mg/kg per day IV divided qid, not to exceed 4 g/d).

GONOCOCCEMIA

Gonococcemia is a severe bacterial infection characterized by fever, chills, scanty acral pustules, and septic polyarthritis.

Synonyms Disseminated gonococcal infection (DGI), gonococcal arthritis-dermatitis syndrome.

EPIDEMIOLOGY

Age Adolescents, young adults.

Gender M = F.

Race Whites > blacks.

Incidence Uncommon.

Etiology *Neisseria gonorrhoeae,* a gram-negative diplococcus that seeds the blood from infected mucosal sites.

Transmission Gonococcus is sexually transmitted. About 1% of patients with untreated mucosal gonococcal infection develop bacteremia.

PATHOPHYSIOLOGY

Gonorrhea is sexually transmitted to a mucosal surface and with menses or other process enters the bloodstream to reach the skin, joints, and other organs. Most signs and symptoms of gonococcemia are manifestations of immune complex formation and deposition.

HISTORY

Gonorrhea is a sexually transmitted mucosal infection that begins with fever, anorexia, malaise, and shaking chills. Three to 21 days later, skin lesions appear as erythematous and hemorrhagic papules over the distal joints with systemic migratory polyarthralgias.

PHYSICAL EXAMINATION

Skin Findings

Type Macules evolving to hemorrhagic pustules (Fig. 20-16A). Centers at times hemorrhagic and necrotic. Rarely, large hemorrhagic bullae.

Size 1 to 5 mm.

Color Erythematous to purple to black.

Distribution Acral, arms more often than legs, near small joints of hands or feet (Fig. 20-16B). Face spared.

Number of Lesions 3 to 20.

Mucous Membranes Usually asymptomatic colonization of oropharynx, urethra, anorectum, or endometrium with *N. gonorrhoeae.*

General Examination

Fever 38° to 39°C, tenosynovitis, septic arthritis, ± infection at other sites/organs (hepatitis, perihepatitis, Fitz–Hugh–Curtis syndrome, myopericarditis, endocarditis, meningitis, perihepatitis. Rarely, pneumonitis, adult respiratory distress syndrome, or osteomyelitis).

DIFFERENTIAL DIAGNOSIS

The diagnosis of gonococcemia is made on clinical findings and confirmed by culture of *N. gonorrhoeae* from mucosal sites. Gonococcemia can be confused with other bacteremias, meningococcemia, endocarditis, infectious arthritis, infectious tenosynovitis, Reiter's syndrome, psoriatic arthritis, or SLE.

LABORATORY EXAMINATIONS

Dermatopathology Immunofluorescence of skin lesion biopsy or skin smear shows *N. gonorrhoeae* in 60% of cases.

Gram's Stain or Bacterial Culture From the male urethra or female cervix may show gonococci. Mucosal sites yield 80 to 90% positive cultures. Skin biopsy, joint fluid, blood only has a 10 to 30% chance of positive culture.

COURSE AND PROGNOSIS

Untreated skin and joint lesions of gonococcemias often gradually resolve; endocardial in-

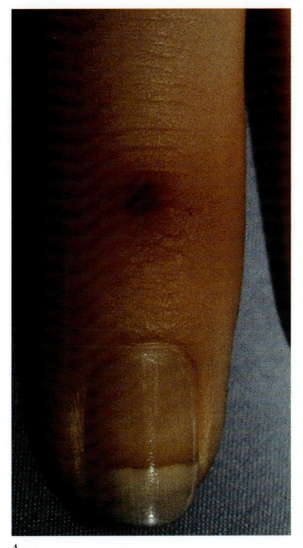

A

Figure 20-16   Gonococcemia   *(A) Hemorrhagic macule over the joint of a young female patient infected with gonococcus.*

volvement of gonococcus is usually fatal or can become chronic disease.

MANAGEMENT

Hospitalization is recommended for initial therapy, especially for patients who cannot reliably comply with treatment, have uncertain diagnoses, or have purulent synovial effusions or other complications. Patients should be examined for clinical evidence of endocarditis or meningitis.

Recommended regimens include:

1. Ceftriaxone 1 g, IM or IV, every 24 h **or**
2. Ceftizoxime 1 g, IV every 8 h **or**
3. Cefotaxime 1 g, IV, every 8 h.

Alternative regimen for patients allergic to β-lactam drugs is spectinomycin 2 g IM every 12 h.

When the infecting organism is proven to be penicillin-sensitive, parenteral treatment may be switched to ampicillin 1 g every 6 h.

Reliable patients with uncomplicated disease may be discharged 24 to 48 hours after all symptoms resolve and may complete the therapy with an oral regimen of:

1. Cefuroxime axetil (500 mg PO bid × 7 d).
2. Amoxicillin with clavulanic acid (500 mg PO tid × 7 d).

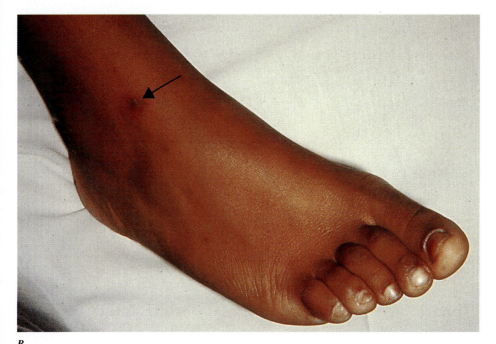

B

Figure 20-16 (continued)   Gonococcemia   (*B*) *Hemorrhagic papule on the foot of a young man infected with gonococcus.*

CAT-SCRATCH DISEASE

Cat-scratch disease is a benign, self-limiting zoonotic infection characterized by a skin or conjunctival lesion(s) following cat scratches or contact with a cat and subsequent chronic tender regional lymphadenopathy.

Synonyms Cat-scratch fever, benign lymphoreticulosis, nonbacterial regional lymphadenitis.

EPIDEMIOLOGY

Age < 21 years.

Gender M > F.

Etiology *Bartonella henselae, B. quintana.*

Transmission History of kitten > cat contact (scratch, bite, lick) in 95% of cases.

Season Late fall, winter, or early spring in cooler climes; in July and August in warmer climes.

HISTORY

Seven to 12 days after cat contact (typically a kitten < 6 months of age), red papules develop at the scratch site. Systemically, mild fever, malaise, chills, general aching, and nausea may be present. One to 4 weeks later, chronic lymphadenitis and regional lymphadenopathy can be found.

PHYSICAL EXAMINATION

Skin Findings

Type Innocuous-looking small papule, vesicle, or pustule at the inoculation site; may ulcerate. Residual linear cat scratch may be detectable.

Color Color of skin to pink to red.

Size 5 to 15 mm.

Palpation Firm, hot, tender to touch.

Distribution of Lesions Primary lesion on exposed skin of head, neck, or extremities.

Mucous Membranes If portal of entry is the conjunctiva, 3- to 5-mm whitish-yellow granulation on palpebral conjunctiva associated with tender preauricular and/or cervical lymphadenopathy is present (referred to as the oculoglandular syndrome of Parinaud).

Other Skin Findings In < 5% of cases, dermatologic manifestations include urticaria, transient maculopapular eruption, vesiculopapular lesions, erythema nodosum, or annular erythema.

General Examination

Regional lymphadenopathy evident within a few days to a few weeks after the primary lesion. Nodes are usually solitary, moderately tender, freely movable. Nodes may suppurate (Fig. 20-17). Generalized lymphadenopathy or involvement of the lymph nodes of more than one region is unusual. Less commonly, systemic disease with encephalitis, pneumonitis, thrombocytopenia, osteomyelitis, hepatitis, or abscesses in liver or spleen may be present.

DIFFERENTIAL DIAGNOSIS

The diagnosis is made with the clinical finding of regional adenopathy, a history of cat exposure and demonstration of small, pleomorphic bacilli in Warthin–Starry-stained sections of the skin lesions, conjunctiva, or lymph nodes. The differential diagnosis of cat-scratch disease includes suppurative bacterial lymphadenitis, atypical mycobacteria, sporotrichosis, tularemia, toxoplasmosis, infectious mononucleosis, tumors, sarcoidosis, lymphogranuloma venereum, and coccidioidomycosis.

LABORATORY EXAMINATIONS

Dermatopathology Skin biopsy of the primary skin lesion will show mid-dermal areas of frank necrosis surrounded by necrobiosis and palisaded histiocytes; multinucleated giant cells and eosinophils may also be seen. Warthin-Starry stain may demonstrate the gram-negative bacillus.

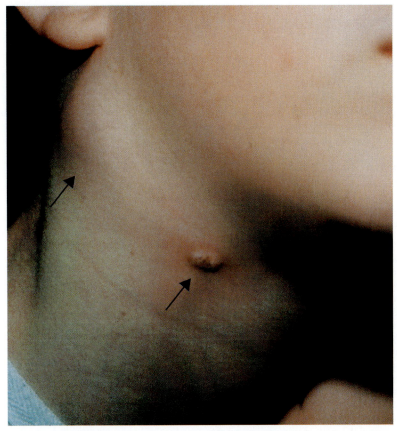

Figure 20-17   Cat-scratch disease   *Suppurative nodule in a child with cat-scratch exposure, with adjacent enlarged lymph node.*

Bacterial Culture   The skin or lymph node may grow *Afipia felis* in special conditions.

COURSE AND PROGNOSIS

Cat-scratch disease has a good prognosis and usually resolves in 2 to 4 months. In rare cases, it may persist for a longer duration.

MANAGEMENT

Cat-scratch disease is self-limited and seems unresponsive to antibiotics. Cefotaxime, genta-micin, amikacin, tobramycin, rifampin, bactrim, and erythromycin have been used and, if started early in the disease, may be of slight benefit.

Aspiration and drainage of supportive, fluctuant nodes will give symptomatic relief. Rarely is surgical removal of lymph nodes necessary. Of note, the disease is self-limited in the cat as well, thus declawing or removing the animal is not necessary.

MYCOBACTERIAL INFECTIONS

LEPROSY

Leprosy is a chronic infection caused by *Mycobacterium leprae*, an organism that has a predilection for the skin and nervous system. The clinical manifestations, course, and prognosis of leprosy depend on the patient's degree of immunity to *M. leprae*.

Synonym Hansen's disease.

CLASSIFICATION

1. *Tuberculoid (TT):* highest host resistance, mildest clinical disease with few skin lesions and few organisms.
2. *Borderline tuberculoid (BT):* numerous, larger skin lesions, peripheral nerve involvement.
3. *Borderline borderline (BB):* "indeterminant"; features both TT and LL, many bacilli are present.
4. *Borderline lepromatous (BL):* multiple skin lesions, leonine facies, late neural lesions.
5. *Lepromatous (LL):* no host cell-mediated immunity. Most severe clinical disease generalized involvement of skin, mucous membranes, respiratory tract, etc. Numerous bacilli.

EPIDEMIOLOGY

Age Any age, peaks at 10 to 20 years of age.

Gender M > F.

Prevalence About 2500 persons infected in the United States. Worldwide, 5.5 million people are estimated to have leprosy. Two to 3 million have significant disabilities from the disease. Endemic leprosy is reported in 53 countries.

Etiology *Mycobacterium leprae,* a slender acid-fast bacillus 3.0×0.5 μm.

Hosts Humans are the main reservoir for *M. leprae*. Wild armadillos (Louisiana), mangabey monkeys, and chimpanzees can also be infected.

Transmission Likely respiratory via aerosolized droplets with organisms.

Geography Africa, Southeast Asia, South and Central America. Disease is endemic in Louisiana, Hawaii, and California.

HISTORY

The incubation period from time of exposure can be anywhere from 2 to 6 years. Childhood leprosy begins with small hyperemic self-resolving macules that, after 18 to 24 months, disappear with a wrinkled, hypopigmented scar. There is a quiescent period until adolescence or adulthood when the more typical skin lesions and neural involvement becomes apparent.

PHYSICAL EXAMINATION

Skin Findings

Type Hypopigmented anesthetic macules (TT) to papules, plaques, nodules, and diffuse skin thickening with loss of hair (LL).

Color Hypopigmented or erythematous.

Size Few mm to several cm.

Shape Annular, oval, round (Fig. 20-18).

Sites of Predilection Face—"leonine" facies due to thick nodular and plaque-like distortions of the face. Mucous membranes—tongue: nodules, plaques, fissures.

Eye Anterior chamber can be involved with resultant glaucoma and cataract formation (LL). Corneal damage and uveitis can also occur.

Testes May be involved with resultant hypogonadism (LL).

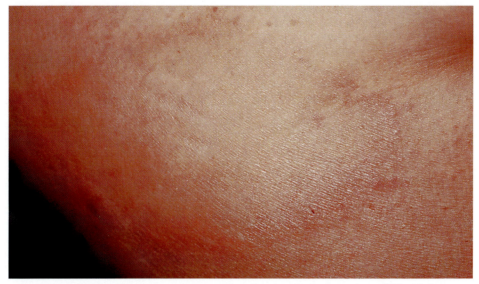

Figure 20-18 Borderline lepromatous leprosy *Annular, anesthetic plaque in a child with leprosy.*

DIFFERENTIAL DIAGNOSIS

Leprosy should be suspected if a patient is from a leprosy-endemic area and presents with chronic skin lesions, skin anesthesia, thickened nerves, or eye complaints. The differential diagnosis is broad given the wide spectrum of clinical disease. Leprosy can be mistaken for tinea corporis, pityriasis alba, tinea versicolor, seborrheic dermatitis, vitiligo, morphea, granuloma annulare, sarcoidosis, leishmaniasis, syphilis, lupus erythmatosus, annular erythema, CTCL, or cutaneous tuberculosis.

LABORATORY EXAMINATIONS

Slit Skin Smear A small skin incision (from earlobes or skin lesions) is made and the site is scraped for tissue fluid and organisms visualized with Ziehl–Neelsen stainings.

Dermatopathology Skin biopsy of TT lesion will show perimeural granuloma formation. Acid-fast bacilli will be sparse or absent. LL lesional biopsy shows an extensive cellular infiltrate separated from the epidermis by a narrow zone of normal collagen. Skin appendages are destroyed. Macrophages are loaded with *M. leprae* (lepra cells or Virchow cells).

COURSE AND PROGNOSIS

Leprosy may be complicated by reactional phenomena.

1. *Lepra type 1 reactions:* the skin lesions become inflamed and painful with severe edema of the hands, feet, and face.
2. *Lepra type 2 reactions (ENL):* painful red nodules appear on the face and limbs and form abscesses or ulcerate.
3. *Lucio's reaction:* irregularly shaped erythematous plaques appear and may ulcerate or become necrotic.

After drug therapy, the main complications are neurologic: contractures of the hands and feet.

MANAGEMENT

Sulfones are the treatment of choice if there is no G6PD deficiency.

1. Dapsone (1 to 2 mg/kg per d PO qd, not to exceed 100 mg/d) is recommended starting with a low dose to avoid negative side effects.

2. Because of dapsone resistance, rifampin (10 to 20 mg/kg per d PO qd, not to exceed 600 mg/d) should be given in conjunction with dapsone for 6 months for the treatment of TT and BT.

3. Clofazamine (1 mg/kg per d PO qd) should be added for treatment of BB, BL, and LL disease and continued for at least 2 years and until skin smears are negative.

CUTANEOUS TUBERCULOSIS

Cutaneous tuberculosis is highly variable in its clinical presentation depending on the route of mycobacterial inoculation and the host response.

CLASSIFICATION

Exogenous infection:

1. Primary tuberculosis complex (PTb) is percutaneous inoculation in a nonimmune host.
2. Tuberculosis verrucosa cutis (TbVC) is percutaneous inoculation in a previously exposed host.

Endogenous spread:

1. Lupus vulgaris (LV).
2. Scrofuloderma (SD).
3. Metastatic tuberculosis (MTb).
4. Acute miliary tuberculosis (AmTb).
5. Orificial tuberculosis (Otb).

Tuberculosis secondary to BCG vaccination.

EPIDEMIOLOGY

Age   Any age. AmTb and PTb more common in infants. SD more common in adolescents/adults. LV affects all ages.

Gender   LV: F > M. TbVC: M > F.

Incidence   LV, SD more common in Europe. LV more common in tropics. TbVC common in third-world countries.

Etiology   *M. tuberculosis,* an obligate human pathogenic mycobacteria. Can also be seen with *M. bovis* or bacille Calmette-Guérin (BCG).

Transmission   Exogenous, auto-inoculation or endogenous.

PATHOPHYSIOLOGY

The clinical presentation of *M. tuberculosis* depends upon the inoculation route, mode of spread, and host cellular immune response.

PHYSICAL EXAMINATION

Skin Findings

Type   Papule at inoculation site to ulcer (PTb chancre; Fig. 20-19) that at late form crusts, plaques that become hyperkeratotic (LV), subcutaneous nodules (SD), fistula formation (MTb), or diffuse macular–papular exanthem (AmTb).

Color   Red to red-brown. Diascopy (i.e., glass slide pressing down on lesion) reveals an "apple jelly" yellow-brown coloration.

Distribution   Exposed skin sites, hands, feet, and knees (TbVC); head and neck (LV); parotid, submandibular, supraclavicular areas (SD); on mucous membranes (Otb) or disseminated (AmTb).

DIFFERENTIAL DIAGNOSIS

The diagnosis of cutaneous tuberculosis should be made by history and clinical presentation and confirmed by collection of *M. tuberculosis* on culture. The differential diagnosis is broad given the wide spectrum of clinical disease. *M. tuberculosis* can be confused with syphilis, cat-scratch disease, sporotrichosis, *M. marinum,* deep fungal infection, sarcoidosis, lymphoma, lupus erythematous, leprosy, leishmaniasis, or panniculitis.

LABORATORY EXAMINATIONS

Dermatopathology

1. *PTb:* nonspecific inflammation followed by epithelioid cells. Langerhans cells, lymphocytes, and caseation necrosis.
2. *AmTb:* nonspecific inflammation and vasculitis.
3. *All other forms:* pseudoepitheliomatous hyperplasia and abscesses. *M. tuberculosis* is demonstrable in PTb, SD, AmTb, MTb, and Otb but difficult to find in LV and TbVC.

Culture   Mycobacteria yield highest in LV and TbVC lesions.

PCR   Detects *M. tuberculosis* DNA in tissue.

Skin Testing   Intradermal skin test converts from negative to positive in PTb. It is negative

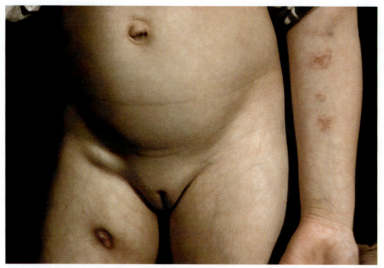

Figure 20-19 Cutaneous Tuberculosis *Primary inoculation site on the thigh with associated inguinal lymphadenopathy and a positive tuberculin test demonstrated on the arm.* (Reproduced with permission from TB Fitzpatrick et al., Color Atlas and Synopsis of Clinical Dermatology, 4th edition. New York: McGraw-Hill, 2001).

in AmTb, positive in LV and TbVC, and may be either negative or positive in SD, Mtb, and Otb.

COURSE AND PROGNOSIS

The course of cutaneous tuberculosis is variable. PTb without treatment self-resolves in 1 year. Tuberculosis from BCG vaccination may appear like PTB, LV, or SD.

MANAGEMENT

The treatment for cutaneous tuberculosis is like pulmonary Tb. Isoniazid and rifampin supplemented with ethambutol, streptomycin, or pyraizinamid can be used for 9 to 12 months. Shorter courses can be attempted with a four-drug regimen.

ATYPICAL MYCOBACTERIA: *M. MARINUM*

Atypical mycobacteria are commonly found in the water and soil and have low grade pathogenicity. *M. marinum* infection follows traumatic inoculation in a fish tank, swimming pool, or brackish water.

Synonyms   Swimming pool granuloma, fish tank granuloma.

EPIDEMIOLOGY

Age   All ages.

Gender   M = F.

Incidence   Uncommon.

Etiology   *Mycobacteria marinum.*

Transmission   Traumatic inoculation and exposure to fish tank, swimming pool, or other aquatic environment.

HISTORY

Red papules appear at the site of inoculation. Over a period of 3 weeks, the papules grow to be about 1 cm nodules and breakdown into ulcers or plaques and may remain as a single lesion or spread proximally (sporotrichocal spread). Systemic symptoms are absent.

PHYSICAL EXAMINATION

Skin Findings

Type   Papule at inoculation site (Fig. 20-20), developing into nodules, plaques. Surface may become hyperkeratotic or ulcerate.

Color   Red to red-brown.

Size   2 mm to 1 cm.

Arrangement   Usually solitary lesion at site of inoculation. Linear arrangement may occur in a "sporotrichoid pattern" up the arm or leg.

General Findings

Regional lymphadenopathy.

DIFFERENTIAL DIAGNOSIS

M. marinum infection is diagnosed by history, physical examination, and culture confirmation of the bacillus. The differential diagnosis includes a wart, sporotrichosis, blastomycosis, *M. tuberculosis,* leishmaniasis, syphilis, foreign body reaction, or tumor.

LABORATORY EXAMINATIONS

Dermatopathology   Skin biopsy of an early lesion will show dermal inflammation with lymphocytes, neutrophils, and histiocytes. Older lesions show epithelial cells and Langerhans giant cells. AFB stain demonstrates *M. marinum* in only 50% of cases. Smears of exudates can also demonstrate AFB.

Bacterial Culture   *M. marinum* will grow at 32°C in 2 to 4 weeks on Lowenstein–Jensen medium and is photochromogenic, differentiating it from the other atypical mycobacteria (i.e., *M. ulcerans* or *M. fortuitum*).

COURSE AND PROGNOSIS

M. marinum lesions tend to heal spontaneously in 1 to 2 years.

MANAGEMENT

Systemic antibiotics have been used with some degree of success.

1.   Tetracycline (25 to 50 mg/kg per day PO divided bid, not to exceed 3 g/d).
2.   Minocycline (2 mg/kg per day PO divided bid, not to exceed 200 mg/d).
3.   Doxycycline (5 mg/kg per day PO divided qd–bid, not to exceed 200 mg/d).
4.   Bactrim (8 to 10 mg TMP/kg per day PO divided bid).
5.   Rifampin (10 to 20 mg/kg per day PO divided qd–bid).

Surgery is not recommended.

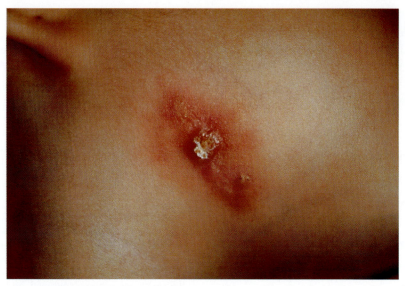

Figure 20-20 Mycobacterial infection *Erythematous plaque with central pustule on the neck of a child exposed to* M. marinum.

LYME BORRELIOSIS

Lyme borreliosis is a spirochetal infectious disease transmitted to humans by the bite of an infected tick. Lyme disease, the syndrome occurring early in the infection, is characterized by a transient annular rash (erythema migrans), followed by late involvement of the joints, nervous system, and/or heart.

EPIDEMIOLOGY

Age All ages; highest attack rate seen in children ages 0 to 14 years and >30 years old.

Gender M = F. There is a slight male predominance in the 10 to 19 year-old age group.

Incidence Common. In endemic areas, 1 to 3% of the population may be affected annually. The number of annually reported cases in the U.S. has increased 25-fold since national surveillance began in 1982. A mean number of 12,500 cases annually were reported to the CDC from 1993 to 1997.

Etiology The spirochete *Borrelia burgdorferi* is responsible for Lyme disease in the United States. *B. burgdorferi* also occurs in Europe, but the two dominant genospecies there are *B. garinii* and *B. afzelii*.

Transmission *B. burgdorferi* is transmitted by the bite of deer ticks (*Ixodes scapularis*) and western black-legged ticks (*Ixodes pacificus*). The deer tick is responsible for transmitting Lyme disease bacteria to humans in the Northeast and Central United States. The western black-legged tick is responsible for Lyme disease on the Pacific Coast. In Europe, the vector tick is *Ixodes ricinus*. *Borrelia* is transmitted to humans following biting and feeding of the tick or nymphs (Fig. 20-21).

Season 80% of Lyme borreliosis occurs in June and July in the Midwestern and Eastern U.S.; January through May in the Northwestern U.S.

Geography Reported from at least 19 countries on three continents. In United States, has been reported from all 50 states with indigenous cases occurring in all but 7 states. Indigenous cases concentrated along Northeast coast (Massachusetts, Rhode Island, Connecticut, New York, New Jersey, Pennsylvania, Delaware, Maryland), Midwest (Minnesota, Wisconsin), and West (California, Oregon, Nevada, Utah). In Europe, Lyme borreliosis occurs widely throughout the continent and Great Britain. It also occurs in Australia.

PATHOPHYSIOLOGY

Lyme borreliosis begins with the rash of erythema migrans, which occurs at the site of entry of the spirochete soon after inoculation. Secondary lesions occur following hematogenous dissemination to the skin. The late joint manifestations appear to be mediated by immune-complex formation. Meningitis results from direct invasion of the cerebrospinal fluid. The pathogenesis of cranial and peripheral neuropathies in Lyme disease is unknown, but might also result from immune mechanisms.

HISTORY

Lyme borreliosis has an incubation period of 1 to 36 d (median, 9 d) after the tick bite. Of note, only 14% of Lyme borreliosis cases are aware of a preceding tick bite. Early Lyme disease is characterized by malaise, fatigue, lethargy, headaches, fever, chills, a stiff neck, arthralgias, myalgias, backaches, anorexia, sore throat, nausea, dysesthesia, vomiting, abdominal pain, and photophobia; 75% of patients will have an associated erythema chronicum migrans rash. Early Lyme disease symptoms disappear by 1 to 2 months. Late Lyme disease can occur in 15% of untreated cases after several weeks to months. Late sequelae include joint, neurologic, and cardiac complications.

PHYSICAL EXAMINATION

Skin Findings in Early Lyme Disease

Type Initial macule or papule enlarges within days to form an expanding annular plaque, at the bite site (Fig. 20-22). Center may become indurated, vesicular, or necrotic.

Size 2 cm to several cm (range, 3 to 70 cm, median 15 cm in diameter).

Number of Lesions Erythema chronicum migrans is typically a solitary lesion. Multiple secondary lesions develop in 17% of cases, ranging in number from 2 to >100. Secondary lesions resemble EM but are smaller, migrate less, and lack central induration.

Other Cutaneous Findings Malar rash, diffuse urticaria, subcutaneous nodules (panniculitis).

Color Erythematous evolving to violaceous.

Arrangement At time concentric rings form. When occurring on the scalp, only a linear streak may be evident on the face or neck.

Distribution Trunk and proximal extremities, especially the axillary and inguinal areas, most common sites. Secondary lesions can occur at any site except the palms and soles and can become confluent.

Mucous Membranes Red throat, conjunctivitis.

Skin Findings in Late Lyme Disease

Lymphocytoma Cutis Synonyms: Lymphadenosis benigna cutis, pseudolymphoma of Spiegler and Fendt. An infiltrative cutaneous disorder, characterized most often by solitary (may be grouped) nodules or plaques; occasionally translucent; red to brown to purple in color; located on the head, especially ear lobes, nipples, scrotum, and extremities; 3 to 5 cm in diameter; usually asymptomatic.

Acrodermatitis Chronica Atrophicans (ACA) Begins with diffuse or localized erythema, usually on one extremity, accompanied by mild to prominent edema, most commonly involving the extensor surfaces and periarticular areas. Asymptomatic dull-red infiltrated plaques arise on the extremities, more commonly on lower legs than forearms, which slowly extend centrifugally over several months to years, leaving central areas of atrophy. Veins and subcutaneous tissue become prominent, easily lifted and pushed into fine accordion-like folds ("cigarette paper" or "tissue paper" skin). Lesions may be single or multiple. Plaque(s) slowly extends centrifugally with an active inflammatory advancing border and a smooth, hairless, tissue paper-like atrophic central area with dull-red, poikilodermatous skin.

Sclerotic or Fibrotic Plaques and Bands Localized fibromas and plaques are seen as subcutaneous nodules around the knees and elbows; may involve the joint capsule with subsequent limitation of movement of joints in hand, feet, or shoulders.

General Findings in Early Lyme Disease

High persistent fever, lymphadenopathy, right upper quadrant tenderness, arthritis, hepatosplenomegaly, muscle tenderness, periorbital edema, and abdominal tenderness.

General Findings in Late Lyme Disease

Arthritis Occurs in 60% of untreated cases, 4 to 6 weeks after the tick bite (range, 1 week to 22 months); sudden in onset, involves one or a few joints. Knee (89%), shoulder (9%), hip (9%), ankle (7%), and elbow (2%).

Neurologic Involvement Occurs in 10 to 20% of untreated cases, 1 to 6 weeks (or longer) following the tick bite. Manifested by meningitis (excruciating headache, neck pain); encephalitis (sleep disturbances, difficulty concentrating, poor memory, irritability, emotional lability, dementia); cranial neuropathies (unilateral or bilateral; optic neuropathy, sixth nerve palsy, facial or Bells's palsy, eighth nerve deafness); sensory and motor radiculopathies (severe radicular pain, dysesthesias, subtle sensory loss, focal weakness, loss of reflexes).

Cardiac Abnormalities Occur in 6 to 10% of untreated cases, usually within 4 weeks. AV block, myopericarditis, and left ventricular dysfunction. Usually transient and not associated with long-term sequelae.

Variants

Lyme disease occurring in Europe is reportedly milder than in United States, with more secondary EM-like skin lesions and fewer arthritic complications, probably due to strain differences in *B. burgdorferi*.

DIFFERENTIAL DIAGNOSIS

The diagnosis of Lyme disease can be made with history and characteristic clinical findings in a person living in or having visited an endemic area. The diagnosis can be confirmed by specific serologic tests. The differential diagnosis of Lyme disease, specifically the rash of erythema chronicum migrans, includes tinea corporis, herald patch of pityriasis rosea, insect (e.g., brown recluse spider) bite, cellulitis, ur-

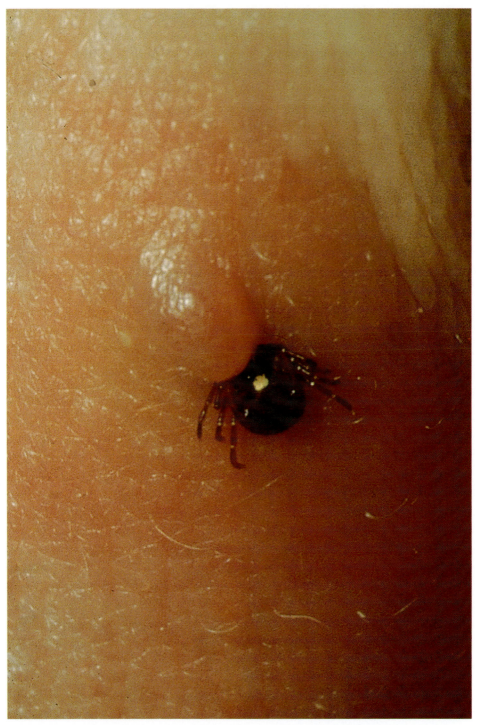

Figure 20-21 **Lyme borreliosis** *A blood-distended nymph* Ixodes scapularis *feeding on human skin. Borrelia transmission usually occurs after prolonged attachment and feeding (36 h).*

ticaria, erythema multiforme, fixed drug eruption, and secondary syphilis.

LABORATORY EXAMINATIONS

Dermatopathology A skin biopsy will show a deep and superficial perivascular and interstitial lymphohistiocytic infiltrate containing plasma cells. Spirochetes can be demonstrated in up to 40% of skin biopsy specimens.

Serology Indirect immunofluorescence antibody (IFA) and ELISA are used to detect antibodies to *B. burgdorferi*. Initial antibody response is with IgM antibodies followed by IgG. Early in Lyme disease, when only the rash has occurred, as few as 50% of patients, have positive serologies; adequate treatment may block seroconversion. Virtually all cases with late manifestations are seropositive with a titer of 1:256 or greater.

COURSE AND PROGNOSIS

The skin lesions in untreated early Lyme disease fade in a median time of 28 d. Both EM and secondary lesions can fade and recur for months. However, following adequate treatment, early lesions resolve within several days and late manifestations are prevented. Late manifestations identified early usually clear following adequate antibiotic therapy; however, delay in diagnosis may result in permanent joint, neurologic, or cardiac disabilities.

MANAGEMENT

Prevention

- Wearing long-sleeved shirts and tucking pants into socks or boot tops may help keep ticks from reaching the skin.
- Insect repellents (such as DEET or permethrin) applied to clothes and exposed skin can help reduce the risk of tick attachment, but should be used sparingly to avoid systemic toxicity.
- Transmission of *B. burgdorferi* from an infected tick usually takes 36 h of tick attach-

ment; thus daily checks for ticks and prompt removal will prevent infection.
- Ticks should be removed with a fine-tipped tweezer by grasping the tick near the skin and pulling it off.
- Petroleum jelly, a hot match, nail polish, or other home remedies are NOT recommended.

Early Lyme Disease

- In children >8 years old, the treatment of choice is (1) tetracycline (250 mg PO qid for 21 d), (2) doxycycline (100 mg PO bid for 21 d), (3) amoxicillin (500 mg PO tid for 21 d), or (4) cefuroxime axetil (500 mg PO qd for 7 d).
- For younger children, the treatment of choice is (1) penicillin V (50 mg/kg per d for 21 d) or (2) amoxicillin (25 to 50 mg/kg per d divided tid to a maximum of 2 g/d for 21 d).
- In penicillin-allergic patients, erythromycin (30 mg/kg per d divided tid to a maximum of 250 mg/d for 21 d) is recommended.

Late Lyme Disease

- For Bell's palsy alone, oral regimens for early disease suffice.
- Neurologic complications can be treated with (1) ceftriaxone (50 to 100 mg/kg per d not to exceed 2 g/d IM or IV for 14 to 28 d); (2) for children >8 years old, doxycycline (100 mg PO or IV bid for 14 to 28 d) or (3) IV PCN (200,000 to 300,000 units/kg for 14 to 28 d).
- Lyme arthritis can be treated with (1) amoxicillin and probenicid (20 to 40 mg/kg per d divided tid, not to exceed 500 mg PO tid for 30 d); (2) ceftriaxone (50 to 100 mg/kg per d not to exceed 2 g/d IM or IV for 14 to 28 d); (3) penicillin IM (2 to 4 million units/week for 2 to 3 weeks); or (4) IV penicillin G (20 million units/d for 2 to 3 weeks).
- Cardiac disease can be treated with (1) amoxicillin (20 to 40 mg/kg per d divided tid, not to exceed 500 mg PO tid for 21 d); (2) ceftriaxone (50 to 100 mg/kg per d not to exceed 2 g/d IM or IV for 14 to 28 d); (3) for children >8 years old, doxycycline (100 mg PO or IV bid for 14 to 28 d) or (4) IV penicillin G (20 million units/d for 14 d).

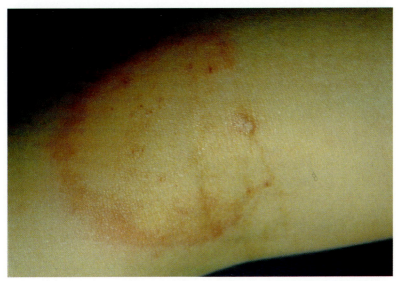

Figure 20-22 Lyme borreliosis, erythema migrans *Solitary enlarging annular plaque on the leg at the site of an asymptomatic tick bite.*

Lyme Disease Vaccination

1. Currently, LYMErix can be considered for individuals aged 15 to 70 who reside, work, or recreate in areas of high or moderate risk. Three IM doses (0.5 mL, 30 μg of purified rOspA lipidated protein) are administered; the second and third doses should be spaced 1 month and 12 months after the initial dose.

2. The safety and immunogenicity of LYMErix has not been established for children <15 years old, pregnant women, immunocompromised individuals, persons with musculoskeletal disease, or persons with a complicated past history of Lyme disease. Thus the vaccine is NOT recommended for these individuals at this time.

CUTANEOUS FUNGAL INFECTIONS

SUPERFICIAL FUNGAL INFECTIONS

Dermatophytes are a unique group of fungi that are capable of infecting nonviable skin including the hair and nails. The three major genera are *Trichophyton, Microsporum,* and *Epidermophyton.* The term "tinea" is used to denote fungal infection and is typically modified by site (e.g., tinea capitis, tinea corporis).

Candida is a normal inhabitant of the oropharynx and gastrointestinal tract. Moist, wet conditions favor *Candida* overgrowth and can lead to superficial infection of the skin.

DERMATOPHYTOSES

TINEA CAPITIS

Tinea capitis is a fungal infection of the scalp and hair characterized by follicular inflammation with painful, boggy nodules that drain pus and result in hair loss.

Synonym   Scalp ringworm.

EPIDEMIOLOGY

Age   Children ages 2 to 10; rarely seen in infants or adults.

Gender   M > F, 5:1.

Race   More common in blacks than in whites.

Incidence   Common. Most common fungal infection in childhood. Affects 3 to 8% of the pediatric population.

Etiology   *Trichophyton tonsurans* is the cause of 90% of the cases of tinea capitis in the U.S. and Western Europe. *Microsporum audouinii* (child to child, via barber, hats, theater seats), *M. canis* (young pets to child and then child to child), *T. verrucosum,* and others can also be seen. *T. violaceum* is the cause of tinea capitis in Eastern and Southern Europe and North Africa.

HISTORY

Two to four days after exposure, scaly slightly pruritic patches appear in the scalp with associated hair loss. Untreated, the lesions can become larger and can be more painful and unsightly. Systemic symptoms may include cervical lymphadenopathy, mild malaise, or low-grade fever, more commonly. A systemic allergy to fungal elements can be seen (see "Tinea and Id reaction" on page 520).

PHYSICAL EXAMINATION

Skin Lesions and Hair Changes

Classification

1.   Ectothrix (infection on the outside of the hair shaft).

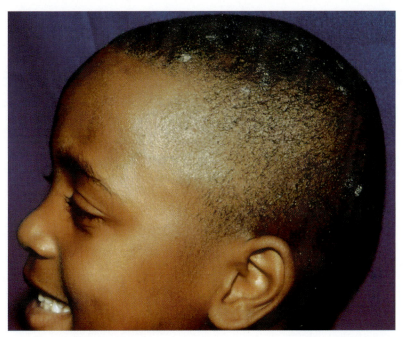

Figure 21-1 Tinea capitis, "gray patch" type *Well-delineated scaly patches scattered on the scalp of a child with "ringworm."*

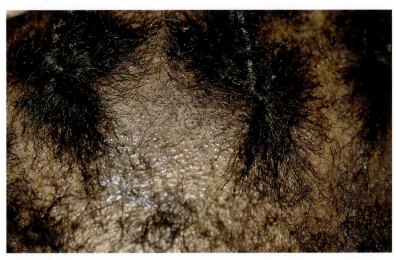

Figure 21-2 Tinea capitis, "black-dot" type *Asymptomatic patch of alopecia on the frontal scalp of a 4-year-old child with a* Trichophyton tonsurans *infection.* (Reproduced with permission from TB Fitzpatrick et al., Color Atlas and Synopsis of Clinical Dermatology, 4th edition. New York: McGraw-Hill, 2001).

a. *Gray patch ringworm.* Brittle hair; shafts break off close to scalp surface. Caused by *M. audouinii* and *M. canis* (Fig. 21-1).

2. Endothrix (infection on the inside of the hair shaft).

   a. *Black dot ringworm.* Broken-off hairs near surface give appearance of dots. Tends to be diffuse and poorly circumscribed. Caused by *T. tonsurans* and *T. violaceum* (Fig. 21-2).

   b. *Kerion.* Boggy, elevated, purulent, inflamed nodule which is painful and drains pus. Hairs do not break off but fall out easily. Heals with residual hair loss. (Fig. 21-3).

   c. *Favus.* Cutaneous atrophy, scar formation, and scarring alopecia are typical of favus, due to infection with *T. schoenleinii.* Scutula (yellowish adherent crusts) are present on the scalp (Fig. 21-4). Favus is now uncommon in Western Europe and North America. In some parts of the world (Middle East, South Africa), however, it is still endemic.

Fluorescence Examination with Wood's Lamp
Examination of scalp with a Wood's lamp reveals bright green hair shafts in scalp infections caused by *M. audouinii* and *M. canis. T. schoenleinii* fluorescence is grayish green. *T. tonsurans,* however, does not exhibit fluorescence.

LABORATORY EXAMINATIONS

Direct Microscopic Examination with 10% KOH   Spores can be seen within (*T. tonsurans* and *T. violaceum*) or surrounding (*Microsporum*) the hair shaft.

Fungal Culture   Infected hair or scalp scale can be inoculated on Sabouraud's agar or other DTM media and the causative organism can be identified in several weeks time.

MANAGEMENT

1. Tinea spreads on brushes, combs, towels, pillowcases, and hats. Children with scalp ringworm should not share these items.

2. Tinea can also be spread by close contact with infected children. The current recommendation is that infected children may attend school once treatment has begun.

3. Antifungal shampoos (ketoconazole 2% or selenium sulfide 2.5%) decrease shedding of fungal elements and thus decrease spread of infection. Patients should be instructed

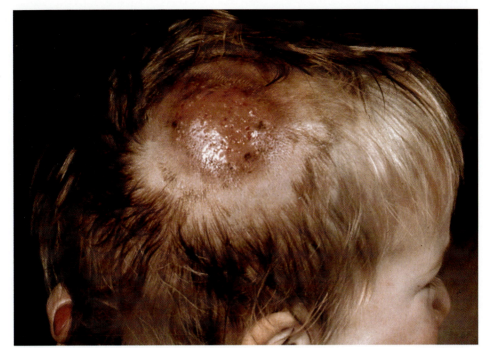

Figure 21-3 Tinea capitis, "kerion" type *Large boggy, erythematous nodule on the scalp of a child.* (Reproduced with permission from TB Fitzpatrick et al., Color Atlas and Synopsis of Clinical Dermatology, 4th edition. New York: McGraw-Hill, 2001).

to lather the shampoo and let it sit on the scalp for 5 to 10 min before rinsing 2 to 3 ×/week.

Systemic Therapies Topical treatments are not effective in treating the hair bulb; thus oral antifungal treatment is needed:

1. Oral griseofulvin (15 mg/kg per d for 6 to 8 weeks) is the gold standard for tinea capitis in children. Refractory cases may need higher doses (20 to 25 mg/kg/per d for 6 to 8 weeks). Known side effects include headaches and gastrointestinal upset.
2. Fluconazole (5 mg/kg per d × 4 to 6 weeks OR 6 mg/kg per d × 20 d OR 8 mg/kg per week × 4 to 6 weeks). Side effects include nausea, vomiting, and LFT abnormalities.

3. Newer antifungal agents are efficacious and safe in children, but none of these agents have yet been officially approved by the FDA; all current use is strictly off label:
   a. Itraconazole (5 mg/kg per d × 4 to 6 weeks OR 5 mg/kg per d × 1 week each month for 2 to 3 months). Side effects include nausea, vomiting, and LFT abnormalities.
   b. Terbinafine. For children < 20 kg, 62.5 mg/d × 2 to 4 weeks. For children 20 to 40 kg, 125 mg/d × 2 to 4 weeks. For children > 40 kg, 250 mg/d × 2 to 4 weeks. Side effects include GI upset and rarely, Stevens–Johnson syndrome or toxic epidermal necrolysis.

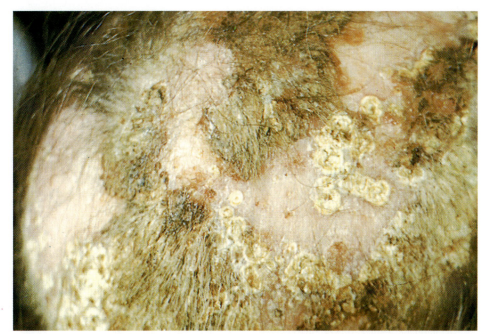

Figure 21-4 **Tinea capitis, "favus" type** *Yellowish adherent crusts and scales called "scutula" on a child with a* Trichophyton schoenleinii *infection.* (Reproduced with permission from IM Freedberg et al., Dermatology in General Medicine, 5th edition. New York: McGraw-Hill, 1999).

TINEA FACIEI

Tinea faciei is a superficial fungal infection on the face, characterized by a well-circumscribed erythematous enlarging plaque.

Synonyms Tinea faciale, tinea facialis, ringworm of the face.

EPIDEMIOLOGY

Age Most common in children.

Incidence Common.

Etiology *Trichophyton mentagrophytes, T. rubrum* most commonly; also *Microsporum audouinii, M. canis.*

Predisposing Factors Animal exposure, especially puppies or kittens.

HISTORY

An asymptomatic papule slowly enlarges to a plaque. The lesion is asymptomatic or mildly pruritic. No systemic symptoms are present.

PHYSICAL EXAMINATION

Skin Findings

Type Well-circumscribed macule to plaque of variable size; elevated border. Scaling often is minimal (Fig. 21-5).

Color Pink to red. In dark skin, hyperpigmentation.

Distribution Any area of face.

DIFFERENTIAL DIAGNOSIS

Tinea faciei is the most commonly misdiagnosed fungal infection. It is often mistaken for seborrheic dermatitis, contact dermatitis, erythema chronicum migrans, lupus erythematosus, polymorphic light eruption, photodrug eruption, or a lymphocytic infiltrate.

LABORATORY EXAMINATIONS

KOH Direct Microscopic Examination Examination of scraping shows hyphae. Scrapings from patients who have used topical corticosteroids show massive numbers of hyphae.

Fungal Culture Skin scrapings taken from the area and inoculated on Sabouraud's agar or other DTM media will grow the causative dermatophyte in a few weeks.

MANAGEMENT

Topical antifungals are effective for tinea faciei. They should be applied bid at least 2 cm beyond the advancing edge of the skin lesion until the lesion clears (typically 6 weeks). It is recommended to continue the topical medication for one more week after clinical clearing to ensure clinical cure. The topical agents are as follows:

1. Substituted pyridone.
    a. Ciclopirox (Loprox).
2. Naphthiomates.
    a. Tolnaftate (Tinactin).
3. Imidazoles.
    a. Clotrimazole (Lotrimin, Mycelex).
    b. Econazole (Spectazole).
    c. Miconazole (Micatin).
    d. Ketoconazole (Nizoral).
    e. Oxiconizole (Oxistat).
4. Allylamines.
    a. Terbinafine (Lamisil).
    b. Naftifine (Naftin).

Affected household members or pets should also be treated.

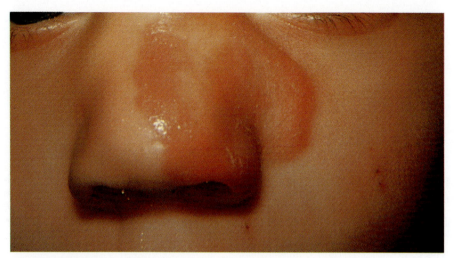

Figure 21-5 Tinea faciei *Sharply marginated, enlarging plaque with a raised annular border on the face of a child.*

TINEA CORPORIS

These scaling papular lesions occur in an annular arrangement with peripheral enlargement and central clearing on the trunk, limbs, or face ("ringworm").

Synonyms   Ringworm, tinea corporis gladiatorum.

EPIDEMIOLOGY

Age   All ages.

Incidence   Common.

Exposure   Animals, especially puppies and kittens.

Etiology   *Microsporum canis > M. audouinii, Trichophyton mentagrophytes, T. rubrum.*

PHYSICAL EXAMINATION

Skin Findings

Type   Small to large, scaling, sharply marginated plaques with or without pustules or vesicles.

Size   1 to 10 cm.

Color   Pink to red.

Shape and Arrangement   Peripheral enlargement and central clearing, producing an annular configuration (Fig. 21-6).

Distribution   Single and occasionally scattered multiple lesions.

Sites of Predilection   Exposed skin of forearm, neck.

DIFFERENTIAL DIAGNOSIS

Tinea is diagnosed by the demonstration of hyphae in a cutaneous lesion. It is often mistaken for annular erythemas, psoriasis, contact dermatitis, eczema, pityriasis rosea, seborrhea, granuloma annulare, or lupus erythematosus.

LABORATORY EXAMINATIONS

KOH Direct Microscopic Examination   Examination of scales from the advancing border should demonstrate hyphae, arthrospores, or budding yeasts. One cannot identify the type of dermatophyte but can note its presence or absence.

Fungal Culture   Skin lesion scrapings can be inoculated on Sabouraud's agar or other media, and specific dermatophyte types will grow and can be identified in a matter of weeks.

MANAGEMENT

Topical Antifungal Treatment
See page 508 for details.

Oral Antifungal Treatment
See page 506 for details.

Prophylaxis   Affected household members or pets should also be treated.

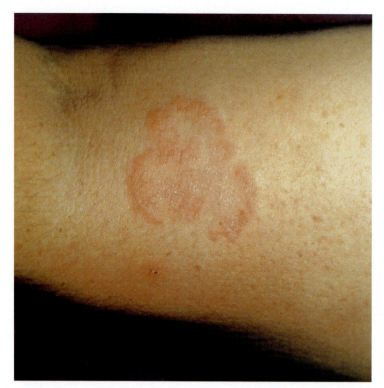

Figure 21-6   Tinea corporis   *Well-demarcated enlarging plaque with a raised annular border on the forearm.*

TINEA CRURIS

Tinea cruris is a subacute or chronic fungal infection of the upper thigh or groin area, usually caused by *Epidermophyton floccosum* or *Trichophyton rubrum*.

Synonym   Jock itch.

EPIDEMIOLOGY

Age   Adolescents and young adults.

Gender   M > F.

Predisposing Factors   Concomitant tinea pedis, warm, humid environment, tight clothing, obesity.

Etiology   *Trichophyton rubrum* and *T. mentagrophytes*.

PATHOPHYSIOLOGY

Most patients with tinea cruris have concomitant tinea pedis. The fungal infection on the feet typically precedes the groin infection. The fungal elements are spread when underclothes are dragged over the infected feet up to the groin area.

HISTORY

Often seen in athletes, tinea cruris begins as erythema and mild pruritus in the groin area. Occlusive, wet clothing (tight clothes, exercise outfits, bathing suits) aggravates the condition and it slowly spreads.

PHYSICAL EXAMINATION

Skin Findings

Type   Well-demarcated plaques with papules, scaling, occasional pustules, and central clearing.

Color   Dull red to brown.

Distribution   Bilateral intertriginous areas, upper thighs and buttock (Fig. 21-7). Scrotum is rarely involved (in contrast to candidiasis).

DIFFERENTIAL DIAGNOSIS

The diagnosis of tinea cruris is made by demonstration of a fungal organism on KOH or fungal culture. The differential diagnosis includes erythrasma, intertrigo, seborrheic dermatitis, psoriasis, irritant dermatitis, and contact dermatitis.

LABORATORY EXAMINATIONS

KOH Direct Microscopic Examination   Examination of scrapings will show hyphae, arthrospores, or budding yeasts.

Fungal Culture   Skin scrapings taken from the area and inoculated on Sabouraud's agar or other DTM media will grow causative dermatophyte in a few weeks.

MANAGEMENT

Topical Antifungal Treatment
See page 508 for details.

Oral Antifungal Treatment
See page 506 for details.

Measures to prevent recurrence include:

1. Less occlusive clothing.
2. Shower shoes in public or home bathroom floor.
3. Antifungal foot (Zeasorb AF) powder.
4. Concomitant treatment of tinea pedis (athlete's foot) if present.
5. Patients should be instructed to put on their socks before their underwear to avoid dragging the fungal elements from the floor or their infected feet up to their groin area.

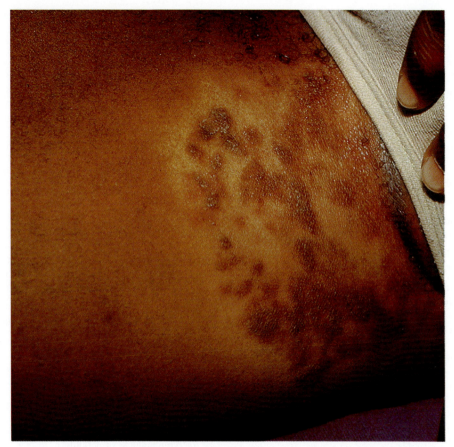

Figure 21-7 Tinea cruris *Enlarging pruritic plaque in the groin area worsening on topical steroids.*

TINEA PEDIS

Tinea pedis is an itchy, scaly fungal infection of the feet seen in adolescents or adults, but rarely in young children.

Synonym Athlete's foot.

EPIDEMIOLOGY

Age Adolescents and adults; rare in children.

Gender M = F.

Incidence Most common fungal infection in adolescents and adults.

Etiology *Trichophyton rubrum, T. mentagrophytes > Epidermophyton floccosum.*

Predisposing Factors Hot, humid weather; occlusive footwear.

HISTORY

Tinea pedis usually begins as interdigital scaling and fissuring, especially between the fourth and fifth toes. It can then spread to affect both plantar aspects of the feet but rarely involves the dorsa. One or two palms may also become involved. Systemic symptoms are rare. A systemic allergic response can be seen (see "Tinea and Id Reaction" later in the chapter).

PHYSICAL EXAMINATION

Skin Findings

Type Scaling, plus maceration, and vesicles or bullae (Fig. 21-8).

Color Pink to red; opaque white scales.

Distribution Common in the webspace between third and fourth toes and the plantar aspect of the feet, especially in the arch. Rarely spreads to involve the dorsa of the feet.

DIFFERENTIAL DIAGNOSIS

The diagnosis of tinea pedis is made by history, clinical presentation, and demonstration of fungal elements by KOH or culture. Tinea pedis, although common in adolescents and adults, is *uncommon* in children. Most instances of "athlete's foot" in children are actually foot eczema or a shoe dermatitis.

LABORATORY EXAMINATIONS

KOH Direct Microscopic Examination Examination of the webspace or scaly areas reveals hyphae, arthrospores, or budding yeasts.

Fungal Culture Skin scrapings inoculated on Sabouraud's agar or DTM media will show fungal growth in a few weeks.

COURSE AND PROGNOSIS

Tinea pedis tends to be chronic and recurrent with exacerbations in hot weather or with exercise. Macerated skin may provide portal of entry for lymphangiitis or cellulitis.

MANAGEMENT

Tinea pedis is difficult to treat and is prone to recurrences. Acute episodes can be treated with open wet compresses (Burrow's solution 1:80) and topical antifungal creams. (See page 508 for details). They should be applied bid over both feet up to the ankles bilaterally until the lesions clear (typically 2 to 6 weeks). It is recommended to continue the topical medication for one more week after clinical clearing to ensure clinical cure.

Oral Antifungal Treatment
See page 506 for details.
 Keeping the feet dry will help prevent relapses and can be achieved with open footwear or absorbent socks/foot powder (Zeasorb AF).

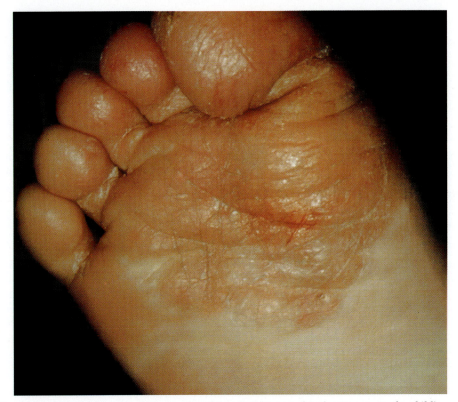

Figure 21-8 Tinea pedis *Erythema, scale, and vesiculation on the plantar aspect of a child's foot. KOH scraping demonstrated hyphae.*

TINEA MANUUM

Tinea manuum is a chronic dermatophytosis of the hand(s), often unilateral, and most commonly on the dominant hand. There is almost invariably a preexisting tinea pedis, with or without nail involvement (onychomycosis).

Synonym   Tinea manus.

EPIDEMIOLOGY

Age   Adolescents and adults. Uncommon in children.

Gender   M = F.

Incidence   Common.

Etiology   *Trichophyton rubrum, T. mentagrophytes > Epidermophyton floccosum.*

HISTORY

Tinea manuum usually presents as unilateral palmar scaling in an individual with chronic or intermittent preexisting tinea pedis or onychomycosis. Like tinea pedis, it tends to have a chronic and relapsing course.

PHYSICAL EXAMINATION

Skin Findings

Type   Hyperkeratosis, scaling papules, and vesicles in clusters (Fig. 21-9).

Color   Pink to red.

Distribution   Diffuse hyperkeratosis of the palms or patchy scaling on the dorsa and sides of fingers; 50% of patients have *unilateral* involvement.

DIFFERENTIAL DIAGNOSIS

The diagnosis of tinea manuum is made by history and demonstration of fungal organisms by KOH or culture. It is often mistaken for psoriasis, lichen planus, allergic contact or irritant dermatitis, or dyshidrotic eczema.

LABORATORY EXAMINATIONS

KOH Direct Microscopic Examination   Examination of scales taken from the advancing edge will show hyphae elements.

Fungal Culture   Skin scrapings can be inoculated on Sabouraud's agar or DTM media and will grow the causative dermatophyte in several weeks time.

COURSE AND PROGNOSIS

When combined with tinea capititis, onychomycosis, tinea pedis, or tinea corporis, tinea manuum may recur following treatment, and this can be a frustrating problem.

MANAGEMENT

Acute episodes of tinea manuum can be treated with open wet compresses (Burrow's solution 1:80) and topical antifungal creams. (See page 508 for details.)

Oral Antifungal Treatment
See page 506 for details.
   Eradication of other concomitant tinea infections (e.g., tinea capitis, onychomycosis) needs to occur to prevent further recurrences.

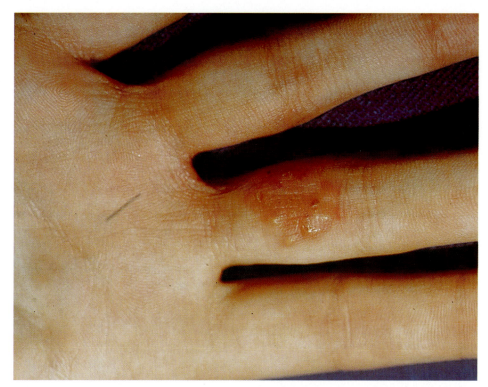

Figure 21-9 Tinea manuum *Clustered erythematous papules on the hand of a child. KOH scraping demonstrated hyphae.*

TINEA UNGUIUM (ONYCHOMYCOSIS)

Onychomycosis is a common, unsightly fungal infection of the toenails and/or fingernails.

Synonym Tinea unguium.

EPIDEMIOLOGY

Age Adolescents and adults, rarely children.

Incidence Common in adolescents and adults, especially those chronically affected with tinea pedis or tinea manuum.

Etiology *Trichophyton rubrum, T. mentagrophytes,* and *Epidermophyton floccosum.* Onychomycosis due to nondermatophytes is usually caused by *Candida* species.

HISTORY

Onychomycosis typically is seen in individuals with chronic tinea pedis or tinea manuum. However, onychomycosis can also superinfect diseased nails as seen in psoriasis or eczema. The onset is slow and insidious, and typically affects the toenails more often than the fingernails. Topical treatments are ineffective and oral regimens, while efficacious, do not prevent relapses.

PHYSICAL EXAMINATION

Nail Lesions

Distal Subungual Onychomycosis Whitish-brownish-yellow discoloration of the free edge of the nail. Subungual hyperkeratosis leads to separation of nail plate and nail bed with subungual accumulation of friable keratinous debris.

White Superficial Onychomycosis Appears as white, sharply outlined area on the nail plate (of toenails). Surface of nail friable, rough. This presentation occurs relatively commonly in HIV-infected patients in both toenails and fingernails.

Proximal Subungual Onychomycosis Rare. Starts as whitish-brown area on the proximal part of the nail plate. May enlarge to affect the whole nail plate.

Candida Onychomycosis Affects both toenails and fingernails in chronic mucocutaneous candidiasis. Thickening of nail plate, which is rough, furrowed, and eventually disintegrates into a hyperkeratotic, brittle, and fissured horny mass.

Distribution Characteristically, infected nails coexist with normal-appearing nails (Fig. 21-10). Toenails more frequently involved than fingernails. In chronic immunosuppression, there is a tendency towards involvement of all 20 nails (seen in chronic mucocutaneous candidiasis and acrodermatitis enteropathica).

DIFFERENTIAL DIAGNOSIS

The diagnosis of onychomycosis can be made by history, clinical presentation and demonstration of hyphae with KOH, fungal nail culture or histologic PAS staining of a nail specimen. The differential diagnosis includes nail psoriasis, eczema, trauma, photo-onycholysis, and pachonychia congenita.

LABORATORY EXAMINATIONS

KOH Direct Microscopic Examination Examination of nail scrapings reveals hyphae.

Fungal Culture Nail clippings taken and inoculated on Sabouraud's agar or other DTM media will grow the causative dermatophyte in a few weeks.

Dermatopathology A PAS stain of an infected nail clipping will reveal hyphae.

MANAGEMENT

Topical treatment for onychomycosis is not successful. Oral antifungals are the treatment of choice.

Oral Antifungal Treatment
See page 506 for details. Oral griseofulvin may not be as effective as fluconazole, itraconazole, or terbinafine for toenail clearance.

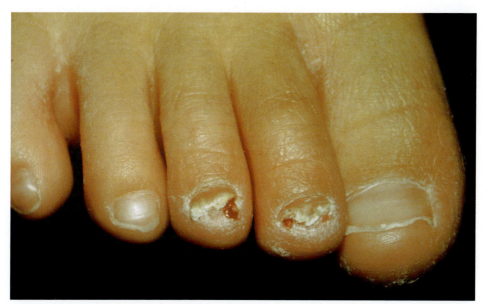

Figure 21-10 Onychomycosis *Onycholysis of the second and third toenails. Fungal culture of the nail grew* Trichophyton rubrum.

TINEA AND ID REACTION

The "id" reaction to tinea is an allergic reaction to fungal elements characterized by a vesicular eruption on the trunk and extremities.

Synonym Dermatophytid reaction.

EPIDEMIOLOGY

Age Any age.

Gender M = F.

Incidence Uncommon.

Etiology Unclear.

PATHOPHYSIOLOGY

An id reaction is thought to be a hypersensitivity reaction to some fungal element that occurs as the fungus is being cleared from the body. The exact mechanism is unclear.

HISTORY

An id reaction is an uncommon generalized vesicular eruption that appears after the primary focus of tinea (tinea capitis, faciei, corporis, pedis or manuum) has been present for a while and clearance has started.

PHYSICAL EXAMINATION

Skin Findings

Type Diffuse papules and vesicles, edema (Fig. 21-11A).

Color Pink to red.

Size 2 to 5 mm.

Distribution Trunk and extremities (Fig. 21-11B).

Sites of Predilection Palms and sides of fingers.

Other Concomitant tinea infection elsewhere on the body.

General Findings

Usually none. Mild lymphadenopathy may be present.

DIFFERENTIAL DIAGNOSIS

An id reaction is diagnosed if a primary tinea infection is identified and subsequent generalized skin vesicles are KOH negative. Id can be confused with a drug hypersensitivity reaction, viral exanthem, dyshidrotic eczema, or generalized tinea infection.

LABORATORY EXAMINATIONS

Dermatopathology Skin biopsy shows nonspecific epidermal spongiotic vesicles without eosinophils.

KOH of Vesicular Lesions Negative for hyphae or spores.

Fungal Culture Culture of vesicular lesions will be negative for organisms.

COURSE AND PROGNOSIS

Once the primary tinea infection has been cleared, the id reaction disappears.

MANAGEMENT

Eradication of the primary fungal infection is the best way to treat an id reaction. Symptomatic relief can be obtained with a short course of topical steroids. Topical steroids are effective if used in appropriate strengths. (See page 48 for more details.)

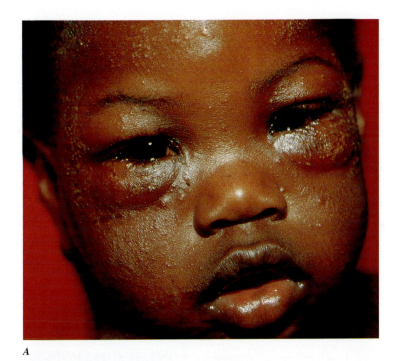

A

B

Figure 21-11   Tinea and id reaction   *(A) Diffuse vesicular rash in a child being treated for tinea capititis. (B) Diffuse vesicular lesions on the arm of the same child.*

CANDIDIASIS

ORAL CANDIDIASIS

Oral candidiasis is characterized by the presence of painful, white, milk-like removable plaques on the oral mucosa.

Synonyms   Moniliasis, thrush, mycotic stomatitis, *Candida* leukoplakia.

EPIDEMIOLOGY

Age   Newborns, not apparent until day of life 8 or 9.

Gender   M = F.

Incidence   Common in newborns and infants. In adults, it may be a marker for immunodeficiency.

Etiology   *Cundida albicans,* most commonly.

Transmission   *Candida* is present in the mouth and intestinal tract of 30 to 50% of the normal population and > 20% of the genital tract in normal women. *Candida* is transmitted to the infant at the time of delivery during passage through the vaginal canal.

PATHOPHYSIOLOGY

C. albicans is part of the normal oral and vaginal flora. Oral thrush is transmitted to the baby during passage through the birth canal.

HISTORY

In newborns and infants, the white curd-like plaques appear at day of life 8 to 9 and are usually asymptomatic.

PHYSICAL EXAMINATION

Skin Findings

Type of Lesion   Friable white plaques on any mucosal surface; mechanical removal with a dry gauze pad leaves an erythematous or bleeding mucosal surface.

Size   Few mm to several cm.

Color   White to creamy.

Palpation   Plaques are friable and removable with dry gauze.

Distribution of Lesions   Dorsum of tongue, buccal mucosa, hard and soft palate, and pharynx (Fig. 21-12).

DIFFERENTIAL DIAGNOSIS

Oral thrush is diagnosed by clinical impression; the soft plaques can be scraped away with a piece of gauze. A KOH preparation of scraping from mucosal surface can confirm the diagnosis. The differential diagnosis includes oral hairy leukoplakia, condyloma acuminatum, geographic tongue, hairy tongue, lichen planus, and a bite irritation.

LABORATORY EXAMINATIONS

KOH Preparation   Scraping of the white plaque shows *Candida* pseudohyphae as well as budding yeast forms.

Yeast Cultures   Buccal or tongue plaques scraped and cultured will grow species of *Candida*.

COURSE AND PROGNOSIS

Oral candidiasis is benign and usually asymptomatic. It responds nicely to topical treatment, but may intermittently recur. In adults, chronic recurrent oral candidiasis may be a sign of immunosuppression.

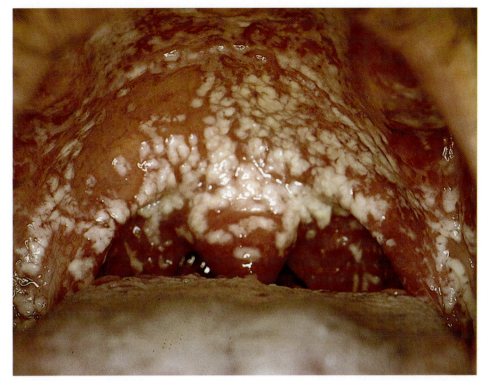

Figure 21-12   Oral Candidiasis   *White plaques on the hard palate representing colonies of* Candida *that can be removed by rubbing the area with gauze.* (Reproduced with permission from TB Fitzpatrick et al., Color Atlas and Synopsis of Clinical Dermatology, 3rd edition. New York: McGraw-Hill, 1997).

MANAGEMENT

For mild cases, nystatin suspension (applied with a Q-tip to the mucosal lesions 4 ×/d until clinical clearing is noted. Refractory or recurrent cases may require:

1. Nystatin suspension (2 mL PO qid for 2 days beyond clinical clearing).
2. Other anticandidal agents are efficacious, but none of these agents have yet been officially approved by the FDA; all current use is strictly off label:
   a. Clotrimazole troches (10 mg dissolved slowly on oral mucosa 5 ×/d).
   b. Itraconazole suspension (1 to 2 mg/kg per d PO qd × 7 to 10 d). Side effects include nausea, vomiting, and LFT abnormalities.
   c. Fluconazole (5 to 8 mg/kg per day × 2 wks).

CUTANEOUS CANDIDIASIS

Cutaneous candidiasis is a superficial infection occurring on moist cutaneous sites and mucosal surfaces; many patients have predisposing factors such as increased moisture at the site of infection, diabetes, antibiotic therapy, or alteration in systemic immunity.

Synonyms   Moniliasis, candidosis.

EPIDEMIOLOGY

Age   Any age. Infants (diaper area, mouth).

Gender   M = F.

Incidence   Common.

Etiology   *Candida albicans;* uncommonly other candidal species. *C. albicans* is a normal inhabitant of the oropharynx and GI tract, *not* of the skin.

Other Predisposing Factors   Diabetes, obesity, hyperhidrosis, heat, maceration, immunologic defects (depressed T-cell function), polyendocrinopathies, systemic antibacterial agents, systemic and topical corticosteroids, chronic debilitation (carcinoma, leukemia), chemotherapy.

CLASSIFICATION

Candida in occluded skin occurs where occlusion creates a warm, moist environment for *Candida* to thrive.

1.   Intertrigo.
     a.   Body folds (neck, groin, intergluteal, axilla, inframammary).
     b.   Webspaces: fingers, toes (erosio interdigitalis blastomycetica) associated with frequent wetting of hands/feet. May be also associated with candidal paronychia.
2.   Genital.
     a.   Balanoposthitis or balanitis.
     b.   Vulvitis.
3.   Occluded skin, other.
     a.   Diaper dermatitis (Fig. 21-13).
     b.   Dressings (extremity in a cast).
     c.   Other (back of nonambulatory hospitalized patient).

Chronic Mucocutaneous Candidiasis   A group of rare, immunologic (e.g., T-cell defects) or endocrinologic disorders (e.g., hy-poparathyroidism, hypoadrenalism, hypothyroidism, diabetes) that lead to recurrent or persistent mucosal, cutaneous, or nail *C. albicans* infections.

HISTORY

Areas of candida overgrowth tend to be moist and warm with frequent episodes of wetness (from sweating, water exposure). The areas usually start off pink and sometimes slightly pruritic. They progress to red, macerated, sore, painful, irritated skin.

PHYSICAL EXAMINATION

Skin Findings

Type   Erythematous papules and pustules coalescing into plaques with erosions; oozing, scattered satellite pustules are evident.

Color   Beefy red areas with thickened white skin or exudates.

Distribution   Any body fold, webspaces between fingers (Fig. 21-14), toes, genital area.

DIFFERENTIAL DIAGNOSIS

The diagnosis of *Candida* is made by history and exam, and can be confirmed by demonstration of *Candida* yeast forms by KOH or culture. The differential diagnoses include psoriasis, erythrasma, atopic dermatitis, irritant dermatitis, seborrheic dermatitis, or other fungal infection.

LABORATORY EXAMINATIONS

Microscopic Examination   Skin scrapings stained with Gram stain or 10 to 30% KOH preparation shows pseudohyphae and yeast forms.

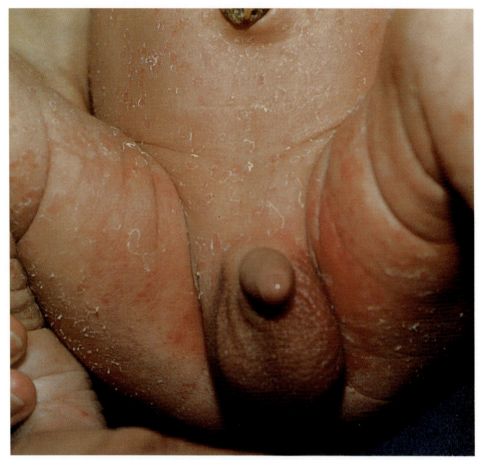

Figure 21-13 Candidiasis, diaper dermatitis *Beefy, red, Candida diaper dermatitis with character-istic "satellite pustules."* (Slide courtesy of Karen Wiss).

Fungal Culture Skin scrapings inoculated on Sabouraud's agar will grow *Candida*.

MANAGEMENT

Prevention Keeping intertriginous areas dry and open to air as much as possible will help. Daily application of topical powders (Nystatin powder) or creams can help.

Topical Antifungal Treatment
Topical antifungals are effective for *Candida*. They should be applied bid to the affected areas until the lesion clears (typically 6 weeks). It is recommended to continue the topical medication for one more week after clinical clear-

ing to ensure clinical cure. The topical agents are as follows:

1. Nystatin (Mycostatin, Nystex).
2. Amphotericin B (Fungizone).
3. Substituted pyridone.
   a. Ciclopirox (Loprox).
4. Imidazoles.
   a. Clotrimazole (Lotrimin, Mycelex).
   b. Econazole (Spectazole).
   c. Miconazole (Micatin).
   d. Ketoconazole (Nizoral).
   e. Oxiconizole (Oxistat).
   f. Sulconazole (Exelderm).
5. Antifungals and steroid combinations are effective for *Candida* treatment, but have a

---

strong steroid component and thus should be used sparingly:

a. Nystatin + triamcinolone (Mycolog).
b. 1% clotrimazole + betamethasone dipropionate (Lotrisone).

Oral Antifungal Treatment

If extensive or resistant to topical treatment, oral antifungal treatment may be needed.

1. Fluconazole (5 to 8 mg/kg per d PO qd × 2 to 3 weeks). Side effects include nausea, vomiting, and LFT abnormalities.
2. Ketoconazole (for < 20 kg, 50 mg PO qd; for 20 to 40 kg, 100 mg PO qd; for > 40 kg, 200 mg PO qd × 2 to 3 weeks). Side effects include nausea, vomiting, and LFT abnormalities.
3. Newer antifungal agents are efficacious and safe in children, but they have yet to be officially approved by the FDA; all current use is off-label:
   a. Itraconazole (5 mg/kg per d PO × 2 to 3 weeks). Side effects include nausea, vomiting, and LFT abnormalities.
4. For fluconazole-resistant candidiasis:
   a. Amphotericin B (0.25 to 1 mg/kg per d IV qd or qod × 2 to 3 weeks). Side effects include renal tubular acidosis, hypokalemia, hypomagnesemia, fever, chills, delirium, phlebitis, nausea, vomiting, hypotension, hypertension, renal failure, bone marrow depression.

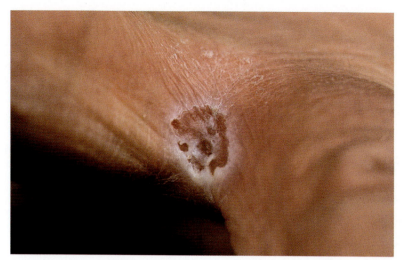

Figure 21-14   Candidiasis, interdigital   *Eroded and macerated area of candidal overgrowth in the* *webspace of the hand.* (Reproduced with permission from TB Fitzpatrick et al., Color Atlas and Synopsis of Clinical Dermatology, 3rd edition. New York: McGraw-Hill, 1997).

PITYRIASIS VERSICOLOR

Pityriasis versicolor is a common asymptomatic superficial fungal infection of the trunk, characterized by white or brown scaling macule and associated with the overgrowth of *Pityrosporum ovale*.

Synonym   Tinea versicolor.

EPIDEMIOLOGY

Age   Can be seen in children. More common in adolescents, young adults.

Gender   M = F.

Incidence   Common.

Etiology   *Pityrosporum ovale* (also known as *P. orbiculare* and *Malassezia furfur*), a lipophilic yeast that is a normal inhabitant of skin. *Pityrosporum* infections are not contagious, but an overgrowth of resident cutaneous form under certain favorable conditions. Seborrheic dermatitis and *Pityrosporum* folliculitis are thought to be other cutaneous manifestations of *P. ovale* overgrowth, and all three conditions can be seen concomitantly.

Predisposing Factors   High humidity or sebum on the skin can cause *P. ovale* overgrowth. Application of oils (e.g., cocoa butter, bath oil) on children leads to *P. ovale* overgrowth.

Prevalence/Seasons   In temperate zones, occurs in 2% of population, especially during summer months. In tropical zones, occurs in up to 40% of the population. In athletes, rash may persist year round.

PATHOPHYSIOLOGY

Pityrosporum ovale is a normal inhabitant of the skin. Favorable conditions (e.g., sweat, sebum, oils) allows for overgrowth. The pigmentary changes are due to dicarboxylic acids formed by enzymatic oxidation of fatty acids in skin surface lipids inhibiting tyrosinase in epidermal melanocytes.

HISTORY

The rash of pityriasis versicolor begins insidiously and spreads over months to years. It is typically asymptomatic or mildly pruritic. The resultant blotchy pigmentation is what usually brings the patient into the office.

PHYSICAL EXAMINATION

Skin Lesions

Type   Macule, sharply marginated, with fine scaling that is easily scraped off with the edge of a glass microscope slide.

Color   In light skin types, lesions are typically darker (tan to brown). In dark skin types, lesions are typically light (off-white to white; Fig. 21-15).

Size   5 mm to several cm.

Shape   Round or oval.

Distribution   Scattered discrete lesions.

Sites of Predilection   Upper trunk, upper arms, neck, abdomen, axillae, groin, thighs, genitalia. Rarely on the face.

DIFFERENTIAL DIAGNOSIS

Tinea versicolor is recognized by the distribution and shape of the lesions and is easily identified by examination of the scales for fungus. The differential diagnosis includes vitiligo, pityriasis rosea, pityriasis alba, postinflammatory hypopigmentation, tinea corporis, seborrheic dermatitis, guttate psoriasis, and nummular eczema.

LABORATORY EXAMINATIONS

Dermatopathology   Skin biopsy will show budding yeast and hyphae forms in the most superficial layers of the stratum corneum. PAS stain will stain *P. ovale* very bright pink.

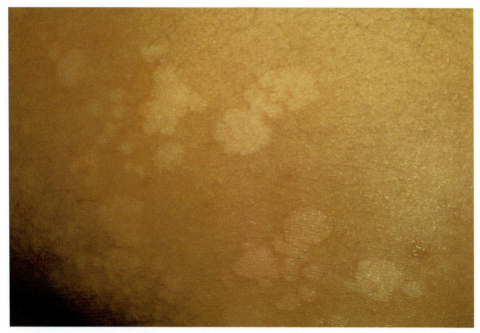

Figure 21-15 Pityriasis versicolor *Scaly, hypopigmented macules of pityriasis versicolor on the chest of a child.*

KOH Prep Scraping of scaly macules put in 10 to 20% KOH will show filamentous hyphae and spores (a so-called spaghetti-and-meatballs appearance; Fig. 21-16).

Wood's Lamp Examination Faint yellow-green fluorescence of scales may be detected.

COURSE AND PROGNOSIS

Pityriasis versicolor has a benign but chronic/relapsing course. Skin or systemic symptoms are rare, but the pigmentary changes can be very noticeable and cosmetically unappealing.

MANAGEMENT

Pityriasis versicolor responds well to topical agents:

1. Antifungal shampoos can be lathered on the body and left on for 10 to 15 min followed by a shower or bath qd for 1 to 2 weeks.
   a. Selenium sulfide shampoo (Selsun).
   b. Ketoconazole 2% shampoo (Nizoral).
2. Imidazole creams can be used to small, localized areas bid for 1 to 2 weeks:
   a. Clotrimazole (Lotrimin, Mycelex).
   b. Econazole (Spectazole).
   c. Miconazole (Micatin).
   d. Ketoconazole (Nizoral).
   e. Oxiconizole (Oxistat).
   f. Sulconazole (Exelderm).
3. For chronic, recurrent, or severe involvement:
   a. Ketoconazole (for < 20 kg, 50 mg PO qd; for 20 to 40 kg, 100 mg PO qd; for > 40 kg, 200 mg PO qd × 2 to

3 weeks). Side effects include nausea, vomiting, and LFT abnormalities.

b. Newer antifungal agents are efficacious and safe in children, but they have yet to be officially approved by the FDA; all current use is strictly off-label. Itraconazole (5 mg/kg per d PO qd × 2 to 3 weeks). Side effects include nausea, vomiting, and LFT abnormalities.

It is important to warn the patient about likely recurrences and predisposing factors (sweat and/or topical oils). In athletes, treatment may need to be repeated prophylactically. Additionally, even when *P. ovale* is cleared, the pigmentary changes of pityriasis versicolor can persist for months and do not represent therapeutic failure.

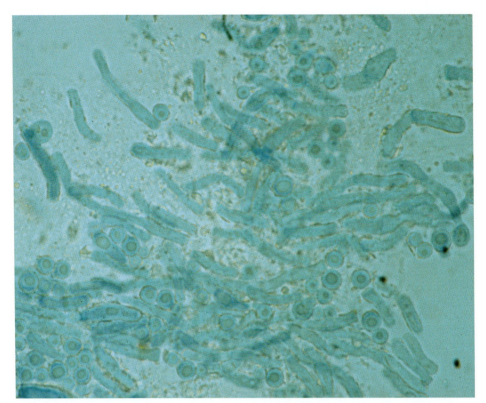

Figure 21-16   Pityriasis versicolor, potassium hydroxide (KOH) preparation   *Potassium hydroxide (KOH) preparation demonstrating filamentous hyphae and spores ("spaghetti-and-meatballs") appearance characteristic of pityriasis versicolor.*

DEEP FUNGAL INFECTIONS

SPOROTRICHOSIS

Sporotrichosis is a deep fungal infection that follows accidental inoculation of the skin and is characterized by ulceration and/or nodule formation at the inoculation site, followed by subcutaneous nodule formation along the course of lymphatic drainage.

Synonym Sporotrichum infection.

EPIDEMIOLOGY

Age Any age.

Gender M > F.

Etiology *Sporothrix schenckii,* a dimorphic fungus commonly found in soil. In the tissue, the organism looks like a cigar-shaped yeast.

Transmission Commonly, subcutaneous inoculation by a contaminated thorn, rock, glass, barb, splinter, cat scratch, or other sharp item. Rarely inhalation, aspiration, or ingestion causes systemic infection. Most cases are isolated. Epidemics do occur. In Uruguay, 80% of cases occur following an armadillo scratch. There are also reports that cats can transmit sporotrichosis.

Geography Ubiquitous, worldwide. More common in temperate, tropical zones. Present on rose and barberry thorns, wood splinters, sphagnum moss, straw, marsh hay, soils.

PATHOPHYSIOLOGY

Following subcutaneous inoculation, *S. schenckii* grows locally and slowly spreads along the draining lymphatics. Secondary skin lesions develop along the lymphatic chain. In rare instances after inhalation, the organism can cause a granulomatous pneumonitis.

HISTORY

Three days to 12 weeks after trauma, inoculation of the fungal organism, an asymptomatic or slightly painful nodule will appear at the inoculation site followed by erythematous nodule formation extended proximally along the path of lymphatic drainage.

PHYSICAL EXAMINATION

Skin Findings

Type of Lesion

1. Lymphocutaneous sporotrichosis is the most common clinical manifestation seen in 25% of cases. Lesion follows lymphatic extension of local cutaneous type. Proximal to local cutaneous lesion, intervening lymphatics become indurated, nodular, thickened, with occasional ulcer formation (Fig. 21-17).
2. Fixed cutaneous sporotrichosis occurs in 20% of cases and is characterized by a subcutaneous papule, pustule, nodule, ulcer, or plaque appearing at inoculation site several weeks after puncture wound. The patient is previously sensitized to sporotrichosis; thus there is no lymphatic spread.
3. A third, rare chancriform form of sporotrichosis (Fig. 21-18) can be seen in < 8% of cases with associated lymphadenopathy proximally.
4. A final, rare disseminated form of sporotrichosis can be seen in < 1% of cases in the immunocompromised host. Primary skin or pulmonary inoculation with sporotrichosis can lead to hematogenous spread with resultant disease in the liver, spleen, pancreas, thyroid, myocardium, or CNS.

Arrangement Primary nodules with enlarged regional lymph nodes in a linear arrangement described as "sporotrichoid" spread.

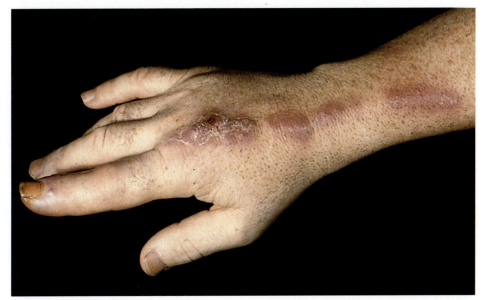

Figure 21-17 Sporotrichosis, sporotrichoid type *Inoculation site on the dorsa of the hand with a linear arrangement of dermal and subcutaneous nodules extending along the lymphatic vessels on the arm.* (Reproduced with permission from TB Fitzpatrick et al., Color Atlas and Synopsis of Clinical Dermatology, 4th edition. New York: McGraw-Hill, 2001).

Distribution Primary lesion most common on dorsum of hand or finger with chronic nodular lymphangitis up arm. In fixed cutaneous type, the face and trunk are most commonly involved in children. Upper extremities are more commonly involved in adults.

DIFFERENTIAL DIAGNOSIS

The diagnosis of sporotrichosis is based upon clinical suspicion and confirmed by isolation of the organism on culture. The differential diagnosis includes tuberculosis, atypical mycobacterial infection, anthrax, tularemia, cat-scratch disease, primary syphilis, leishmaniasis, herpes simplex virus infection, staphylococcal lymphangitis, histoplasmosis, coccidioidomycosis, blastomycosis, and cryptococcosis.

LABORATORY EXAMINATIONS

Dermatopathology Granulomatous, Langerhans'-type giant cells, pyogenic microabscesses. Organisms rare, difficult to visualize. Yeast, if visible, appear as 1 to 3 μm by 3 to 10 μm cigar-shaped forms.

Fungal Culture A fluorescent antibody is available to help detect the *S. schenckii* organism in vitro. Organism can be isolated within a few days after culture of skin aspirate of lesional biopsy specimen.

COURSE AND PROGNOSIS

Sporotrichosis shows little tendency to resolve spontaneously. The deep fungal infections respond well to systemic therapy, but relapses are possible.

MANAGEMENT

Oral antifungal agents are effective in sporotrichosis. The various regimens should be taken 4 to 6 weeks beyond resolution of the lesions:

1. Fluconazole (5 to 8 mg/kg per d PO qd × 2 to 3 weeks). Side effects include nausea, vomiting, and LFT abnormalities.
2. Ketoconazole (for < 20 kg, 50 mg PO qd; for 20 to 40 kg, 100 mg PO qd; for > 40 kg, 200 mg PO qd × 2 to 3 weeks). Side effects include nausea, vomiting, and LFT abnormalities.

3. Newer antifungal agents are efficacious and safe in children, but have not yet been officially approved by the FDA; all current use is strictly off-label:
   a. Itraconazole (5 mg/kg per d PO qd × 2 to 3 weeks). Side effects include nausea, vomiting, and LFT abnormalities.

For severe or systemic disease, especially in immunocompromised hosts:

Amphotericin B (0.25 to 1 mg/kg per d IV qd or qod × 2 to 3 weeks). Side effects include renal tubular acidosis, hypokalemia, hypomagnesemia, fever, chills, delirium, phlebitis, nausea, vomiting, hypotension, hypertension, renal failure, and bone marrow depression.

In the past, there has also been reported success with saturated solution of potassium iodide, SSKI (1 or 2 drops/year of age PO tid to a maximum of 120 drops/d given for 4 to 6 weeks beyond clinical resolution of cutaneous lesions).

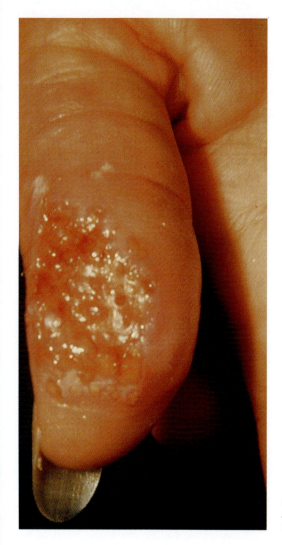

Figure 21-18   Sporotrichosis, chancriform
An ulcerated nodule at the site of inoculation with sporotrichosis.

CRYPTOCOCCOSIS

Cryptococcosis is a deep fungal infection acquired by the inhalation of *Cryptococcus neoformans,* causing a primary pulmonary infection that can lead to hematogenous dissemination, and spread of infectionges, kidneys, and/or skin.

Synonyms   Torulosis, European blastomycosis.

EPIDEMIOLOGY

Age   All ages, even neonates. Does occur in children but more commonly seen in adults age 30 to 60.

Gender   M > F, 3:1.

Incidence   Rare.

Etiology   *Cryptococcus neoformans,* a yeast. Serotypes A, B, C, and D can cause disease in humans. In tissue, cryptococcus looks like a budding yeast form with a capsule.

Transmission   Possible transplacental transmission seems possible. Cryptococcus may also inhabit the female genital tract leading to inoculation of the infant as it passes through the birth canal. More commonly the cryptococcal organism is accidentally inhaled from infected dust of avian feces (pigeons, parakeets, and canaries).

Geography   Worldwide, ubiquitous. Less incidence in U.S. compared to Europe or South America.

PATHOPHYSIOLOGY

C. neoformans is inhaled in dust and causes a primary pulmonary focus of infection with subsequent hematogenous dissemination to meninges, kidneys, and skin; 10 to 15% of patients have skin lesions. Immune deficiency is an important factor in pathogenesis in many patients.

HISTORY

Often, cryptococcal disease remains localized to the lungs with absent or minimal symptoms. In rare instances, especially in immunosuppressed individuals, hematogenous dissemination leads to CNS infection with headache (80%), mental confusion, and visual disturbances for months. Thirty percent of disseminated cases are associated with malignancy (usually Hodgkin's disease).

PHYSICAL EXAMINATION

Skin Findings

Type   Well-demarcated papules, pustules, developing into plaques, nodules, ulcers. Umbilicated papules are often mistaken for molluscum lesions (Fig. 21-19).

Color   Pink to red, bluish.

Distribution   Any site.

Site of Predilection   Face (especially around nose and mouth), scalp.

General Findings

CNS symptoms (headache, behavioral disturbance, seizures), pulmonary symptoms, hepatomegaly, splenomegaly, lymphadenopathy may be present.

DIFFERENTIAL DIAGNOSIS

The diagnosis of cryptococcus is made by history, physical exam, and demonstration of the 5-μm thick-walled round-oval organism in the skin, CNS, sputum, or tissues. The differential diagnosis includes blastomycosis, histoplasmosis, molluscum contagiosum, and other bacterial or systemic fungal infections.

LABORATORY EXAMINATIONS

Dermatopathology   Thick-walled organisms 5 by 20 μm should be visible in the skin biopsy. Special stains with methylene blue, alcian blue, or mucicarmine will brightly stain the polysaccharide capsule.

Indirect Immunofluorescence   Available to detect cryptococcal organism in body fluids of tissue specimens.

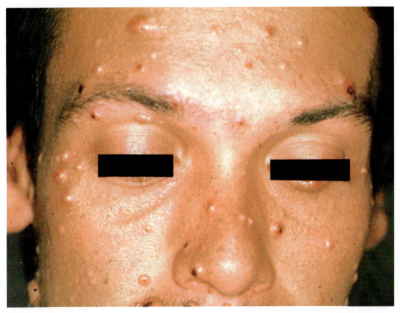

Figure 21-19   Cryptococcosis, disseminated   *Umbilicated nodules on the face of an HIV patient with disseminated cryptococcosis.* (Reproduced with permission from IM Freedberg et al., Dermatology in General Medicine, 5th edition. New York: McGraw-Hill, 1999).

Fungal Culture   Cryptococcus from body fluids or tissues can be grown on Sabouraud's agar.

CXR   Focal pneumonia, patchy infiltrates, solitary nodules, abscesses, or pleural effusions may be present.

COURSE AND PROGNOSIS

Untreated cryptococcosis is fatal in 90% of cases. Appropriate antifungal treatment leads to an 80% cure rate even in disseminated forms of disease.

MANAGEMENT

The treatment of choice for cryptococcus is amphotericin B (0.1 to 0.3 mg/kg per d IV and intrathecally qd, not to exceed 30 mg/kg for 2 months). Side effects include renal tubular acidosis, hypokalemia, hypomagnesemia, fever, chills, delirium, phlebitis, nausea, vomiting, hypotension, hypertension, renal failure, and bone marrow depression.

Another effective medication is flucytosine (100 to 150 mg/kg administered qid for 2 months). But since flucytosine-resistant strains

of *Cryptococcus* are possible, combination therapy with amphotericin B is still recommended. Side effects include nausea, headache, diarrhea, rash, anemia, leukopenia, thrombopenia, LFT abnormalities, confusion, and sedation.

In unresponsive disease, adjuncts to amphotericin B may be required, with:

1.   Miconazole (20 to 40 mg/kg per d IV divided tid for 2 months). Side effects include nausea, vomiting, diarrhea, phlebitis, pruritus, headache, anemia, hyperlipidemia, arrhythmias, and anaphylaxis.
2.   Ketoconazole (for < 20 kg, 50 mg PO qd; for 20 to 40 kg, 100 mg PO qd; for > 40 kg, 200 mg PO qd × 2 months). Side effects include nausea, vomiting, and LFT abnormalities.
3.   Fluconazole (5 to 8 mg/kg per d PO qd × 2 months). Side effects include nausea, vomiting, and LFT abnormalities.
4.   Newer antifungal agents are efficacious and safe in children, but they have yet to be officially approved by the FDA; all current use is off-label:
     a.   Itraconazole (5 mg/kg per d PO qd × 2 to 3 weeks). Side effects include nausea, vomiting, and LFT abnormalities.

HISTOPLASMOSIS

Histoplasmosis is a common, highly infectious systemic fungal infection caused by *Histoplasma capsulatum* and characterized by pulmonary disease.

Synonyms   Darling's disease, cave disease, Ohio Valley disease.

EPIDEMIOLOGY

Age   All ages; infects infants and children as well as adults.

Gender   M = F.

Incidence   Common.

Etiology   *Histoplasma capsulatum* exists in the soil as a saprophyte, mostly form children droppings or feathers, other bird or bat feces.

Transmission   *H. capsulatum* is spread by aerosolized droplets and is acquired by inhalation of spores in soil contaminated with bird or bat droppings.

Geography   Disease is endemic in the Mississippi and Ohio River valleys of the United States (Kentucky, Illinois, Indiana, Missouri, Ohio, Tennessee, and Western New York).

HISTORY

Histoplasmosis exists as self-limited pulmonary infection in 75% of cases, which are asymptomatic. Flu-like pulmonary symptoms (fever, malaise, cough, and chest pain) develop in 25% of cases and < 1% of patients progress to disseminated histoplasmosis (fever, hepatosplenomegaly, anemia, and weight loss).

PHYSICAL EXAMINATION

Skin Findings

Cutaneous lesions in histoplasmosis are rare but may be seen in the disseminated form (Fig. 21-20).

Type   Papules, plaques, pustules, purpura, nodules, abscesses, or ulcers.

Color   Pink, red.

Distribution   Any site, mucosa surface.

General Findings

May be associated with fever, cough, dyspnea, chest pain, hepatosplenomegaly, and weight loss.

DIFFERENTIAL DIAGNOSIS

The diagnosis of histoplasmosis is made by identification of the organism on skin smears, sputum, blood, or tissue biopsies. The differential diagnosis includes miliary tuberculosis, coccidioidomycosis, cryptococcosis, leishmaniasis, and lymphoma.

LABORATORY EXAMINATIONS

Dermatopathology   Skin biopsy of an active lesion may show small intracellular yeast-like organism.

Touch Preparation   Lesional skin biopsy touched to glass slide and stained with Giemsa stain will show *H. capsulatum*.

Fungal Culture   Tissue or blood inoculated on Sabouraud's agar may grow *H. capsulatum*.

Histoplasmosis Skin Test   In infants, a positive reaction 2 to 3 weeks after infection indicates active, current infection; but in endemic populations, up to 90% of children and adults react positively, signifying past or present infection.

Serology   Immunodiffusion, agar gel precipitin, yeast phase complement fixation, collodion, or latex particle agglutination can be performed on blood samples. Titers greater than 1:32 are highly suggestive of active histoplasmosis disease.

CXR   Interstitial infiltrates and/or hilar adenopathy.

COURSE AND PROGNOSIS

In 99% of cases, histoplasmosis is a benign and self-limited disease. The disseminated form of untreated does have a high mortality rate.

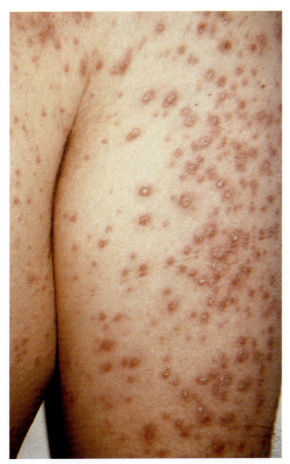

Figure 21-20 Histoplasmosis, disseminated *Scattered erythematous papules and pustules in an HIV-infected individual with disseminated histoplasmosis.* (Reproduced with permission from TB Fitzpatrick et al., Color Atlas and Synopsis of Clinical Dermatology, 4th edition. New York: McGraw-Hill, 2001).

▎MANAGEMENT

If bird or bat droppings are to be cleared in an endemic area for *H. capsulatum*, protective equipment (respirators, goggles, and so forth) should be worn. Most cases of histoplasmosis do not require therapy. In severe cases of disseminated disease, systemic antifungals may be necessary. (See page 504 for more details.) Refractory cases or for meningeal involvement may require amphotericin B (0.25 to 1 mg/kg per d IV qd or qod × 12 weeks). Side effects include renal tubular acidosis, hypokalemia, hypomagnesemia, fever, chills, delirium, phlebitis, nausea, vomiting, hypotension, hypertension, renal failure and bone marrow depression.

RICKETTSIAL INFECTION

ROCKY MOUNTAIN SPOTTED FEVER

Rocky Mountain spotted fever (RMSF), the most severe of the rickettsial infections, is characterized by sudden onset of fever, severe headache, myalgia, and a characteristic acral exanthem; it is associated with significant mortality.

EPIDEMIOLOGY

Age   Any age.

Gender   M > F.

Incidence   Uncommon.

Etiology   Caused by *Rickettsia rickettsii*.

Transmission   Occurs through bite of an infected tick or inoculation through abrasions contaminated with tick feces or tissue juices. The reservoirs and vectors are the wood tick (*Dermacentor andersoni*) in the Western U.S., the dog tick (*D. variabilis*) in the Eastern U.S., and the lone star tick (*Amblyomma americanum)* in the Southern U.S. Patient either lives in or has recently visited an endemic area; *however, only 62% have knowledge of a recent tick bite.*

Season   April to September in the U.S. (95% of patients).

Geography   Occurs only in the Western Hemisphere. In the United States, the highest endemic areas are centered around Virginia, North Carolina, South Carolina, Georgia, Kansas, Oklahoma, Texas, and New York City.

PATHOPHYSIOLOGY

Following inoculation, there is an initial local replication of the organism in endothelial cells followed by hematogenous dissemination. Focal infection of vascular smooth muscle causes a generalized vasculitis. Hypotension, local necrosis, gangrene, and DIC may follow. The petechial rash results from extravasated blood after vascular necrosis.

HISTORY

The incubation period for RMSF after tick exposure ranges from 5 to 7 d. The rash, present in 84% of cases, begins on d 3 or 4 on the extremities and spreads proximally. By day 6 or 7 the rash is generalized. Systemic symptoms include abrupt onset of fever (94%); severe headache (94%); generalized myalgia, especially the back and leg muscles (87%); a sudden shaking rigor; photophobia; prostration; and nausea with occasional vomiting.

PHYSICAL EXAMINATION

Skin Findings

Type   Early lesions are macular, becoming papular in 1 to 3 d. Rarely an eschar (round crusted ulcer) may be present at the site of the tick bite. With DIC, the skin infarcts and gangrene occurs.

Color   Pink, evolving to deep red, violaceous, and purpuric macules and papules (Fig. 22-1).

Size   2 to 6 mm.

Distribution of Lesions   Characteristically, rash begins to wrists, forearms, and ankles, and somewhat later on palms and soles. Within 6 to 18 h, rash spreads centripetally to the arms, thighs, trunk, and face (Fig. 22-2). Gangrene occurs in acral areas.

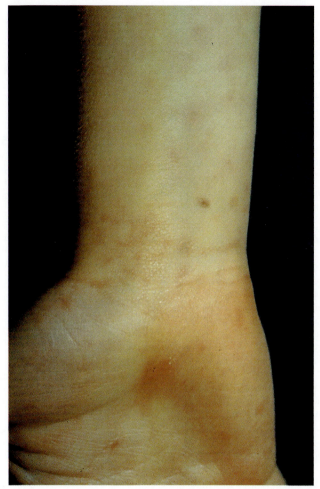

Figure 22-1   Rocky Mountain spotted fever   *Scattered pink, red and purpuric macules and papules on the forearm of a child.*

General Findings

Fever to 40°C. Patient may become hypotensive. Hepatomegaly, splenomegaly, GI hemorrhages, altered consciousness, transient deafness, incontinence, oliguria, and secondary bacterial infections of the lung, middle ear, and parotid gland may occur. Septic shock may ensue.

Variants

Spotless Fever Accounts for 13% of cases. Associated with higher mortality because diagnosis is overlooked.

Abdominal Syndrome Can mimic acute abdomen, acute cholecystitis, acute appendicitis.

DIFFERENTIAL DIAGNOSIS

The diagnosis of RMSF should be entertained in patients who live or have traveled to endemic areas, and who appear severely ill with the generalized purpuric RMSF-like exanthem. The diagnosis must be made clinically and confirmed later. The differential diagnosis includes meningococcemia, *Staphylococcus aureus* septicemia, other rickettsioses (ehrlichiosis, murine typhus, epidemic typhus, rickettsialpox), leptospirosis, typhoid fever, viral exanthem (measles, varicella, rubella, enterovirus), drug reaction, and an immune-complex-mediated vasculitis.

LABORATORY EXAMINATIONS

Dermatopathology Skin biopsy will show a necrotizing vasculitis. *Rickettsia* can at times be demonstrated within the endothelial cells.

Direct Immunofluorescence Can stain for specific *R. rickettsii* antigen within endothelial cells.

Serology Immunofluorescent antibody test (IFA) can be used to measure both IgG and IgM antibodies against *R. rickettsii*. A fourfold rise in titer between acute and convalescent stages of the disease is diagnostic.

COURSE AND PROGNOSIS

Untreated, the fatality rate for RMSF is 20%. With adequate therapy, the mortality decreases to 3%. Severely affected patients may experience DIC, purpura fulminans, permanent cardiac, and/or neurologic sequelae. The most important prognostic factor is early diagnosis and treatment even if this means starting antibiotics before confirmatory study results are available.

MANAGEMENT

Either tetracycline or chloramphenicol is the treatment of choice for RMSF.

1. Oral or IV tetracycline (usually not recommended for children <9 years, 20 to 40 mg/kg per d divided qid, not to exceed 2 g/d) for 7 to 10 d, is recommended.
2. In severe refractory cases, IV chloramphenicol (50 to 100 mg/kg per d, not to exceed 4 g/d), is recommended.

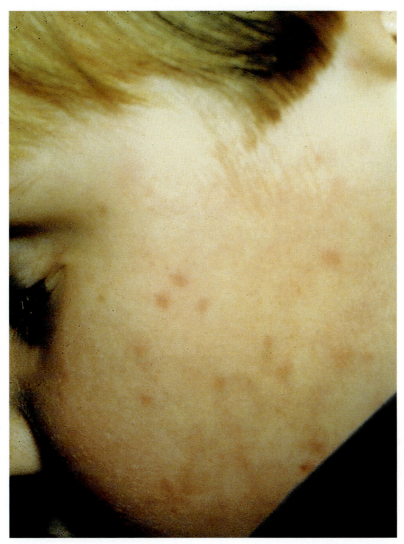

Figure 22-2   Rocky Mountain spotted fever   *Later face involvement of the rash is seen in the same child.*

CUTANEOUS VIRAL INFECTIONS

HERPES SIMPLEX VIRUS

HERPETIC GINGIVOSTOMATITIS

Primary herpetic gingivostomatitis is the most common herpetic infection in children. It is typically caused by herpes simplex virus 1 (HSV-1) and characterized by vesicular lesions of the mouth.

Synonyms   Herpes, herpes simplex, cold sore, fever blister, herpes febrilis, herpes labialis.

EPIDEMIOLOGY

Age   Seen in children ages 1 to 5 years of age.

Gender   M = F.

Incidence   By adulthood, > 85% of the population has serologic evidence of HSV-1.

Etiology   Herpes simplex virus 1 (HSV-1) >> type 2 (HSV-2).

Transmission   Herpes virus is transmitted by mucosal or skin contact.

PATHOPHYSIOLOGY

Transmission and primary infection of HSV occurs through close contact with a person shedding virus at a peripheral site, mucosal suface, or secretion. HSV is inactivated promptly at room temperature so aerosolized or fomitic spread is unlikely. Infection occurs via inoculation onto susceptible mucosal surface or break in skin. Subsequent to primary infection at inoculation site, HSV ascends peripheral sensory nerves and enters the sensory or autonomic nerve root ganglia, where latency is established. Latency can occur after both symptomatic and asymptomatic primary infection. Recrudescences may be clinically symptomatic or asymptomatic (see "Recurrent Facial–Oral Herpes" on page 548).

HISTORY

Two to twenty days after exposure, the symptoms of primary herpetic gingivostomatitis may be mild and unapparent to severe with high fever, sore throat, and lymphadenopathy. The pain may be so debilitating that hospitalization is necessary for intravenous hydration.

PHYSICAL EXAMINATION

Skin Findings

Type   An erythematous plaque is often noted initially, followed soon by grouped, often umbilicated, vesicles, which may evolve to pustules. Erosions enlarge to ulcerations, which may be crusted or moist and heal in 2 to 4 weeks, often with resultant postinflammatory hypo- or hyperpigmentation. Scarring is uncommon. The area of involvement may be circumferential around the mouth (Fig. 23-1).

Arrangement   Herpetiform (grouped) vesicles.

Distribution   Oral mucosa minimally to extensively involved in primary HSV gingivo-

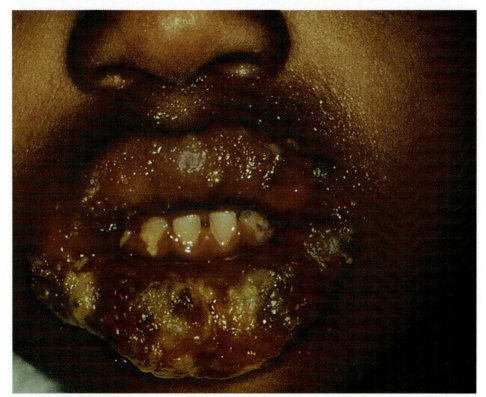

Figure 23-1 Herpetic gingivostomatitis *Severe circumferential perioral erosions and ulcerations that prevent the child from being able to eat or drink.*

stomatitis, with vesicles that quickly slough to form erosions at any site in the oropharynx.

General Findings

Fever and lymphadenopathy are often present during symptomatic primary herpetic gingivostomatitis. Signs of aseptic meningitis may be present: headache, fever, nuchal rigidity, CSF pleocytosis with normal sugar content, and positive HSV CSF culture.

DIFFERENTIAL DIAGNOSIS

The clinical suspicion of herpes stomatitis can be confirmed by Tzanck smear, direct immunofluorescence antibody (DFA), or viral culture. The differential diagnosis includes aphthous stomatitis, hand-foot-and-mouth disease, herpangina, erythema multiforme, or Behçet's disease.

LABORATORY EXAMINATIONS

Tzanck Smear Cells from the base of an intact vesicle are smeared thinly on a microscope slide, dried, and stained with either Wright's or Giemsa's stain. Tzanck smear is positive if multinucleated giant keratinocytes are detected (Fig. 23-2). The Tzanck smear is positive in 75% of early cases, but does not differentiate HSV-1 from HSV-2 or VZV.

Direct Immunofluorescence (DFA) Cells from the base of an intact vesicle can be smeared on a glass slide and immunofluorescent antibodies can be used to stain for the presence of HSV-1.

Dermatopathology Ballooning and reticular epidermal degeneration, acanthosis, and intraepidermal vesicle formation. Intranuclear inclusion bodies, multinucleate giant keratinocytes, and multilocular vesicles may be present.

Electron Microscopy Can detect HSV particles.

Viral Culture Cultures are easily available and helpful. HSV can be cultured from vesicle fluid or from scraping the base of an erosion. Culture must be done early in the course of the outbreak and prior to acyclovir treatment. Documents the presence of HSV-1 in 1 to 10 d.

Serology Primary HSV-1 infection can be documented by demonstration of seroconversion.

COURSE AND PROGNOSIS

Episodes of primary herpetic gingivostomatitis are self-limiting but can range in severity from mild asymptomatic infection to severe debilitating disease requiring hospitalization.

MANAGEMENT

The treatment of choice for herpetic gingivostomatitis is oral or IV acyclovir (5 mg/kg every 8 h for 5 to 7 d or until clinical resolution occurs) and symptomatic measures. Acetaminophen and 2% viscous lidocaine can be used for oral pain and IV fluids may be needed to prevent dehydration.

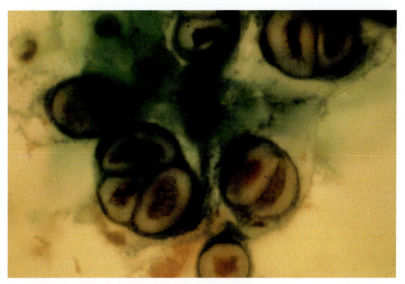

Figure 23-2   Herpetic infection, Tzanck smear   *Giemsa stain of vesicle contents demonstrating multinucleated giant cells (fused virally infected keratinocytes) are indicative of a herpetic infection.*

RECURRENT FACIAL–ORAL HERPES

Recurrent facial–oral herpes is a reactivation of latent herpetic infection typically caused by herpes simplex virus 1 (HSV-1) and characterized by localized blisters of the mouth (particularly the vermillion border) or body.

Synonyms   Cold sores, fever blisters, herpes, herpes simplex, herpes labialis.

EPIDEMIOLOGY

Age   Any age. Most common in young adults.

Gender   M = F.

Prevalence   Estimated one-third of the U.S. population experiences recurrent HSV-1.

Incidence   By adulthood, $> 85\%$ of the population has serologic evidence of HSV-1 infection.

Transmission   Herpes virus is transmitted by skin-to-skin, skin-to-mucosa, or mucosa-to-mucosa contact.

Precipitating Factors   Sunlight, stress, illness, or local trauma may precipitate blistering episodes.

Etiology   Herpes simplex virus 1 and 2.

PATHOPHYSIOLOGY

Subsequent to the primary HSV-1 infection, HSV ascends the peripheral sensory nerves and enters the trigeminal ganglion, where latency is established. Recurrences occur at the same site each time and may be clinically asymptomatic or symptomatic.

HISTORY

Recurrent HSV-1 episodes are typically heralded by a prodrome of tingling, itching, or burning sensation, which usually precedes any visible skin changes by 24 h. The skin then flares with a small, localized crop of blisters followed by healing. Systemic symptoms are usually absent.

PHYSICAL EXAMINATION

Skin Findings

Type   Often a plaque of erythema with grouped vesicles that heal in 1 to 2 weeks (Fig. 23-3).

Color   Erythematous plaque.

Size   1- to 2-cm plaque.

Arrangement   Herpetiform (i.e., grouped) vesicles.

Distribution   May occur at any mucocutaneous site.

Sites of Predilection   Most common sites are perioral, cheek, nose tip, distal finger. Periocular localization requires examination of the cornea.

General Findings

Regional lymphadenopathy may be present. Fever in recurrent herpes is unusual.

DIFFERENTIAL DIAGNOSIS

The diagnosis of recurrent facial–oral herpes can be confirmed by Tzanck smear, direct immunofluorescence (DFA), or viral culture. The differential diagnosis includes varicella zoster, aphthous ulcers, and contact dermatitis.

LABORATORY EXAMINATIONS

Same as for herpetic gingivostomatits. (See page 544 for more details.)

Serology   Recurrent HSV-1 can only be ruled out if patient is seronegative for HSV-1 antibodies. The presence of HSV-1 antibodies cannot differentiate a primary infection from a recurrent episode.

COURSE AND PROGNOSIS

Recurrent facial–oral herpetic outbreaks are localized and self-limited. Outbreaks typically number 1 to 4/year and are typically milder and of shorter duration than the primary infection. They tend to become less frequent as the individual gets older. Oral antiviral agents, if used early (during prodromal period), may abort or minimize symptoms.

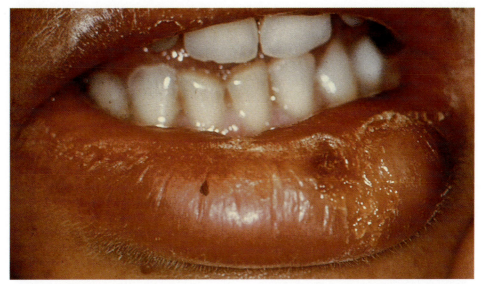

Figure 23-3 Recurrent facial–oral herpes *Localized recurrent lesion that begins with vesicles and heals with crusting on the lower lip.*

MANAGEMENT

In recurrent facial–oral herpes, some patients who start antiviral therapy at the beginning of the prodrome or within 2 days after onset of lesions may benefit from therapy, although this has not been proved. The antiviral regimen recommended is:

1. Acyclovir (30 mg/kg per d, not to exceed 200 mg PO 5 times a day for 5 d).

2. Topical pencyclovir cream (Denavir cream, q2h to the lesion topically). If a patient is having frequent recurrent outbreaks (> 6 in one year), daily treatment can reduce the frequency of recurrences by 75%. After 1 year of continuous daily suppressive therapy, acyclovir should be discontinued so that the patient's recurrence rate may be reassessed. The antiviral dosage recommended for suppressive therapy is acyclovir (30 mg/kg per d divided bid or tid).

ECZEMA HERPETICUM

Eczema herpeticum is a widespread herpes simplex virus type infection superimposed on diseased skin (most commonly atopic dermatitis or Darier's disease). It is characterized by widespread vesicles and erosions, fever, and malaise, and can be a recurrent problem.

Synonym   Kaposi's varicelliform eruption.

EPIDEMIOLOGY

Age   Children > adults.

Etiology   Herpes simplex virus (HSV-1), less commonly type 2 (HSV-2).

Transmission   Commonly from parental recurrent facial–oral herpes.

Risk Factors   Most commonly, eczema herpeticum is superimposed on atopic dermatitis, and more serious infections occur in erythrodermic atopic dermatitis. Also, Darier's disease, thermal burns, pemphigus vulgaris, ichthyosis vulgaris, and mycosis fungoides.

PATHOPHYSIOLOGY

On abnormal skin (atopic dermatitis or Darier's disease) the barrier function of the skin is impaired and viral or bacterial superinfection can easily become widespread. In the case of eczema herpeticum, frequently a child with atopic dermatitis becomes inoculated with HSV-1 from a parent with a clinical or subclinical case of recurrent oral–facial herpes. The disease then becomes widespread because of the infant's uncontrolled scratching, auto-inoculation and impaired skin barrier function.

HISTORY

Herpetic skin lesions begin on impaired skin and may extend peripherally for several weeks during the primary infection. Systemic symptoms include fever, malaise, and irritability.

PHYSICAL EXAMINATION

Skin Findings

Type   Umbilicated vesicles evolving into "punched-out" erosions (Fig. 23-4). Vesicles are first confined to the impaired skin areas and are, in contrast to primary or recurrent HSV eruptions, not grouped but widespread. Erosions may become confluent, producing large denuded areas. Larger crusted lesions and follicular pustules occur with staphylococcal superinfection (Fig. 23-5). Successive crops of new vesiculation may occur.

Shape of Individual Lesions   Dome-shaped vesicle or punched out lesions.

Arrangement of Multiple Lesions   Widespread on impaired skin areas.

Distribution of Lesions   Common sites: face, neck, trunk.

General Examination

Widespread disease often associated with fever and lymphadenopathy.

DIFFERENTIAL DIAGNOSIS

The diagnosis of eczema herpeticum can be made in an individual with known chronic skin disease and a slow-onset, widespread, painful vesicular rash. The diagnosis can be confirmed by Tzanck test, direct immunofluorescence (DFA), or HSV culture. The differential diagnosis includes varicella zoster with dissemination, disseminated (systemic) HSV infection, widespread bullous impetigo, staphylococcal folliculitis, pseudomonal (hot-tub) folliculitis, and *Candida* folliculitis.

LABORATORY EXAMINATIONS

HSV-1 or HSV-2 can be detected by Tzanck, skin biopsy, or serology. (See page 544 for more details.)

Skin Culture   Will be positive for herpes virus (1 > 2). Frequently, superinfection with *Staphylococcus aureus/Streptococcus pyogenes* is present.

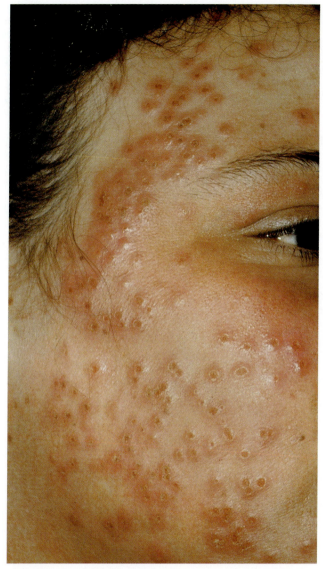

Figure 23-4 Eczema herpeticum *Widespread punched-out lesions on a child with atopic dermatitis and superimposed herpes simplex infection.*

COURSE AND PROGNOSIS

Eczema herpeticum self-resolves in 2 to 6 weeks. Recurrent episodes tend to be milder and not associated with as severe systemic symptoms. The risk of systemic dissemination is possible, especially in immunocompromised patients.

MANAGEMENT

Preventative measures aimed at controlling the underlying chronic dermatosis (atopic dermatitis or Darier's disease) will improve the skin's barrier function and prevent widespread cutaneous viral and bacterial infection.

Mild cases of eczema herpeticum can be managed on an outpatient basis with acyclovir (30 mg/kg per d not to exceed 200 mg PO 5 ×/d for 5 to 10 d) and topical pencyclovir cream (Denavir cream, to affected areas q2h).

For localized, uncomplicated bacterial superinfection, topical bactroban ointment (bid to tid to the affected areas).

In more severe cases with high fever or marked prostration, hospitalization may be needed with:

1. Systemic acyclovir (1 to 3 g/m^2 per d IV divided tid for 7 d).
2. CBC and blood cultures.
3. Systemic antibiotics if indicated:
   a. Dicloxacillin (25 to 50 mg/kg per d PO divided qid for 7 to 10 d).
   b. Cephalexin (Keflex 25 to 50 mg/kg per d PO divided qid, not to exceed 4 g/d for 7 to 10 d).

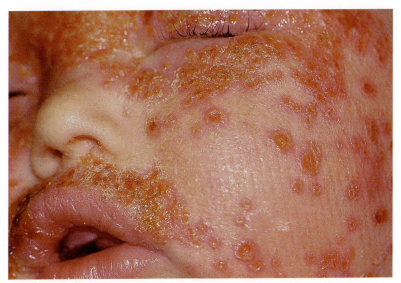

Figure 23-5   Eczema herpeticum   *Widespread crusted lesions on a child with atopic dermatitis kissed by a parent with active HSV-1 recurrent oral–facial herpes with resultant eczema herpeticum. Clinical picture is complicated by* Staph. aureus *superinfection causing yellow-brown crusted appearance.*

HERPETIC WHITLOW

Herpetic whitlow is a cutaneous herpetic infection of the distal fingertip, usually caused by recurrent oral–facial HSV-1 inadvertently inoculated onto the hand.

EPIDEMIOLOGY

Age   Any age.

Gender   M = F.

Incidence   Common.

Transmission   Herpetic whitlow is typically seen in physicians, dentists, dental hygienists, and nurses who examine the mouth or genital regions of patients and inadvertently become inoculated with herpes on their hands.

PATHOPHYSIOLOGY

HSV-1, typically from a patient's mouth with clinical or subclinical recurrent oral–facial herpes, gets inoculated onto a health care worker's finger, and herpetic whitlow ensues. After the primary infection, the herpes virus becomes dormant in the nerve and can recur in the same location.

HISTORY

Two to eight days following exposure, painful vesicular lesions appear on one or more fingertips of the infected individual. Systemic symptoms are rare but can include fever and regional lymphadenopathy. Lesions take 1 to 3 weeks to resolve and recurrences are possible.

PHYSICAL EXAMINATION

Skin Findings

Type   Grouped vesicles.

Color   Whitish-red or blue lesions on an erythematous base (Fig. 23-6).

Size   2- to 4-mm vesicles.

Arrangement   Herpetic (grouped vesicles).

Distribution   Distal fingertips.

DIFFERENTIAL DIAGNOSIS

The diagnosis of herpetic whitlow can be made by history and physical exam. Tzanck, direct immunofluorescence (DFA), or viral culture confirmation is possible. The differential diagnosis includes dyshidrotic eczema, contact dermatitis, or other paronychial infection.

LABORATORY EXAMINATIONS

HSV-1 or HSV-2 can be identified by Tzanck, viral culture, DFA, or skin biopsy. (See page 544 for more details.)

COURSE AND PROGNOSIS

Herpetic whitlow will self-resolve without treatment, but recurrences are possible.

MANAGEMENT

Much of the treatment of herpetic whitlow is symptomatic with:

1. Analgesics for pain.
2. Topical pencyclovir cream (Denavir cream, to affected areas q2h).
3. Topical antibiotics (bactroban, bacitracin, polysporin, or neosporin) for crusted lesions with evidence of bacterial superinfection.

In severe cases, systemic therapy may be indicated with acyclovir (30 mg/kg per d not to exceed 200 mg PO 5 ×/d for 5 to 10 d).

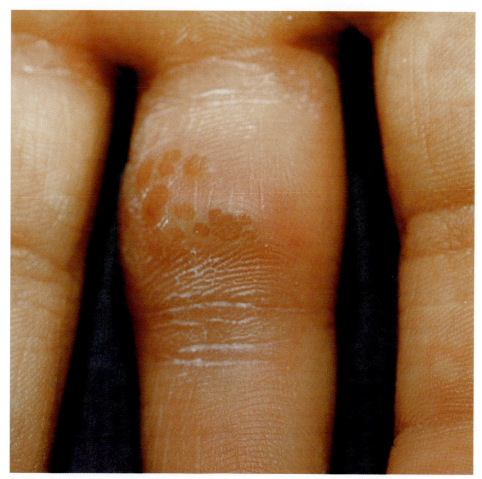

Figure 23-6 Herpetic whitlow *Painful grouped red-blue vesicles on the middle finger of a child.*

HERPES GLADIATORUM

Herpes gladiatorum is a herpetic infection seen primarily in contact sports players (e.g., wrestlers, rugby players) who abrade their skin and come into contact with an active HSV infection on their opponent.

EPIDEMIOLOGY

Age   Any age.

Gender   M > F.

Incidence   Common. HSV-1 among wrestlers and rugby players is as high as 67%.

Etiology   Herpes simplex virus 1 (HSV-1) >> HSV-2.

Transmission   Skin-to-skin or mucous membrane-to-skin contact.

PATHOPHYSIOLOGY

HSV-1 is transmitted to the opponent during infected skin-to-skin exposure in rough contact sports. Of note, studies have shown negative oropharyngeal swabs for active mucosal HSV-1; thus saliva seems not to be a major source of infection. The virus then becomes latent in the sensory nerve ganglia, and recurrences at the ectopic site are possible.

HISTORY

Two to eight days after contact, herpetic lesions can occur at atypical sites (head, trunk, extremities) and are often associated with edema, pain, and regional lymphadenopathy.

PHYSICAL EXAMINATION

Skin Findings

Type   Group vesicles.

Color   Clear to white vesicles on an erythematous base (Fig. 23-7).

Size   2 to 5 mm.

Number   Typically one lesion seen from exposure, but in more severe cases there can be HSV-1 inoculated onto several different sites.

Distribution   Any site.

Sites of Predilection   Head (73%), trunk (28%), and extremities (47%).

General Findings

May be associated with fever, malaise, and regional lymphadenopathy.

DIAGNOSIS AND DIFFERENTIAL DIAGNOSIS

The diagnosis of herpes gladiatorum is a clinical one and is often misdiagnosed because of the atypical location of the herpetic lesion and/or incomplete history. The differential diagnosis includes contact dermatitis and varicella zoster.

LABORATORY EXAMINATIONS

HSV-1 or HSV-2 can be detected by Tzanck, DFA, viral culture, or skin biopsy. (See page 544 for more details.)

COURSE AND PROGNOSIS

The primary episode of herpes gladiatorum may last 2 to 6 weeks but does self-resolve. Recurrences are less painful and resolve more quickly.

MANAGEMENT

Wrestlers, rugby players, parents, and coaches need to be made aware of the transmission of HSV-1, and active lesions should be covered to prevent spread.

Primary herpes gladiatorum can be treated with:

1. Topical pencyclovir cream (Denavir cream to affected areas q2h).
2. Acyclovir (30 mg/kg per d not to exceed 200 mg PO 5 ×/d for 5 to 10 d).

For localized, uncomplicated bacterial superinfection, topical bactroban ointment (bid to tid to the affected areas).

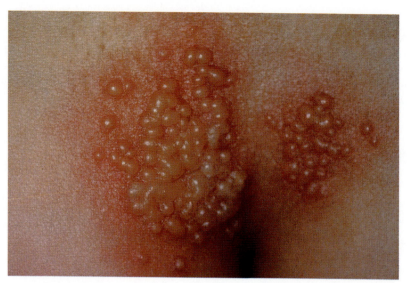

Figure 23-7   Herpes gladiatorum   *Grouped vesicles on an erythematous base on the buttocks of an infant.*

DISSEMINATED HERPES SIMPLEX INFECTION

Disseminated herpes simplex infection is a potentially fatal, systemic HSV infection, characterized by widespread mucocutaneous vesicles, pustules, erosions, and ulcerations. It is associated with signs of pneumonia, encephalitis, and hepatitis, as well as involvement of other organ systems. It usually occurs in an immunocompromised host.

EPIDEMIOLOGY

Age   Any age.

Etiology   Herpes simplex virus (HSV) type 1 or type 2.

Incidence   Uncommon, but incidence rising due to organ transplantation, chemotherapy, and AIDS.

Risk Factors   Disseminated herpes can occur in immunocompromised states (organ transplantation, cancer chemotherapy, corticosteroid therapy), hematologic and lymphoreticular malignancies, and in severe malnutrition.

PATHOPHYSIOLOGY

Sixty to 80% of HSV seropositive transplant recipients and patients undergoing chemotherapy for hematologic malignancies will reactivate HSV. Following viremia, disseminated cutaneous or visceral HSV infection may follow. Factors determining whether severe localized disease, cutaneous dissemination, or visceral dissemination will occur are not well defined.

HISTORY

Disseminated herpes simplex infection is typically seen in hospitalized patients with underlying disease. It presents as tender and painful mucocutaneous erosions with systemic fever, malaise, and organ involvement.

PHYSICAL EXAMINATION

Skin Findings

Type   *Recurrent herpetic lesion* (site from which systemic dissemination of HSV occurs) may be present: grouped vesicles, crusts, erosion, ulcers; ulcers may be large (10 to 20 cm in diameter). With mucocutaneous dissemination, vesicles and pustules often hemorrhagic with inflammatory halo; quickly rupture, resulting in "punched-out" erosions. Lesions may be necrotic and then ulcerate. Ulcers may become confluent with polycyclic well-demarcated borders; edges may be slightly raised and rolled. Infarctive skin lesions if complicated by purpura fulminans.

Distribution   Generalized, disseminated (Fig. 23-8). Site of recurrent HSV infection (labial, oropharyngeal, esophageal) may be apparent.

Mucous Membranes   Oropharyngeal erosion, HSV tracheobronchitis with erosions.

General Examination

HSV pneumonitis, hepatitis, or encephalitis may be present.

DIFFERENTIAL DIAGNOSIS

The diagnosis of disseminated HSV is based on clinical suspicion confirmed by Tzanck preparation, direct immunofluorescence, or HSV cultures. The differential diagnosis includes eczema herpeticum, varicella, and cutaneous disseminated zoster.

LABORATORY EXAMINATIONS

HSV-1 or HSV-2 can be detected by Tzanck, viral culture, or DFA of mucocutaneous erosions or tracheobronchial washings. (See page 546 for more details.)

COURSE AND PROGNOSIS

When widespread, visceral dissemination of HSV may occur to liver, lungs, adrenals, GI tract, and CNS. Severe cases can be complicated by disseminated intravascular coagulation. Untreated, the mortality rate of disseminated HSV with organ involvement is high.

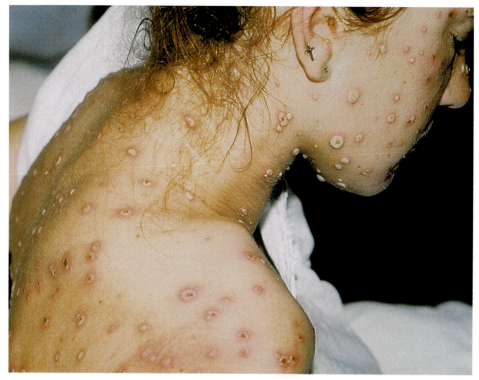

Figure 23-8   Disseminated herpes simplex virus   *Widespread vesicular lesions in an immunocompromised patient.*

MANAGEMENT

Early recognition and treatment are essential in the treatment of disseminated herpes.

Acyclovir Prophylaxis Recommended for seropositive patients undergoing bone marrow transplantation, induction therapy for leukemia, and solid organ transplantation: acyclovir (30 mg/kg per d PO divided tid, not to exceed 200 mg PO 5 ×/d) or acyclovir (1 to 3 g/m² per d IV divided tid). From the day of conditioning, induction or transplantation for 4 to 6 weeks.

For Disseminated HSV Infection

1. Acyclovir (1 to 3 g/m² per d or 5 mg/kg IV divided tid).
2. CBC and blood cultures.
3. Systemic antibiotics if indicated:
   a. Dicloxacillin (25 to 50 mg/kg per d PO divided qid).
   b. Cephalexin (Keflex 25 to 50 mg/kg per d PO divided qid, not to exceed 4 g/d).

VARICELLA ZOSTER VIRUS

VARICELLA

Varicella is a highly contagious primary infection caused by varicella zoster virus, characterized by successive crops of pruritic vesicles that evolve to pustules and crusts, and can heal with scarring. The rash is often accompanied by constitutional symptoms such as fever and malaise.

Synonym Chickenpox.

EPIDEMIOLOGY

Age 90% of cases occur in children <10 years old, less than 5% in persons >15 years old.

Gender M = F.

Incidence Nearly universal; 3,000,000 cases in the United States annually but the annual incidence is declining with the routine administration of the varicella vaccine.

Etiology Varicella-zoster virus (VZV), a herpesvirus.

Transmission Varicella virus is spread via airborne droplets between persons as well as direct contact. Patients are contagious several days before exanthem appears and until the last crop of vesicles crusts over. Once crusted over, the skin lesions are no longer infectious.

Season Metropolitan areas in temperate climates, but varicella epidemics do occur in winter and spring.

Geography Worldwide.

PATHOPHYSIOLOGY

Varicella virus enters through mucosa of upper respiratory tract and oropharynx, followed by local replication and primary viremia. VZV then replicates in the cells of the reticuloendothelial system with subsequent secondary viremia and dissemination of the virus to the skin and mucous membranes. Primary attack usually confers lifelong immunity. Second episodes of varicella have been documented but are rare. As with all herpesviruses, VZV enters a latent phase, residing in sensory ganglia, and reactivation of VZV later in life results in zoster (see "Herpes Zoster" on page 564 for more details).

HISTORY

Varicella is usually transmitted by exposure to a sick contact at daycare, school, an older sibling, or even an adult with zoster. Following an inoculation period of 14 d (range, 10 to 23 d), a mild prodrome of headache, general aches and pains, and malaise may be present. The exanthem appears within 2 to 3 d (Fig. 23-9).

PHYSICAL EXAMINATION

Skin Findings

Type Superficial and thin-walled vesicles on an erythematous base appear as small "drops of water" or "dewdrops on a rose petal" (Fig. 23-10). Vesicles become umbilicated and rapidly evolve to pustules and crusts over an 8- to 12-h period. With subsequent crops, all stages of evolution may be noted simultaneously: papules, vesicles, pustules, crusts. Crusts fall off in 1 to 3 weeks, leaving a pink, somewhat depressed base. Characteristic punched-out permanent scars may persist. Complicated by superinfection by staphylococci or streptococci; impetigo, furuncles, cellulitis, and gangrene may occur.

Color Vesicles are watery yellow. Pustules are filled with creamy white pus. Crusts are brownish-red.

Size 2 to 5 mm.

Number Few to >100 lesions.

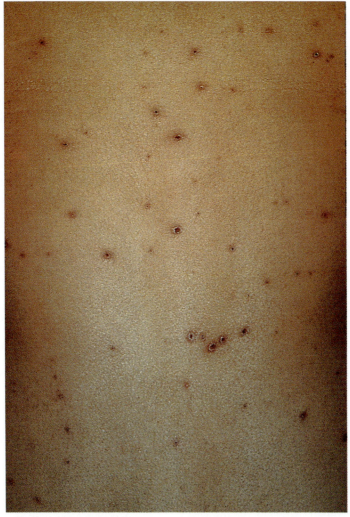

Figure 23-9 **Varicella** *Scattered papules, vesicles, and crusts noted simultaneously in a patient with varicella.*

Distribution of Lesions The initial lesions begin on face and scalp, and then spread to trunk and extremities. Density highest on trunk and face, less on extremities. Palms and soles usually spared.

Mucous Membranes Vesicles (not often observed) and subsequent shallow erosions (2 to 3 mm) most common on palate, but also occur on mucosa of nose, conjunctivae, pharynx, larynx, trachea, GI tract, urinary tract, vagina.

Variants

Varicella gangrenosa occurs in children with leukemia or other severe underlying disease, characterized by gangrenous ulceration. Hemorrhagic varicella can be seen with disseminated intravascular coagulation (purpura fulminans).

General Examination

Low-grade fever. Vesicopustules may rarely occur in the respiratory, GU, and GI tracts.

DIFFERENTIAL DIAGNOSIS

The diagnosis of varicella is made by history and characteristic cutaneous eruption. Exposure to a sick varicella contact can sometimes be elucidated. The diagnosis in atypical cases can be confirmed by Tzanck preparation, direct immunofluorescence test (DFA), viral culture, or serology. The differential diagnosis includes disseminated herpes simplex virus (HSV) infection, cutaneous dissemination of zoster, eczema herpeticum, and the bullous form of impetigo.

LABORATORY EXAMINATIONS

Tzanck Preparation Cytology of scraping from fluid or base of vesicle or pustule shows both giant and multinucleated giant epidermal cells. Tzanck test does not differentiate HSV from VZV.

Electron Microscopy VZV particles can be seen in negative stain preparations but cannot be distinguished from HSV.

Cultures Isolation of virus from skin lesions is possible, but more difficult than with HSV.

Serology Seroconversion, that is, fourfold or greater rise in VZV titers.

COURSE AND PROGNOSIS

The symptoms and rash or varicella typically lasts for 1 to 3 weeks. The primary infection should confer lifelong immunity. If the primary infection occurs at an early age when maternal antibody is still present, a patient may have a second episode of varicella later in life due to incomplete immunity. Varicella in children is a self-limited, benign, but itching and painful eruption. In older or immunocompromised individuals, varicella may have a more severe clinical course, with a higher rate of respiratory or systemic complications.

MANAGEMENT

Vaccination A varicella vaccine is administered to all children as a part of routine well-child care, and the episodes of varicella are steadily decreasing.

Varicella Treatment Varicella is a self-limited cutaneous eruption in children, and treatment usually consists of supportive care:

1. Aveeno oilated oatmeal baths.
2. Topical antipruritic agents (Calamine or Caladryl lotions, Pramasone, or Sarna lotions) can help decrease pruritus.
3. Antipyretic administration is of concern because of a possible link between aspirin and Reye's syndrome in children with varicella.
4. Acyclovir administered within the first 24 h of the exanthem can lessen the severity of outbreak, but higher doses are needed since VZV is not as sensitive to acyclovir as HSV (30 mg/kg per d PO not to exceed 800 mg 5 ×/d for 5 to 10 d).
5. Varicella-zoster immune globulin (VZIG) administration is indicated for individuals with the following illnesses or conditions following significant exposure to VZV: leukemia, lymphoma, cellular immune deficiency, or immunosuppressive treatment.

Localized, Uncomplicated Bacterial Superinfection Topical bactroban ointment (bid to tid to the affected areas).

More Severe Cases In cases complicated by pneumonitis, encephalitis, or varicella occurring in an immunocompromised host, systemic acyclovir (1500 mg/m^2 per d or 30 mg/kg per d IV divided tid for 7 d) or systemic vidarabine (10 to 20 mg/kg per d IV for 7 d) is recommended. Varicella-zoster immune globulin (VZIG) administration may also be helpful.

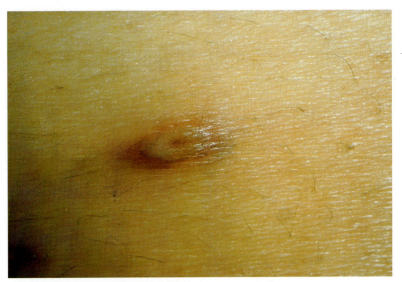

Figure 23-10   Varicella   *Thin-walled vesicle on an erythematous base likened to a "dewdrop on a rose petal" characteristic of varicella infection.*

HERPES ZOSTER

Herpes zoster is an acute localized infection caused by varicella-zoster virus (VZV) and is characterized by unilateral pain and a vesicular or bullous eruption limited to a dermatome innervated by a corresponding sensory ganglion.

Synonym   Shingles.

EPIDEMIOLOGY

Age   Can be seen in any age, but typically seen in persons > 50 years old.

Gender   M = F.

Incidence   300,000 cases (1.4 to 3.4/100,000) annually in the U.S.

Other Factors   Zoster in children is usually seen in immunocompromised settings, especially from lymphoproliferative disorders or chemotherapy. Zoster also can be seen in children who contracted varicella at a young age (< 6 months old). Zoster is about one-third as contagious as varicella, and susceptible contacts can contract varicella.

PATHOPHYSIOLOGY

Varicella-zoster virus, during the course of varicella, ascends along the sensory nerves and in the sensory ganglia, establishes latent infection. It is postulated that humoral and cellular immunity to VZV established with primary infection persists at low levels, and when this immunity ebbs, viral replication within the ganglia occurs. The virus then travels down the sensory nerve, resulting in the dermatomal pain and skin lesions. As the neuritis precedes the skin involvement, pain appears before the skin lesions are visible.

HISTORY

Pain, tenderness, and paresthesia (itching, tingling, burning) in the involved dermatome precedes the eruption by 3 to 5 d. The pain usually persists throughout the eruption, but lessens with time. Systemic symptoms such as headache, malaise, and fever can occur in about 5% of patients.

PHYSICAL EXAMINATION

Skin Findings

Type   Papules (24 h) to vesicles-bullae (48 h) to pustules (96 h) to crusts (7 to 10 d). New lesions continue to appear for up to 1 week.

Color   Clear vesicles on an erythematous base.

Size   2 to 5 mm.

Arrangement   Zosteriform (dermatomal), with herpetiform clusters of lesions. (Fig. 23-11). A few stray lesions outside of the affected dermatome can sometimes be found.

Distribution   Unilateral.

Sites of Predilection   Thoracic (> 50%), trigeminal (10 to 20%), lumbosacral and cervical (10 to 20%).

Mucous Membranes   Vesicles and erosions can occur in mouth, genitalia, and bladder depending on dermatome involved.

Lymphadenopathy   Regional nodes draining the area are often enlarged and tender.

Sensory or Motor Nerve Changes   Detectable by neurologic examination.

Eye   In ophthalmic zoster, nasociliary branch involvement occurs in about one-third of cases and is heralded by vesicles on the side and tip of the nose (Hutchinson's sign). There is usually associated conjunctivitis and occasionally keratitis, scleritis, or iritis. An ophthalmologist should always be consulted in cases of ophthalmic zoster.

DIFFERENTIAL DIAGNOSIS

The prodromal pain of herpes zoster can mimic cardiac or pleural disease, an acute abdomen, or vertebral disease. The rash must be distinguished from herpes simplex virus and contact dermatitis.

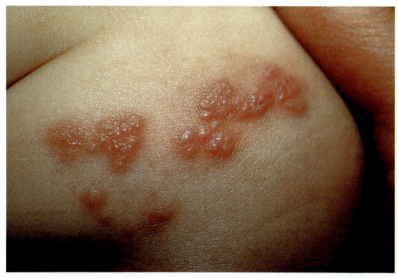

Figure 23-11 Herpes zoster *Grouped vesicles on an erythematous base in a dermatomal distribution on the hip of an infant.*

COURSE AND PROGNOSIS

The rash of zoster is self-limited. The risk of postherpetic neuralgia is around 20 to 40% in adult patients, but less common in children. The highest incidence of postherpetic neuralgia is in ophthalmic zoster. Ophthalmic zoster can lead to keratitis and blindness; thus aggressive treatment should be pursued.

Dissemination of zoster—20 or more lesions outside the affected or adjacent dermatomes—can occur in up to 10% of patients, and is usually seen in immunosuppressed individuals. Motor paralysis occurs in 5% of patients, especially when the virus involves the cranial nerves.

MANAGEMENT

Zoster Treatment Zoster is a self-limited cutaneous eruption in children, and treatment usually consists of supportive care:

1. Aveeno oilated oatmeal baths.
2. Topical antipruritic agents (Calamine or Caladryl lotions, Pramasone, or Sarna lotions) can help decrease pruritus.
3. Antipyretic administration is of concern because of a possible link between aspirin and Reye's syndrome in children with varicella.
4. Acyclovir administered within the first 24 h of the exanthem can lessen the severity of

outbreak, but higher doses are needed since VZV is not as sensitive to acyclovir as HSV (30 mg/kg per d PO not to exceed 800 mg 5 ×/d for 5 to 10 d).
5. Newer agents such as ralacyclovir (Raltrex) or famiciclovir (Famvir) are helpful in adults but pediatric doses are not clear.
6. Varicella-zoster immune globulin (VZIG) administration is indicated for individuals with the following illnesses or conditions following significant exposure to VZV: leukemia, lymphoma, cellular immune deficiency, or immunosuppressive treatment.

Localized, Uncomplicated Bacterial Superinfection Topical bactroban ointment (bid to tid to the affected areas).

Postherpetic Neuralgia Rare in children, postherpetic neuralgia can be treated with topical applications of capsaicin (Zostrix cream tid to qid). Systemic steroids are of more use in older individuals (> 50 years old), but can be considered.

Ophthalmic Zoster or Severe Disseminated VZV Systemic acyclovir (1500 mg/m^2 per d or 30 mg/kg per d IV divided tid for 7 d) or systemic vidarabine (10 to 20 mg/kg per d IV for 7 d). Varicella-zoster immune globulin (VZIG) administration may also be helpful. Topical idoxuridine or vidarabine ophthalmic ointment should be used for any eye involvement, and an ophthalmologic consultation is recommended.

HUMAN PAPILLOMAVIRUS

Warts are discrete benign epithelial proliferations caused by the human papillomavirus (HPV). Different HPV types cause different clinical manifestations. Verruca vulgaris (the common wart) is caused by HPV types 2, 4, 7, 27, and 29. Verruca plana (flat warts) are caused by HPV types 3, 10, 28, and 41. Verruca plantaris (plantar warts) are caused by HPV types 1, 2, and 4.

VERRUCA VULGARIS

Verruca vulgaris are benign keratotic papules typically located on the knees of children.

Synonym Common wart.

EPIDEMIOLOGY

Age Schoolchildren; incidence decreases after age 25.

Gender F > M.

Incidence Common.

Etiology Human papillomavirus (HPV) types 2 and 4, less frequently caused by HPV types 1, 7, and types 27 to 29.

Other Factors Contagion occurs in groups—small (home) or large (school gymnasium). Nail-biters or cuticle-pickers are more prone to periungal lesions.

PHYSICAL EXAMINATION

Skin Findings

Type Firm hyperkeratotic papules (Fig. 23-12), clefted surface, may have a filiform projection.

Size 1 to 10 mm.

Color Skin color, characteristic red dots (thrombosing capillary loops) can be seen with hand lens.

Shape Round, polycyclic.

Arrangement Isolated lesion, scattered discrete lesions.

Sites of Predilection Sites of trauma—hands, fingers, knees.

DIFFERENTIAL DIAGNOSIS

The differential diagnosis of a wart can be made by clinical exam. The papillomatous surface and the red dots (thrombosed capillary loops) are a diagnostic marker for warts. Warts can be confused with nevi, acne, molluscum, or other benign growths.

COURSE AND PROGNOSIS

Warts are slow growing and usually spontaneously disappear after months to years.

MANAGEMENT

In asymptomatic children, warts will often self-resolve without treatment. Enlarging or spreading lesions can be treated with:

1. Liquid nitrogen (in-office cryotherapy, 5 to 10 sec of LN_2 administration to each wart with Q-tips or with a cryotherapy gun).
2. Topical salicylic acid preparations (Compound W, Duofilm, Occlusal HP, Mediplast, Trans-Ver-Sal).
3. Squaric acid in-office sensitization to 2% solution followed by at home application of 0.1% solution qd–qod.

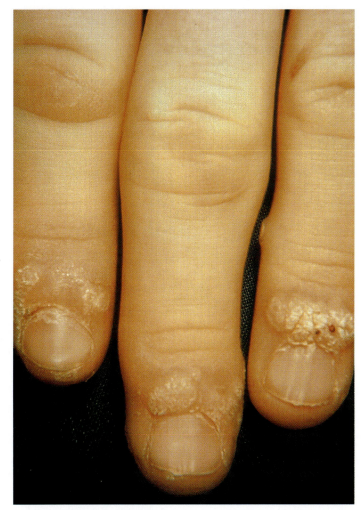

Figure 23-12 **Verruca vulgaris** *Verrucous papules on the periungal region of a child's fingers.*

4. Curettage with local anesthesia.
5. Laser surgery.

Unproven approaches include:

1. Hot-water immersion (113°F for 30 min 3×/week).

2. Hypnosis.
3. Topical Retin-A cream qhs.
4. Topical imiquimod (Aldara cream Monday, Wednesday, and Friday).
5. Duct tape occlusion.

VERRUCA PLANA

Verruca plana are flat-topped, 2- to 5-mm papules, typically scattered on the face, arms, and legs of children.

Synonym   Flat wart.

EPIDEMIOLOGY

Age   Seen most in young children; can also be seen in adults.

Gender   F > M.

Incidence   Common.

Etiology   HPV types 1, 2, 3, 10, and 11.

Other Factors   In adolescents and adults, shaving can spread the lesions.

PHYSICAL EXAMINATION

Skin Findings

Type   Flat-topped papules (Fig. 23-13).

Size   1 to 5 mm.

Color   Skin-colored or light brown.

Shape   Round, oval, polygonal, linear lesions (inoculation of virus by scratching).

Number   Few lesions to hundreds.

Distribution   Any site.

Sites of Predilection   Face, dorsa of hands, shins.

COURSE AND PROGNOSIS

Flat warts tend to self-resolve over time.

MANAGEMENT

In asymptomatic children, flat warts will often self-resolve without treatment. Enlarging or spreading lesions can be treated with:

1. Liquid nitrogen (in-office cryotherapy, 5 to 10 sec of LN_2 administration to each wart with Q-tips or with a cryotherapy gun).
2. Topical salicylic acid preparations (Compound W, Duofilm, Occlusal HP, Mediplast, Trans-Ver-Sal).
3. Curettage with local anesthesia.
4. Laser surgery.

Unproven approaches include:

1. Hot-water immersion (113°F for 30 min 3×/week).
2. Hypnosis.
3. Topical Retin-A cream qhs.
4. Topical imiquimod (Aldara cream applied Monday, Wednesday, and Friday).
5. Duct tape occlusion.

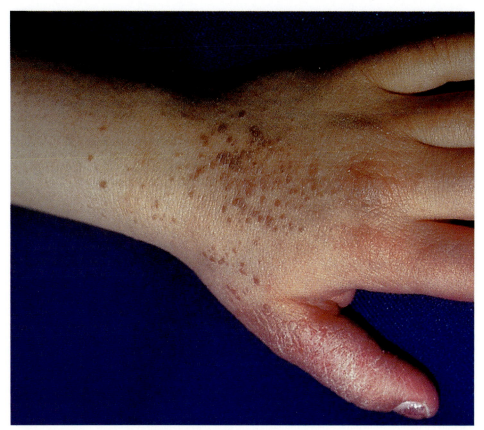

Figure 23-13 Verruca plana *Scattered flat-topped papules increasing in number on the dorsum of a child's hand.*

VERRUCA PLANTARIS

Verruca plantaris are keratotic lesions located on the plantar aspect of the feet. They tend to be the most painful and difficult to treat wart infection.

Synonym Plantar wart.

EPIDEMIOLOGY

Age Any age, typically 5 to 25.

Gender F > M.

Incidence Common.

Etiology HPV 1, 2, and 4.

Other Factors Trauma is a factor, as the lesions often occur on sites of pressure.

PHYSICAL EXAMINATION

Skin Findings

Type Small, shiny, sharply marginated papule. Progresses to plaque with rough hyperkeratotic surface, often covered by a callus-like hyperkeratosis (Fig. 23-14).

Color Skin-colored. To identify diagnostic red dots (thrombosed capillary loops indicative of wart virus infection), many plantar warts must be pared with a scalpel to remove the overlying hyperkeratosis.

Palpation Tenderness may be marked, especially in certain acute types.

Distribution Plantar foot, especially pressure points: heads of metatarsal, heels, and toes.

COURSE AND PROGNOSIS

Untreated, 50% of plantaris warts self-resolve in 6 months. Others persist and can become quite large and/or painful.

DIFFERENTIAL DIAGNOSIS

The diagnosis of a plantar wart is made by clinical findings. Verruca plantaris can be mistaken for corns, calluses, or scars. Paring of the lesion should reveal red dots (thrombosed capillary loops) in verruca, thus distinguishing them from other plantar lesions.

MANAGEMENT

In asymptomatic children, plantar warts will often self-resolve without treatment. Enlarging or spreading lesions can be treated with:

1. Liquid nitrogen (in-office cryotherapy, 5 to 10 sec of LN_2 administration to each wart with Q-tips or with a cryotherapy gun).
2. Topical salicylic acid preparations (Compound W, Duofilm, Occlusal HP, Mediplast, Trans-Ver-Sal).
3. In-office sensitization with 2% squaric acid followed by home application of a 0.1% squaric acid solution qod to qd.
4. Curettage with local anesthesia.
5. Laser surgery.

Unproven approaches include:

1. Hyperthermia using hot water (113°F) immersion for 1/2 to 3/4 h 2 or 3 times weekly for 16 treatments can be effective, as the wart virus is thermolabile.
2. Hypnosis.
3. Topical Retin-A cream qhs.
4. Topical imiquimod (Aldara cream Monday, Wednesday, and Friday).

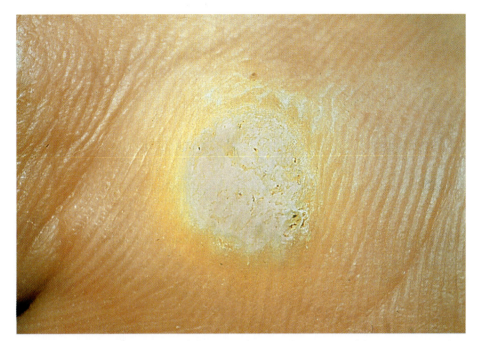

Figure 23-14 Verruca plantaris *Rough keratotic plaque with pinpoint red dots representing dilated blood vessels charactersitc of a plantar wart.*

CONDYLOMA ACUMINATUM

Condyloma are soft, skin-colored, fleshy warts occurring on mucocutaneous junctions and intertriginous areas, resulting from an infection by human papillomavirus (HPV).

Synonyms Genital acuminate or veneral wart, verruca acuminata.

EPIDEMIOLOGY

Age Typically seen in sexually active adults; seen with increased frequency in children.

Gender M = F.

Etiology Human papillomavirus (HPV) types 6, 11 most commonly; also types 16, 18, 31, 33.

Transmission Contagious, nonsexually and sexually transmitted. In infants and children, HPV may be acquired during delivery. The presence of condyloma in the anogenital area should alert one to the possibility of sexual abuse. Nonvenereal transmission is more likely if there are (1) no other signs of sexual abuse, (2) the lesions are distant from the anus or introitus, or (3) warts are present in close contacts (e.g., mother's hands).

Incidence Common. Increased manifold during the past two decades.

HISTORY

Condyloma can appear weeks to years after exposure and tend to spread with local trauma or irritation.

PHYSICAL FINDINGS

Skin Findings

Type Pinhead papules to cauliflower-like papules to plaques (Fig. 23-15).

Color Skin colored, pink, or red.

Palpation Soft.

Shape May be filiform or sessile.

Distribution Rarely few isolated lesions, usually clusters. Perianal/buttock area. May be on the male glans penis, female labia.

Arrangement May be solitary. Grouped into grapelike or cauliflower-like cluster.

DIFFERENTIAL DIAGNOSIS

The diagnosis of condyloma is often made clinically and occasionally confirmed by biopsy. The differential diagnosis of condyloma includes condylomata lata (syphilis), intraepithelial neoplasia, bowenoid papulosis, squamous cell carcinoma, molluscum contagiosum, lichen nitidus, lichen planus, normal sebaceous glands, pearly penile papules, folliculitis, moles, seborrheic keratoses, skin tags, pilar cyst, and scabetic nodules.

LABORATORY EXAMINATIONS

Dermatopathology On skin biopsy, the epidermis shows marked acanthosis and pseudo-epitheliomatous hyperplasia.

Acetowhitening Subclinical lesions can be visualized by wetting the area with gauze soaked with 5% acetic acid for 5 min. Using a 10x hand lens, warts appear as tiny white papules.

COURSE AND PROGNOSIS

Condyloma may clear spontaneously but tend to recur even after appropriate therapy, due to persistence of latent HPV in normal-appearing perilesional skin. The major significance of HPV infection is their oncogenicity later on in life. HPV types 16, 18, 31, and 33 are the major etiologic factors for cervical carcinoma in women. The importance of the annual Pap test must be stressed to women with a history of genital warts. Additionally, genital warts can be transmitted perinatally to the infant.

MANAGEMENT

Condyloma are often difficult to treat and recurrences are frequent. Few cases may self-resolve.

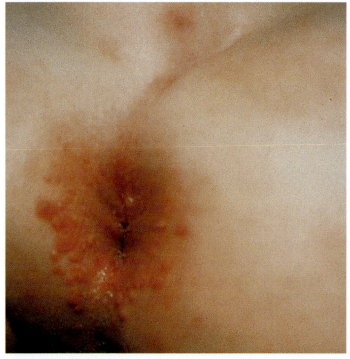

Figure 23-15 Condyloma acuminatum *Perianal verrucous papules in a child. The perianal location should alert one to the possibility of sexual abuse, but often the warts are caused by nonvenereal warts in close family members that bathe or care for the child.*

Spreading lesions can be treated by cryotherapy with liquid nitrogen.

Topical home regimens include:

1. Podofilox (Condolox solution applied 3 consecutive d/week to the area until lesions resolve).

2. Imiquimod (Aldara cream applied 3 ×/ week to the area until the lesions resolve).

Alternative treatments in adolescents or adults include:

1. *Podophyllin* (10 to 25%) in compound tincture of benzoin can be applied in the office and washed off in 1 to 4 h. Mucosal warts are more likely to respond than highly keratinized warts. Podophyllin is contraindicated in pregnancy.

2. *Trichloracetic acid* (80 to 90%) can also be used in the office. The acid is applied only to the warts and then powder, talc, or baking soda is layered on top to remove the excess acid.

3. *Electrodesiccation, electrocautery, or laser surgery* are reserved for the most refractory cases. They are highly effective in destruction of infected tissue and HPV.

Condyloma in children, especially in the anogential region, should alert the physician to the possibility of child abuse. Fortunately, most instances are nonvenereal in transmission and can be explained by nonvenereal warts in close family members. A work-up should be pursued with the help of social services if necessary.

POXVIRUS

MOLLUSCUM CONTAGIOSUM

Molluscum contagiosum is a common viral infection of childhood, characterized by discrete, umbilicated, pearly-white papules.

EPIDEMIOLOGY

Age Children, usually between the age of 3 and 16.

Gender M > F.

Incidence Common.

Transmission Skin to skin contact. In sexually active adults, the primary genital location of the lesions suggests it is spread sexually.

Risk Factors Increased incidence in young children, swimmers, and in children who bathe together. Also, increased incidence in immunosuppressed individuals.

HISTORY

Molluscum lesions typically appear anywhere from 14 days to 6 months after exposure. They can spread by autoinoculation, but typically self-resolve in a few months. The lesions are asymptomatic or mildly pruritic and can look inflamed prior to spontaneous involution. Symptoms are absent.

PHYSICAL EXAMINATION

Skin Findings

Type Papules to nodules with central umbilication.

Size 2 to 5 mm, rarely 10 to 18-mm lesions.

Color Pearly-white or flesh-colored.

Shape Round, oval, hemispherical, umbilicated.

Number Isolated single lesion or multiple scattered discrete lesions.

Sites of Predilection Axillae (Fig. 23-16), antecubital and crural folds.

DIFFERENTIAL DIAGNOSIS

The diagnosis of molluscum contagiosum can be made if characteristic dome-shaped papules with central umbilication are noted (Fig. 23-17). With smaller lesions or atypical cases, molluscum can be confused with nevi, warts, acne, or in adults, basal cell carcinoma.

LABORATORY EXAMINATION

Dermatopathology Skin biopsy will reveal molluscum bodies (epithelial cells with large intracytoplasmic inclusions, aka Henderson–Patterson bodies).

Skin Scrape A simple skin scrape of the central core, obtained by pointed scalpel without local anesthesia, reveals molluscum with Giemsa's staining.

COURSE AND PROGNOSIS

Molluscum are common in children and often self-resolve.

MANAGEMENT

In asymptomatic children, molluscum will often self-resolve without treatment. Enlarging or spreading lesions can be treated with:

1. Liquid nitrogen (in-office cryotherapy, 5 to 10 sec of LN_2 administration to each wart with Q-tips or with a cryotherapy gun).
2. Cantharone (blistering beetle extract which needs to be washed off after 2 to 6 h) can be used.

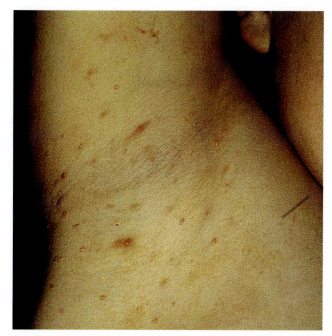

Figure 23-16 Molluscum contagiosum *Scattered umbilicated dome-shaped papules in the axillary region of a child.*

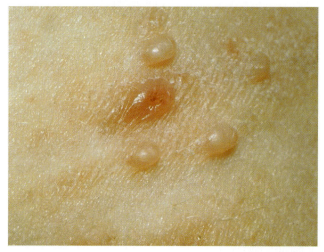

Figure 23-17 Molluscum contagiosum *Close-up of dome-shaped umbilicated papules.*

Unproven approaches include:

1. Topical Retin-A cream QHS.
2. Topical imiquimod (Aldara cream 3×/wk).
3. At home, tape-striping (Scotch tape placed over molluscum at night and peeled off in the morning).

For severe, extensive cases, curettage with local anesthesia, or laser surgery can be considered.

EPSTEIN–BARR VIRUS

INFECTIOUS MONONUCLEOSIS

Infectious mononucleosis is a contagious viral disease caused by Epstein–Barr virus (EBV) and characterized by fever, malaise, tonsillitis, hepatosplenomegaly, lymphadenopathy, +/− a rash. The disease is notorious for its association with debilitating fatigue.

Synonyms   Mono, EBV infection, kissing disease.

EPIDEMIOLOGY

Age   All ages, typically adolescents, ages 13 to 25 years old.

Gender   M = F.

Incidence   Common.

Eitology   Epstein–Barr virus (EBV).

Transmission   Spread via saliva or blood during viremia phase.

HISTORY

Infectious mononucleosis begins 30 to 50 d after exposure with fever, malaise, and a sore throat. A marked tonsillitis and associated cervical lymphadenopathy ensure. Hepatosplenomegaly is common; 10 to 15% of pateints will have a generalized exanthem (macular or papular), 50% of patients will have periorbital edema, 25% of patients have an associated exanthem (petechiae on the palate). Chronic debilitating fatigue is often a hallmark of this disease.

PHYSICAL EXAMINATION

Skin Findings

Type   Macules or papules, edema.

Color   Bright pink or red.

Size   1 to 5 mm.

Distribution   Generalized eruption, periorbital edema.

Mucous Membranes   Petechiae at the junction of the soft and hard palate, marked membranous tonsillitis (Fig. 23-18).

General Findings

Fever (101°F to 104°F), malaise, fatigue, hepatosplenomegaly, and lymphadenopathy.

DIFFERENTIAL DIAGNOSIS

Infectious mononucleosis in children can be very mild and asymptomatic. In adolescents, the disease tends to be more severe and thus easier to recognize. The diagnosis of infectious mononucleosis is made by the triad of clinical findings, leukocytosis (10,000 to 40,000 μm^2), and serologic confirmation (heterophile antibody test). The differential diagnosis includes other viral exanthems, drug eruption, and systemic bacterial infection.

LABORATORY EXAMINATIONS

Monospot Test   A rapid slide test of the patient's blood for the presence of heterophile antibodies can be false negative, especially in children < 4 years old.

Serology   Serologic antibody tests for IgA antibodies angainst the EBV capsid may be helpful.

COURSE AND PROGNOSIS

Most cases of infectious mononucleosis self-resolve in 10 to 20 d. The most severe complication is splenomegaly with the risk of splenic rupture. In rare instances, a more chronic form of the disease has been seen, with relapses and chronic fatigue.

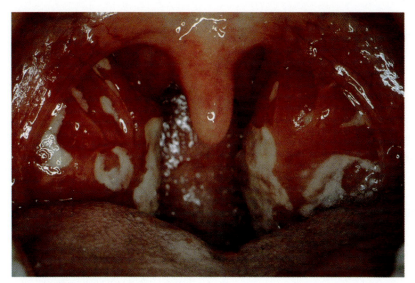

Figure 23-18   Infectious mononucleosis   *Marked white exudate on the tonsils of a child with infectious mononucleosis.*

MANAGEMENT

Infectious mononucleosis will self-resolve with supportive measures. In 25% of cases a concurrent ß-hemolytic strep throat in present and should be treated with penicillin (25 to 50 mg/kg per d divided tid to qid, not to exceed 3 g/d), or erythromycin (30 to 50 mg/kg per d divided qid, not to exceed 2 g/d) Amoxicillin should be avoided since 80 to 90% of patients with infectious mononucleosis if given amoxicillin will erupt in a copper-colored generalized hypersensitivity reaction (this is NOT a true drug allergy, and the patient can use amoxicillin in the future without problems).

If the tonsillitis is severe, the patient may require hospitalization and systemic steroids to reduce soft-tissue swelling (and airway obstruction).

HUMAN PARVOVIRUS B19

ERYTHEMA INFECTIOSUM

Erythema infectiosum is a childhood exanthem caused by parvovirus B19 and characterized by a "slapped-cheek" appearance on the face and a lacy-reticulated rash on the body.

Synonym Fifth's disease.

EPIDEMIOLOGY

Age All ages. Primarily seen in children age 3 to 12 years old.

Gender F > M.

Incidence Common. Up to 60% of adults are seropositive for parvovirus B19 IgG antibodies.

Season Late winter, early spring.

Etiology Human parvovirus B19.

Transmission Spread via aerosolized respiratory droplets during the viremic stage.

HISTORY

Erythema infectiosum begins 6 to 14 d after exposure with fever, malaise, headache, chills, arthritis, and arthralgias. On day 3 to 4 the rash appears as the viremia resolves. Pruritus may be present.

PHYSICAL EXAMINATION

Skin Findings

Type Edematous plaques ("slapped-cheek" appearance; (Fig. 23-19A), macules, and papules.

Color Pink to red.

Shape Round to oral.

Arrangement Coalescing lesions to form a lacy reticulated appearance (Fig. 23-19B).

Distribution "Slapped cheeks." Reticulated lesions on extensor surfaces of extremities, trunk, neck.

Mucous Membranes +/− exanthem.

DIFFERENTIAL DIAGNOSIS

The diagnosis of erythema infectiosum is based on clinical findings. It can be misdiagnosed commonly as other childhood exanthems: rubella, measles, scarlet fever, erythema subitum, enteroviral infections, or drug reactions.

LABORATORY EXAMINATIONS

Serology Blood may show anti-parvoviral B19 IgM antibodies or IgG seroconversion.

COURSE AND PROGNOSIS

By the time the "slapped cheek" and lacy body rash is present, the viremia has resolved. The rash slowly resolves over 1 to 3 weeks and can recur or seem to "flare" with temperature fluctuations, sunlight, or friction. Rarely, there may be an associated arthritis, but this is seen more commonly in adults. In persons with chronic hemolytic anemias (sickle-cell anemia, hereditary spherocytosis, thalassemia, pyruvate kinase deficiency, or autoimmune hemolytic anemia) parvovirus B19 may induce an aplastic crisis with worsening anemia. Similarly, pregnant women have an 8% chance of infection with parvoviral B19 exposure, and the virus could affect erythrocyte precursor cells in the developing fetus, leading to hydrops fetalis and fetal death in 3 to 5%.

MANAGEMENT

Erythema infectiosum is self-limited and no treatment is necessary. By the time the rash is noted, the viremia is over; thus children are no longer contagious and can resume normal activities.

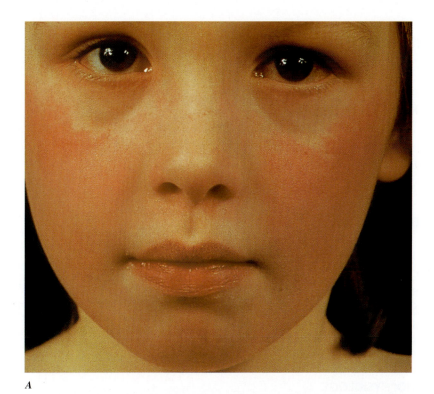

A

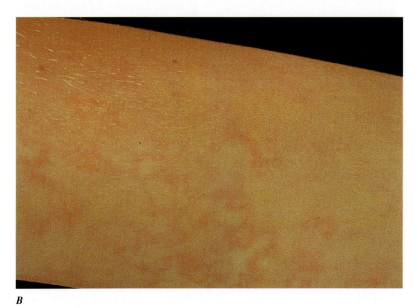

B

Figure 23-19   Erythema infectiosum   *(A) "Slapped-cheek" appearance in a child with parvovirus B19 infection. (B) Lacy, reticulated rash on the body of the same child.*

HUMAN HERPESVIRUS 6

EXANTHEM SUBITUM

Exanthem subitum is a common benign rash of childhood caused by human herpesvirus 6 and characterized by a fever and generalized exanthem in a well-appearing child.

Synonyms Roseola infantum, sixth disease.

EPIDEMIOLOGY

Age Usually children 6 months to 3 years old.

Gender M = F.

Incidence Common.

Etiology Human herpesvirus 6 (HHV-6).

Transmission Unclear. Communicability seems low and seems to be from asymptomatic viral shedding.

PATHOPHYSIOLOGY

87% of infants <1 month old have HHV-6 antibodies (likely passive maternal transplacental transfer). The infants then become seronegative for HHV-6, making them susceptible to infection, and by age 3, 75% of children are seropositive again for HHV-6 antibodies.

HISTORY

Exanthem subitum is characterized by 3 to 5 d of fever followed by a generalized rash for < 1 to 2 d. The hallmark of the infection is a well-appearing infant (Fig. 23-20A) despite the temperature and skin findings.

PHYSICAL EXAMINATION

Skin Findings

Type Macules/papules, edema.

Color Rose pink.

Size 2 to 3 mm.

Distribution Maculopapular rash on trunk (Fig. 23-20B), spreading to neck and extremities, periorbital edema.

General Findings

High fever (and febrile seizures in 6%), then rapid defervescence at time of rash onset.

DIFFERENTIAL DIAGNOSIS

The diagnosis of exanthem subitum is made by the idiosyncratic clinical presentation of a well-appearing playful child with high fever and diffuse rash. The differential diagnosis includes measles, rubella, scarlet fever, erythema infectiosum, and other viral exanthems.

LABORATORY EXAMINATIONS

Hematology Mild leukopenia with relative lymphocytosis.

Serology IgM or a fourfold rise in HHV-6 antibodies can be demonstrated.

COURSE AND PROGNOSIS

Exanthem subitum is self-limited. One attack confers lifelong immunity.

MANAGEMENT

No treatment is necessary, especially since most children are well appearing. Acetaminophen and fluids for fever and other asymptomatic measures may be taken.

CUTANEOUS VIRAL INFECTIONS

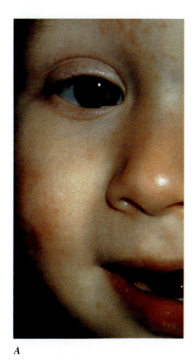

A

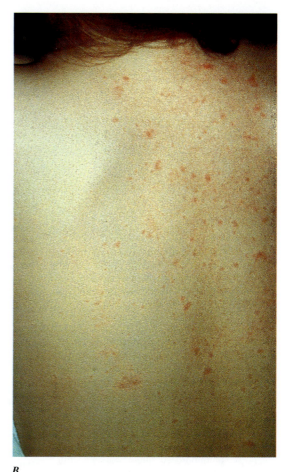

B

Figure 23-20 Exanthem subitum *(A) Well-appearance of a child with HHV-6 infection. **(B)** Maculopapular rash on the body of the same child.*

MEASLES VIRUS

MEASLES

Measles is a highly contagious childhood viral infection characterized by fever, coryza, cough, conjunctivitis, pathognomonic enanthem (Koplik's spots), and an exanthem, and can be complicated, acutely and chronically, by significant morbidity and mortality.

Synonyms Rubeola, morbilli.

EPIDEMIOLOGY

Age Prior to measles immunization, measles was seen in children ages 5 to 9 years in the United States. Since routine vaccination, cases are seen in children >10 years old or infants <15 months old.

Gender M = F.

Incidence United States: Greater than four-fold increase, 1988 to 1989. Worldwide: Hyperendemic in many underdeveloped countries, resulting in >1.5 million deaths annually.

Etiology Measles virus, a paramyxovirus.

Risk Factors Following immunization begun in 1963, incidence has decreased by 98%. Current outbreaks in the United States occur in inner-city unimmunized preschool-age children, school-age persons immunized at early age, and imported cases. Most outbreaks are in primary or secondary schools, colleges, universities, or daycare centers.

Transmission Spread by respiratory droplets aerosolized by sneezing and coughing. Infected persons contagious from several days before onset of rash up to 5 days after lesions appear. Attack rate for susceptible contacts exceeds 90 to 100%. Asymptomatic infection is rare.

Season Prior to widespread use of vaccine, epidemics occurred every 2 to 3 years, in late winter to early spring.

Geography Worldwide.

PATHOPHYSIOLOGY

Measles virus enters cells of the respiratory tract, replicates locally, spreads to local lymph nodes, and disseminates hematogenously to skin and mucous membranes.

HISTORY

Ten to fifteen days after exposure a prodrome of coryza and a *hacking, barklike cough,* photophobia, malaise, and fever may be present. An enanthem (Koplik's spots) appears, followed by the exanthem that begins behind the ears and hairline and spreads downwards.

PHYSICAL EXAMINATION

Skin Findings

Type of Lesion Exanthem: macules and papules. Periorbital edema in prodrome.

Color Initially erythematous, fading to yellow-tan.

Arrangement Initial discrete lesions may become confluent, especially on face, neck, and shoulders (Fig. 23-21A).

Distribution of Lesions Appear on forehead at hairline, behind ears; spread centrifugally and inferiorly to involve the face, trunk (Fig. 23-21B).

Mucous Membranes Enanthem with Koplik's spots: cluster of tiny bluish-white papules with an erythematous areola (Fig. 23-21C), appearing on or after second day of febrile illness, on buccal mucosa opposite premolar teeth. Bulbar conjunctivae: conjunctivitis.

General Examination

Generalized lymphadenopathy common. Otherwise unremarkable.

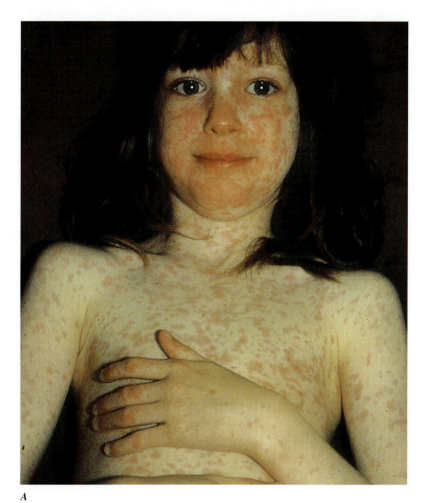

A

Figure 23-21 Measles *(A) Erythematous coalescing macules on face and trunk of a child with measles.*

DIFFERENTIAL DIAGNOSIS

Measles is a clinical diagnosis that can be diagnosed by its head-to-toe progression or by the presence of pathognomonic Koplik's spots. The differential diagnosis includes other viral exanthems, secondary syphilis, scarlet fever, and a morbilliform drug eruption.

LABORATORY EXAMINATIONS

Cultures Isolate virus from blood, urine, and pharyngeal secretions.

Hematology Leukocytosis with a lymphopenia.

Serology Demonstrate fourfold or greater rise in measles titer.

COURSE AND PROGNOSIS

The infection is self-limited but uncommonly can be complicated by pneumonia, otitis media, laryngitis, encephalitis, myocarditis, and/or pericarditits.

MANAGEMENT

Prevention Prophylactic immunization with the live attenuated vaccine is recommended for all children $\geq$ 15 months old.

Acute Infection No specific antiviral therapy is used, but high-dose vitamin A does seem to decrease the morbidity and mortality of hospitalized cases of measles. Otherwise symptomatic treatment and respiratory isolation are recommended.

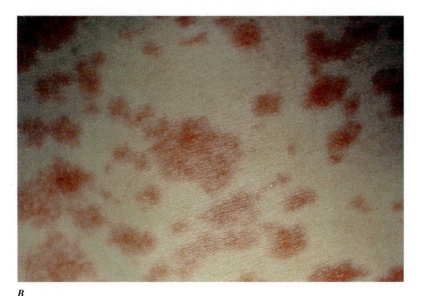

B

Figure 23-21 (continued)   Measles   *(B) Close-up view of erythematous macules coalescing into plaques.*

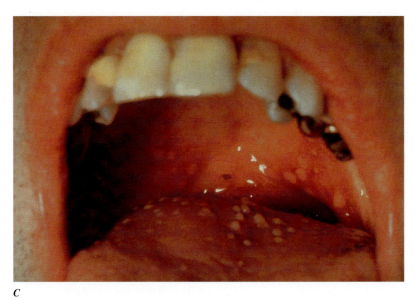

C

Figure 23-21 (continued)   Measles   *(C) White spots (Koplik's spots) on the hard palate of a person with measles.*

RUBELLA VIRUS

RUBELLA

Rubella is a common benign childhood infection manifested by a characteristic exanthem and lymphadenopathy; however, occurring in pregnancy, it may result in the congenital rubella syndrome with serious chronic fetal infection and malformation.

Synonyms   German measles, three-day measles.

EPIDEMIOLOGY

Age   Prior to widespread immunization, rubella was seen in children <15 years. Currently, rubella is seen in young adults.

Gender   M = F.

Incidence   Prior to vaccination, rubella was a common childhood disease. Since vaccine (1969), the incidence of rubella has decreased.

Etiology   Rubella virus.

Transmission   Rubella virus is spread by inhalation of aerosolized respiratory droplets and is moderately contagious. The period of infectivity is from the end of the incubation period to the disappearance of the rash.

Season   In the past, epidemics in the United States occurred every 6 to 9 years, especially in the spring.

Geography   Worldwide. Marked reduction in incidence in developed countries following widespread immunization.

PATHOPHYSIOLOGY

Rubella virus enters the nasopharynx and spreads to the lymphatics. A viremia ensues, followed by the exanthem, which is thought to be due to the antigen–antibody complexes depositing in the skin.

HISTORY

Fourteen to twenty-one days after exposure to the rubella virus, a prodrome of anorexia, malaise, conjunctivitis, headache, low-grade fever, and mild upper respiratory tract symptoms may be present. Inapparent infection is common and can be seen in 50 to 80% of actual infections. The exanthem of rubella begins on the face and moves downward. Lymphadenopathy, arthritis, and arthralgias may be present. Typically older individuals have more severe symptoms than younger ones.

PHYSICAL EXAMINATION

Skin Findings

Type   Macules, papules.

Color   Pink.

Arrangement   Truncal lesions may become confluent, creating a scarlatiniform eruption (Fig. 23-22B).

Distribution of Lesions   Initially on forehead, spreading inferiorly to face (Fig. 23-22A), trunk, and extremities during first day. By second day, facial exanthem fades. By third day, exanthem fades completely without residual pigmentary change or scaling.

Mucous Membranes   Petechiae on soft palate and uvula (Forchheimer's sign; Fig. 23-22C) during prodrome (also seen in infectious mononucleosis).

General Examination

Lymph Nodes   Enlargement noted during prodrome. Postauricular, suboccipital, and posterior cervical lymph nodes enlarged and possibly tender. Mild generalized lymphadenopathy may occur. Enlargement usually persists for one week, but may last for months.

Spleen   May be enlarged.

Joints   Arthritis occurs in adults. Possible effusion.

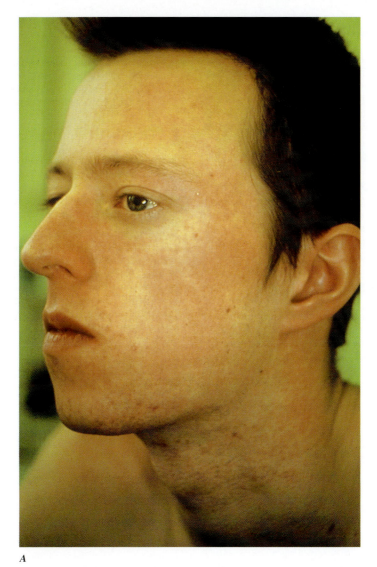

A

Figure 23-22   Rubella   *(A) Confluent erythematous macules on the face of an individual with rubella.*

DIFFERENTIAL DIAGNOSIS

The diagnosis of rubella is made clinically and can be confirmed by serology. The exanthem, enanthem, and lymphadenopathy are not specific and can be seen in other viral infections (enteroviral infections, reoviruses, adenoviruses, measles), scarlet fever, or a drug eruption.

LABORATORY EXAMINATIONS

Hematology   Leukopenia and neutropenia.

Serology   Acute and convalescent rubella antibody titers drawn 2 weeks apart show fourfold or greater rise in titers.

Culture   Virus can be isolated from throat or the joint fluid aspirate.

COURSE AND PROGNOSIS

In most persons rubella is mild and self-limited. However, when rubella occurs in a pregnant woman during the first trimester, the infection can be passed transplacentally to the developing fetus. Approximately half of infants who acquire rubella during the first trimester of intrauterine life will show clinical signs of damage from the virus. Manifestations of the congenital rubella syndrome are congenital heart defects, cataracts, microphthalmia, deafness, microcephaly, and hydrocephaly.

MANAGEMENT

Prophylaxis   Rubella is preventable by immunization with live-attenuated vaccine. Rubella titers should be documented in young women; if anti-rubella antibody titers are negative, rubella immunization should be given.

Acute Infection   No treatment is necessary since rubella is self-limited. Symptomatic treatment with antihistamines or Sarna lotion for pruritus can be used. Infected children should be kept home from school for 5 days after the onset of the rash and pregnant women need to document immunity or avoid exposures, especially during first trimester.

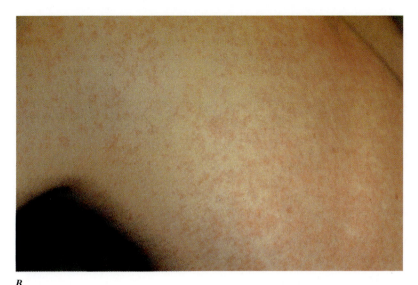

B

Figure 23-22 (continued) **Rubella** *(B) Rash spreading from face to trunk of the same individual.*

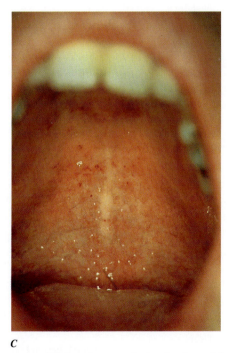

C

Figure 23-22 (continued) **Rubella** *(C) Petechiae on the hard palate of the same individual (Forchheimer's sign).*

COXSACKIE VIRUS

HAND-FOOT-AND-MOUTH DISEASE

Hand-foot-and-mouth disease (HFMD) is a childhood syndrome caused by an enterovirus. It is characterized by ulcerative oral lesions and an exanthem on the distal extremities, in association with a mild febrile illness.

EPIDEMIOLOGY

Age   Usually children <10 years old.

Gender   M = F.

Season   Epidemic outbreaks every 3 years, in temperate climates: seasonal patterns in warmer months.

Etiology   Coxsackie A16 or enterovirus 71; sporadic cases have been reported with coxsackie A4-7, A9, A10, B2 and B5.

Transmission   Highly contagious, spread from person to person by oral–oral and fecal–oral routes.

PATHOPHYSIOLOGY

Enteroviral implantation in the GI tract (buccal mucosa and ileum) leads to extension into regional lymph nodes, and 72 h later a viremia occurs with seeding of the oral mucosa and skin of the hands and feet, causing vesicle formation.

HISTORY

Three to six days after exposure, HFMD causes a prodrome of low-grade fever, malaise, and abdominal pain or respiratory symptoms. Frequently 5 to 10 painful ulcerative oral lesions are present, leading to refusal to eat. Few to 100 cutaneous lesions appear together or shortly after the oral lesions and may be asymptomatic or tender and painful, resolving in 7 to 10 d without scarring.

PHYSICAL EXAMINATION

Skin Findings

Type   Lesions begin as macules or papules, which progress to transient vesicles that rapidly coalesce, ulcerate, and crust over before healing without scarring.

Color   Pink to red.

Shape   Round to oval.

Size   2 to 8 mm.

Distribution   The dorsa of the hands and feet and sides of fingers (Fig. 23-23A) and toes are more often involved than the palms and soles (Fig. 23-23B). Oral lesions are most frequently located on the hard palate, tongue, and buccal mucosa (Fig. 23-23C).

General Findings

Typically, HFMD is accompanied by low-grade fever, malaise, and a sore mouth. In some patients, it may be associated with high fever, severe malaise, diarrhea, and joint pains.

LABORATORY EXAMINATIONS

Histopathology   Epidermal reticular degeneration leads to an intraepidermal vesicle filled with neutrophils, mononuclear cells, and proteinaceous eosinophilic material. The dermis reveals a perivascular mixed-cell infiltrate.

Electron Microscopy   Intracytoplasmic particles in a crystalline array characteristic of coxsackie viral infections.

Serology   In acute serum, neutralizing antibodies may be detected but disappear rapidly. In convalescent serum, elevated titers of complement-fixing antibodies are found.

Tzanck Preparation   Negative for both multinucleated giant cells and inclusion bodies.

Viral Culture   Virus may be isolated from vesicles, throat washings, and stool specimens.

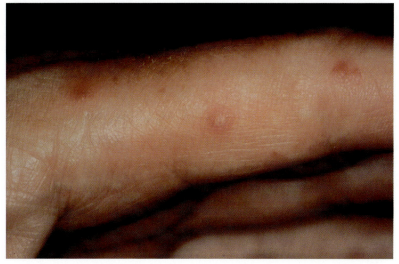

A

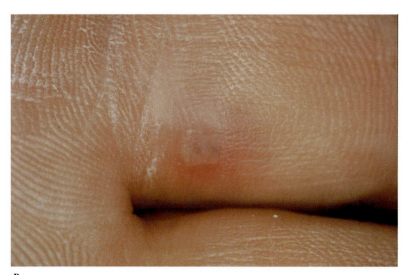

B

Figure 23-23 Hand-foot-and-mouth disease *(A) Vesicular lesions on the sides of the fingers of a patient with HFMD. (B) Vesicular lesion on the foot of the same patient.*

DIFFERENTIAL DIAGNOSIS

A sudden outbreak of oral and distal extremity lesions is pathognomonic for HFMD; however, if only the oral lesions are present, the differential diagnosis would include herpes simplex virus infection, aphthous stomatitis, herpangina, and erythema multiforme major.

COURSE AND PROGNOSIS

Most commonly, HFMD is self-limited, and a rise in serum antibodies eliminates the viremia in 7 to 10 d. A few cases have been more prolonged or recurrent. Serious sequelae rarely occur; however, coxsackievirus has been implicated in cases of myocarditis, meningoencephalitis, aseptic meningitis, paralytic disease, and a systemic illness resembling rubeola. Infection acquired during the first trimester of pregnancy may result in spontaneous abortion.

MANAGEMENT

No treatment for HFMD is needed. Symptomatically, topical application of dyclonine HCl solution (Dyclone), lidocaine (Zylactin L), or benzocaine (Orabase or Oragel) may help reduce oral discomfort.

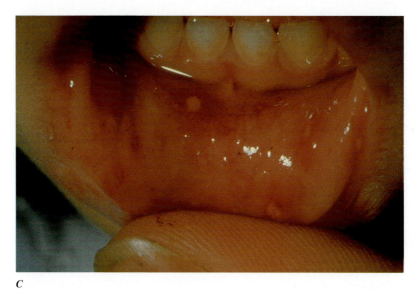

C

Figure 23-23 (continued) Hand-foot-and-mouth disease *(C) Scattered 3- 5-mm ulcers on the buccal mucosa of the same patient.*

GIANOTTI–CROSTI SYNDROME

Papular acrodermatitis of childhood is a rare, self-limited eruption, characterized by the onset of nonpruritic lichenoid papules on the face, buttocks, and extremities, and at times associated with mild constitutional symptoms and acute hepatitis. Historically, an epidemic of the syndrome was associated with hepatitis B surface antigen in Japan (subtype ayw).

EPIDEMIOLOGY

Classification

1. Papular acrodermatitis of childhood. Associated with viral agents such as hepatitis B, Epstein–Barr virus, parainfluenza virus, coxsackie A16, respiratory syncytial virus, poliovirus, CMV, and group A, hemolytic streptococci.
2. Papulovesicular acro-localized syndrome. Unknown etiology, not associated with hepatomegaly, liver function abnormalities, or hepatitis virus infection.

Age   Children between 3 months and 15 years of age; peak incidence between the years of age 1 and 6.

Gender   M = F.

Incidence   Rare.

Etiology   May represent a host response to a variety of infectious agents. Original cases were associated with hepatitis B surface antigenemia.

HISTORY

Often preceded by an upper respiratory infection, papular acrodermatitis begins almost simultaneously with systemic symptoms such as malaise, low-grade fever, and diarrhea. Hepatitis is not always present but can present at the same time or 1 to 2 weeks after the appearance of the rash.

PHYSICAL EXAMINATION

Skin Findings

Type   Monomorphous papules or plaques. Occasionally the rash has a purpuric or coarse-infiltrated tumor-like appearance.

Color   Flesh-colored, pale pink, or coppery red.

Shape   Flat-topped discrete or coalescing lesions.

Size   1 to 10 mm (in infants, 5 to 10 mm; in older children, 1 to 2 mm).

Arrangement   In crops.

Distribution   Usually symmetric, involving the face (Fig. 23-24A), buttocks, extremities, palms, soles, and occasionally the upper back.

Sites of Predilection   Face, elbows (Fig. 23-24B), knees.

General Findings

Low-grade fever, generalized lymphadenopathy (mainly inguinal and axillary), hepatomegaly, splenomegaly, hepatitis.

DIFFERENTIAL DIAGNOSIS

The diagnosis of papular acrodermatitis is suspected by the acute onset of lichenoid papules, constitutional symptoms, ± liver enzyme abnormalities. The differential diagnosis includes drug hypersensitivity, lichen planus, and lichen nitidus.

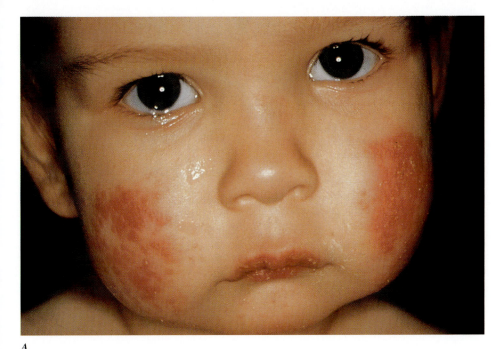

A

Figure 23-24   Gianotti–Crosti syndrome   *(A) Monomorphous papules coalescing into plaques on the cheeks of a child.*

LABORATORY EXAMINATIONS

Histopathology
Liver   May show similar findings to acute viral hepatitis.

Skin   Hyperkeratosis, acanthosis, focal spongiosis, exocytosis, liquefaction and generation of basal cell layer, mixed dermal infiltrate consisting of lymphocytes and histiocytes, dilated dermal capillaries, and swelling of the vascular endothelium.

Hematology   Usually normal CBC and ESR. Leukopenia with a relative increase in monocytes (up to 20%), and mild hypochromic anemia, have been reported.

Chemistry   May have abnormal LFTs (SGOT, SGPT, alkaline phosphatase) with normal bilirubin level.

Serology   May show elevated levels of hepatitis B surface antigen.

COURSE AND PROGNOSIS

Papular acrodermatitis has a self-limited course and the rash resolves spontaneously after a variable period of 2 to 8 weeks (usually 15 to 20 d); lymphadenitis lasts for 2 to 3 months; hepatomegaly persists for 3 months; hepatitis resolves in 2 months and does not progress to chronic liver disease.

MANAGEMENT

No treatment is necessary since the rash and liver abnormalities resolve spontaneously. Symptomatic relief can be obtained with:

1.   Aveeno oilated oatmeal baths.
2.   Topical antipruritic agents (Calamine or Caladryl, Pramasone, or Sarna lotions).

Of note, topical steroids may aggravate the condition.

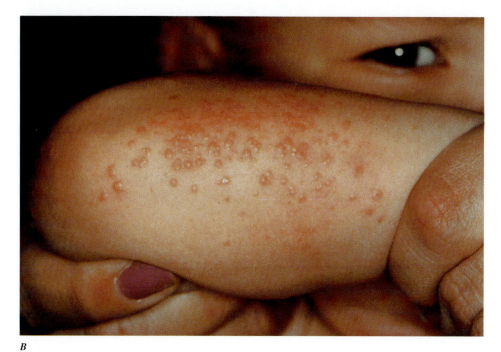

Figure 23-24 (continued)   **Gianotti–Crosti syndrome**   *(B) Erythematous papules on the elbows of the same patient.*

AQUATIC INFESTATIONS

CUTANEOUS LARVA MIGRANS

Cutaneous larva migrans is a skin infestation caused by nematode larvae that penetrate the skin and migrate leaving a characteristic erythematous, serpiginous burrow underneath the skin.

Synonym   Creeping eruption.

EPIDEMIOLOGY

Age   Most common in children and adolescents.

Gender   M = F.

Incidence   Uncommon.

Etiology   Most cases caused by the hookworm larvae of dogs (*Ancylostoma braziliense, A. caninum, Uncinaria stenocephala*) or the hookworm larvae of cats (*Bunostomum phlebotomum*); other parasitic nematodes can be seen.

Geography   Common in warm humid, sandy, coastal areas. In the U.S., hookworm larvae are found in states bordering the Gulf of Mexico or the Atlantic Ocean, extending from Texas to Rhode Island.

PATHOPHYSIOLOGY

Dogs and cats with hookworm can defecate feces infested with hookworm ova. The ova of hookworms are deposited in the sand or soil, and there they hatch into larvae. The larvae can penetrate the skin of humans when they are stepped on with bare feet and proceed to wander serpiginously under the skin; hence the nickname "creeping eruption."

HISTORY

Larvae tend to penetrate the skin and begin to migrate at a rate of 1 to 2 cm/d for 4 weeks to 6 months. After aimless wandering, the larvae typically die and the cutaneous tracts self-resolve. Skin symptoms include pruritus. Systemic symptoms are absent.

PHYSICAL EXAMINATION

Skin Findings

Type   Serpiginous   linear   tracks/burrows (Fig. 24-1).

Color   Flesh colored to pink.

Size   Width 2 to 3 mm, extending at 1 to 2 cm/d.

Number   Several or many tracks.

Distribution   Exposed sites, most commonly the feet, lower legs, buttocks, and hands.

Variant   Larva currens caused by *Strongyloides stercoralis*. Papules, urticaria, and papulovesicles occur at the site of larval penetration and are associated with intense pruritus. The larvae can go from the skin into the blood vessels and migrate to the intestinal mucosa.

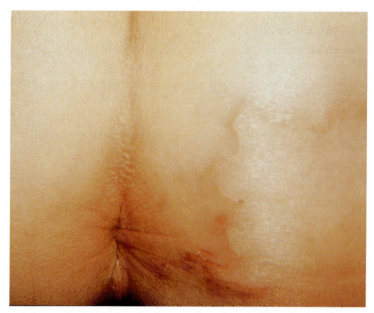

Figure 24-1 Cutaneous larva migrans *Serpiginous lesion on the buttock of an infant infected with hookworm larvae.*

General Findings

Visceral larvae (typically *Toxocara canis, T. cati, A. lumbricoides*) cause peripheral eosinophilia, hepatomegaly, and pneumonitis.

DIFFERENTIAL DIAGNOSIS

The diagnosis of cutaneous larvae migrans is made by the characteristic clinical presentation of slowly curvilinear migrating tracks under the skin. The differential diagnosis includes phytophotodermatitis, erythema chronicum migrans (Lyme borreliosis), jellyfish sting, and granuloma annulare.

COURSE AND PROGNOSIS

Cutaneous larva migrans is typically self-limited because the human skin is a "dead-end" host. Most larvae die after 2 to 4 weeks of aimless wandering underneath the skin, and the skin rash resolves in about 4 to 6 weeks.

MANAGEMENT

Ultimately, the larval eruption will self-resolve in 4 to 6 weeks. Attempts at larval destruction are challenging. Modalities include trichloroacetic acid (TCA) or cryotherapy aimed at a site just beyond the progressing burrow. Oral thiabendazole (25 mg/kg bid for 2 to 4 d, not to exceed 2 to 4 g/d), may be used, but side effects include dizziness, nausea, cramps, and vomiting. Topical thiabendazole (thiabendazole 2% cream) may be better tolerated. Albendazole (400 mg PO qd × 3 d) is also effective. Symptomatic relief with topical steroids ± occlusion until the pruritus self-resolves is the safest, least harmful treatment of choice.

CERCARIAL DERMATITIS

Cercarial dermatitis is an acute allergic pruritic eruption that develops following skin infiltration by *Schistosoma cercariae.*

Synonyms   Swimmers' itch, collector's itch, Schistosome dermatitis, clam-diggers itch.

EPIDEMIOLOGY

Age   Any age.

Gender   M = F.

Incidence   Common.

Etiology   The parasitic cercariae of the *Schistosoma* genus have birds, ducks, and cattle as the usual hosts, with snails as the intermediate host. Humans may become an accidental host by contacting either the fresh water or marine form of the parasite.

Swimmer's Itch   *Trichobilharzia ocellata* and *T. physellae,* common in swamps.

Collector's Itch   *T. stagnicolae,* common in shallow waters.

Geography   Occurs globally but most common in North America, specifically in bathers of the fresh water lakes in the north central United States.

PATHOPHYSIOLOGY

Both the spines and proteolytic enzymes of the cercariae, used to penetrate the skin, incite an acute inflammatory urticarial reaction with subsequent exposure, the rash.

HISTORY

Onset   Initial exposure causes no symptoms. Subsequent exposures incite an allergic response to a protein residue deposited by the invading parasite. At the time of cercarial penetration, an itching sensation (lasting 5 min to 1 h) associated with 1- to 2-mm macules at sites of penetration may be noted. Initial macules persist a few hours and are proceeded (10 to 15 h later) by a more severe pruritic eruption. The eruption may progress to a more severe state, peaking in 2 or 3 d and resolving within 7 d. Systemic symptoms are rare.

PHYSICAL EXAMINATION

Skin Findings

Type   Papules with surrounding areas of erythema and possible progression to edema, vesicles, and urticarial wheals.

Color   Pink to red.

Size   3 to 5 mm.

Distribution   On exposed skin, spares area covered by clothing (Fig. 24-2).

General Findings

Severe cases may have associated fever, nausea, and malaise.

DIFFERENTIAL DIAGNOSIS

The diagnosis of cercarial dermatitis can be made if a history of swimming in fresh water lakes is elicited and a characteristic eruption sparing the bathing-suit area is noted. The differential diagnosis includes seabather's itch, drug eruption, and viral exanthem.

COURSE AND PROGNOSIS

The initial pruritic, macular eruption lasts minutes to hours and is followed by a more extensive papular eruption 10 to 15 h later. This papular eruption generally peaks within 2 to 3 d and self-resolves with no sequelae in 7 to 14 d.

MANAGEMENT

Prevention   Avoidance of prolonged immersion in polluted water. Treatment of polluted water with a mixture of copper sulfate and carbonate, or sodium pentochlorphenate, will prevent the recurrent eruption.

Treatment   Since the cercariae do not dwell within the skin, lesions regress spontaneously. Antihistamines and topical steroids can help relieve symptoms.

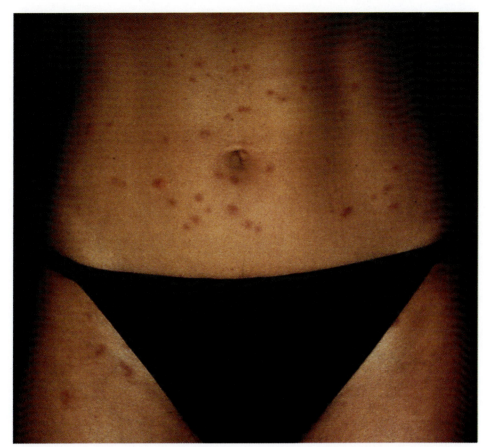

Figure 24-2 Cercarial dermatitis: Swimmer's itch *Erythematous papules on the exposed areas of a swimmer.*

SEABATHER'S ITCH

Seabather's itch is an acute, self-limiting dermatitis, arising shortly after bathing in seawater and characterized by a perifollicular eruption on areas covered by clothing.

Synonyms   Seabather's eruption, marine dermatitis.

EPIDEMIOLOGY

Age   Any age. Children prone to more extensive eruption.

Incidence   Common in those who bathe in the Florida and Cuban salt waters.

Etiology   Typically seabather's itch is caused by the planula larvae of sea anemone (*Edwardsiella lineata*). On the coasts of Florida, it is caused by the planula larva of jellyfish (*Linuche unguiculata*).

HISTORY

Skin lesions develop several hours after bathing in salt water teeming with anemone larvae. Skin lesions may itch or burn and persist for 1 to 2 weeks. Systemic symptoms are uncommon but can include headache, malaise, nausea, vomiting, and fever.

PHYSICAL EXAMINATION

Skin Findings

Type   Macules, papules, or wheals, which may progress to vesiculopapules.

Color   Erythematous.

Size   2 to 3 mm.

Distribution   Areas covered by bathing suit (Fig. 24-3).

DIFFERENTIAL DIAGNOSIS

Seabather's itch is diagnosed by eliciting a history of saltwater exposure and the clinical finding of an eruption limited to the areas covered by a bathing suit. This is in contrast to swimmers' itch, which affects areas *not* covered by a bathing suit.

COURSE AND PROGNOSIS

Initial eruption develops several hours after bathing in salt water, progresses to a vesiculopapular form, crusts, and heals within 7 to 10 d. Systemic symptoms of headache, malaise, nausea, vomiting, and fever may accompany eruption, but are rare. The rash is self-limited and benign.

MANAGEMENT

Prevention   Eruption may be avoided by washing and drying covered areas of the skin immediately after swimming.

Treatment   Symptomatic treatment includes antipruritic lotions, antihistamines, and topical/systemic corticosteroids.

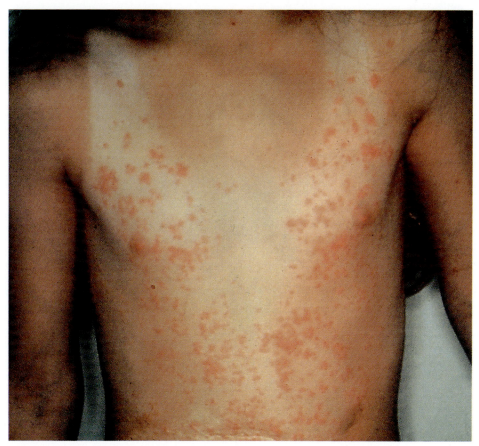

Figure 24-3   Seabather's itch   *Erythematous papules on the unexposed areas of a swimmer.*

SEA URCHIN DERMATITIS

Sea urchins are echinoderms with a flat body covered with long, needle-like spines that contain venom that is released once the spine penetrates the skin.

EPIDEMIOLOGY

Age Any age.

Gender M = F.

Incidence Uncommon.

Etiology Toxins from sea urchin spines and pedicellaria with jaw-like structure are interspersed amongst the spines (Fig. 24-4). Pedicellaria cling to the skin and inject more venom.

HISTORY

Sea urchin dermatitis most commonly occurs when a person accidentally steps on one, although gentle mechanical handling of the sea urchin can also trigger it to sting. Immediate pain and burning locally is followed by muscle and other systemic symptoms.

PHYSICAL EXAMINATION

Skin Findings

Type Puncture site.

Color Surrounding red-purple.

Distribution Commonly on feet or exposed areas that brush against the sea urchin (Fig. 24-5).

General Findings

Extensive pedicellaria stings can lead to short-lived paralysis, aphonia, or respiratory distress.

COURSE AND PROGNOSIS

Sea urchin dermatitis is typically mild and self-limited. Cases in which larger amounts of spine and pedicellaria are left piercing the skin with larger doses of venom administered can have more severe sequelae.

MANAGEMENT

All adherent pedicellaria and spines should be removed as quickly as possible to limit the venom infusion. Symptomatic relief may be achieved with topical soaks, corticosteroids, and analgesics.

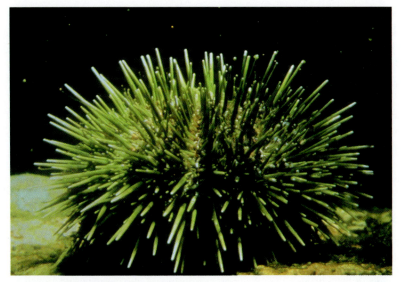

Figure 24-4 **Sea urchin** *Spiny projections of sea urchin.*

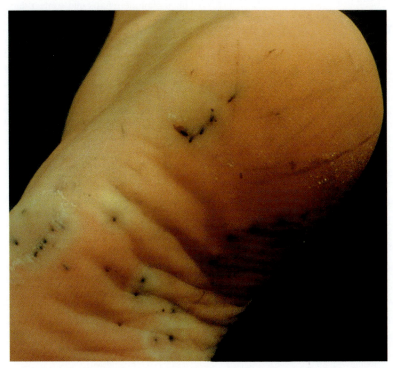

Figure 24-5 **Sea urchin** *Puncture sites on the plantar surface of an individual who stepped on a sea urchin.*

JELLYFISH DERMATITIS

Jellyfish are radial, symmetric animals with body walls enclosing a jelly-like substance and nematocysts (stinging capsules on tentacles that contain venom).

Synonyms *Cnidaria, Coelenterata,* Portuguese man-of-war, hydroids, box jellyfish, sea nettles, sea anemones.

EPIDEMIOLOGY

Age Any age.

Gender M = F.

Incidence Uncommon.

Etiology The rash is caused by jellyfish venom that contains histamine, prostaglandins, kinin-like factors, and other proteins that may be cardiotoxic or neurotoxic.

Geography Jellyfish present in temperate, subtropical, and tropical waters (Fig. 24-6).

HISTORY

Immediately after jellyfish contact, intense burning and stinging occur, followed by pruritus and urticaria. Residual hyperpigmented streaks may last for months. Depending on the jellyfish species, age of the victim, and amount of venom injected, symptoms can range from mild pruritus to severe systemic shock.

PHYSICAL EXAMINATION

Skin Findings

Type Linear streaks or welts (Fig. 24-7) to vesicles and bullae to hemorrhagic lesions to ulcerations and necrosis.

Color Red to purple to brown postinflammatory hyperpigmentation.

Arrangement Linear streaking.

Distribution Any exposed site, most common on the legs and arms.

General Findings

Systemic symptoms range from mild malaise, fever, nausea, vomiting, and muscle aches to severe anaphylaxis and cardiac or pulmonary arrest.

DIFFERENTIAL DIAGNOSIS

The diagnosis of jellyfish stings is made by the history of jellyfish exposure as well as the clinical linear streaking that the tentacles cause on the legs. The differential diagnosis includes phytophotodermatitis and contact dermatitis.

COURSE AND PROGNOSIS

Most jellyfish stings are localized with severe pruritus and burning that gradually self-resolves with mild systemic symptoms. More severe stings can be seen in younger victims with larger affected areas and higher venom injections.

MANAGEMENT

All adherent tentacles or spines should be removed as quickly as possible (with gloves or tweezers) to reduce venom injections. Seawater can be used to try to wash off debris. Topical vinegar or 3% acetic acid left on for 30 min can inactivate the cnidaria. Local or systemic reactions can be treated with antihistamines or corticosteroids. Anaphylactic symptoms can be treated with epinephrine. Antivenoms are available for the most deadly jellyfish (*Chironex fleckeri*) and, if used promptly, are life-saving.

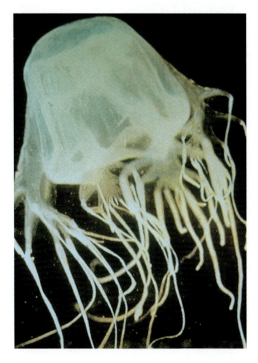

Figure 24-6 Jellyfish dermatitis *Long tentacles of the jellyfish contain venom and are responsible for the streaky dermatitis.*

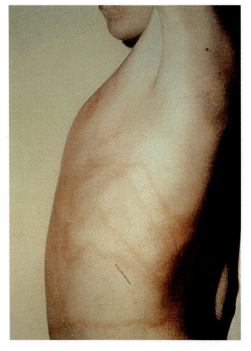

Figure 24-7 Jellyfish dermatitis *Linear hyperpigmented streaks on the side of a child who brushed against the jellyfish tentacles.*

CORAL DERMATITIS

Coral dermatitis is caused by skin accidentally brushing against coral exoskeleton, with resultant laceration, burning, stinging, and foreign body reaction.

Synonyms Fire corals, stony corals.

EPIDEMIOLOGY

Age Any age.

Gender M = F.

Incidence Uncommon.

Etiology Exoskeleton of the coral can be spiny and sharp, cutting into exposed skin.

HISTORY

Corals are located on the floor of the ocean and are accidentally stepped upon or brushed against with a resultant burning, stinging reaction.

PHYSICAL EXAMINATION

Skin Findings

Type Localized papules, pustules.

Color Pink to red.

Arrangement Clustered or linear depending upon exposure pattern.

Distribution Exposed sites, commonly legs and feet (Fig. 24-8).

General Findings

May have mild fever, malaise.

DIFFERENTIAL DIAGNOSIS

The diagnosis is made by the history of coral exposure and localized rash at the site of exposure. The differential diagnosis includes contact dermatitis, sea jellyfish stings, and sea urchin dermatitis.

COURSE AND PROGNOSIS

Coral dermatitis is self-limited and typically resolves in 2 to 4 weeks. Residual hyperpigmentation can persist for months.

MANAGEMENT

No treatment for coral dermatitis is necessary. Symptomatic relief with analgesics and topical steroids can help.

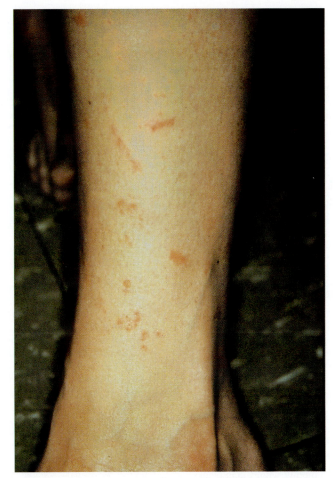

Figure 24-8 Coral dermatitis *Scattered erythematous papules at the sites of skin contact with coral.*

INSECT BITES AND INFESTATIONS

PEDICULOSIS CAPITIS

Pediculosis capitis is an infestation of the scalp by the head louse, which feeds on the scalp and neck and deposits its eggs on the hair.

Synonym Head lice.

EPIDEMIOLOGY

Age More common in children, but all ages.

Gender M = F.

Prevalence Estimated at 6 to 10 million schoolchildren annually in the U.S.

Incidence Common.

Etiology The subspecies of *Pediculus humanus capitis* (1- to 4-mm six-legged, wingless insect; Fig. 25-1). Unlike *P. humanus corporis,* the head louse is not a vector of infectious diseases.

Race More common in whites than blacks.

Transmission Shared hats, caps, brushes, combs; head-to-head contact. Epidemics in schools.

HISTORY

Children are restless and inattentive at school secondary to pruritus of the back and sides of scalp. Scratching and secondary infection associated with occipital and/or cervical lymphadenopathy.

PHYSICAL EXAMINATION

Skin Findings

Type

Head lice identified with eye or with hand lens. The majority of patients have a population of < 10 head lice.

"*Nits,*" or oval grayish-white egg capsules (1 mm long) (Fig. 25-2) firmly cemented to the hairs; vary in number from only a few to thousands. Nits are deposited by head lice on the hair shaft as it emerges from the follicle. With recent infestation, nits are near the scalp; with infestation of long standing, nits may be 10 to 15 cm from scalp. In that scalp hair grows 0.5 mm daily, the presence of nits 15 cm from the scalp indicates that the infestation is approximately 9 months old. New viable eggs have a creamy-yellow color; empty eggshells are white.

Excoriations, crusts, and secondarily impetiginized lesions are commonly seen, and mask the presence of lice and nits; may extend onto neck, forehead, face, and ears. In the extreme, scalp becomes a confluent, purulent mass of matted hair, lice, nits, crusts, and purulent discharge, so-called plica polonica.

Sites of Predilection Head louse nearly always confined to scalp, especially occipital and postauricular regions. Head lice may also infest the beard area or other hairy sites.

DIFFERENTIAL DIAGNOSIS

The diagnosis of pediculosis capitis is made by the clinical findings and confirmed by detection of nits and/or lice. The differential diagnosis includes hair casts, hair lacquer, hair gels, dandruff (epidermal scales), impetigo, seborrheic dermatitis, and tinea capitis.

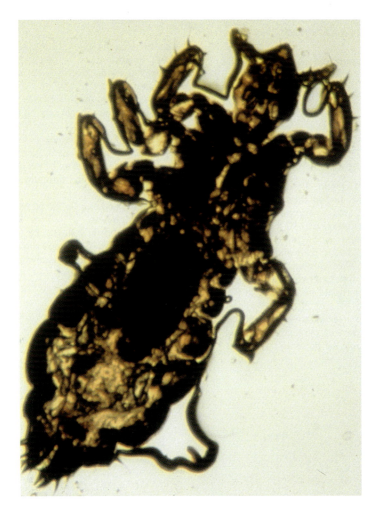

Figure 25-1 Pediculus humanus *Six-legged wingless insect responsible for head lice.*

LABORATORY EXAMINATIONS

Microscopic Examination Of the hair can more clearly show lice and/or nits.

Wood's Light Examination Nits will fluoresce pearly-white and are not movable.

MANAGEMENT

Recommended Regimen

1. Malathion 5% lotion (Ovide) should be used with the fine-toothed metal comb (LiceMeister) and a second application should be performed 8 to 10 d later.
2. Over-the-counter permethrin 1% cream (Nix) rinse applied to scalp and washed off after 10 min. Then combing dead nits out with a metal fine-tooth comb is possible. The treatment should be repeated in 8 to 10 d.
3. If 8 to 10 d after second treatment, nits and eggs are still present, pyrethrin/pyrethroid-resistant lice may be present.

Other

1. Lindane (Kwell) should be avoided in children, because there is potential toxicity associated with overuse or accidental ingestion.
2. Home remedies (such as oils, kerosene, formic acid, and vinegar) are NOT recommended.
3. All other family members should be checked for asymptomatic lice, because epidemics start in the family, not the school.
4. Floors, play areas, and furniture should be vacuumed.
5. Clothes and bedding should be washed and dried on high heat.
6. Combs and brushes should be soaked in pediculocide for 15 min and should not be shared between family members until infection is cleared.

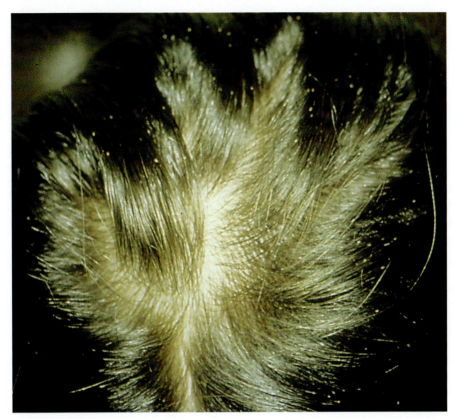

Figure 25-2   Head lice   *Numerous grayish-white lice egg capsules stuck firmly on the hairs in a child with head lice.*

PEDICULOSIS PUBIS

Pediculosis pubis is an infestation of hairy regions, most commonly the pubic area but at times the hairy parts of the chest, axillae, and upper eyelashes. It is manifested clinically by mild to moderate pruritus.

Synonyms   Crabs, crab lice, pubic lice, phthiriasis.

EPIDEMIOLOGY

Age   Most common in adolescents and young adults.

Gender   More extensive infestation in males.

Incidence   Common.

Etiology   *Phthirus or Phthirus pubis,* the crab or pubic louse (1 to 4 mm, six-legged insect, crab-like in appearance; Fig. 25-3). Lives exclusively on humans. Prefers a humid environment; does not tend to wander.

Transmission   Close physical contact such as sexual intercourse; sleeping in same bed; possibly exchange of towels.

HISTORY

Pediculosis pubis may be asymptomatic or pruritic for months. With excoriation and secondary infection, lesions may become tender and be associated with enlarged regional (e.g., inguinal) lymph node.

PHYSICAL EXAMINATION

Skin Findings

Type

Lice appear as 1- to 2-mm, brownish-gray specks in the hairy areas involved. Remain stationary for days; mouth parts embedded in skin; claws grasping a hair on either side (Fig. 25-4). Usually few in number.

Eggs (nits) attached to hair, appear as tiny white-gray specks. Few to numerous.

Papular urticaria (small erythematous papules) noted at sites of feeding, especially periumbilical.

Secondary changes of lichenification, *excoriations, and impetiginized excoriations,* detected in patients with significant pruritus. Serous crusts may be present along with lice and nits when eyelids are infested; occasionally edema of eyelids with severe infestation.

Maculae caeruleae (tâches bleues) are slate-gray or bluish-gray macules, 0.5 to 1.0 cm in diameter, irregular in shape, and nonblanching. Pigment thought to be breakdown product of heme affected by louse saliva.

Distribution   Most commonly found in pubic and axillary areas; also perineum, thighs, lower legs, and trunk, especially in the periumbilical region. In children, eyelashes and eyebrows may be infested without pubic involvement. Maculae caeruleae most common on lower abdominal wall, buttocks, upper thighs.

General Findings

Secondary impetiginization, regional lymphadenopathy.

DIFFERENTIAL DIAGNOSIS

Pediculosis pubis is confirmed by identifying a nit or louse on the hairs. The differential diagnosis includes eczema, tinea, folliculitis, and scabies.

LABORATORY EXAMINATIONS

Microscopy   Lice and nits may be identified with hand lens or microscope.

MANAGEMENT

Recommended Regimen

1. Lindane (Kwell shampoo) applied for 5 min to the infested and adjacent hairy areas and is recommended for affected adolescents or adults. Lindane (Kwell) should be avoided in children because there is potential toxicity associated with overuse or accidental ingestion.

2. All sexual contacts should be checked and treated for pubic lice.
3. Clothes and bedding should be washed and dried on high heat to kill ova and parasites.

4. Pediculosis of the eyelashes can be treated by petrolatum bid to eyelashes × 8 d and mechanical removal.

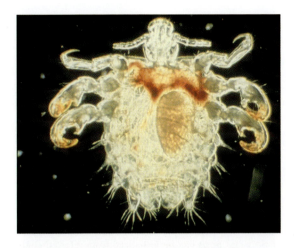

Figure 25-3   Phthirus pubis   *Six-legged crab-like louse responsible for pubic lice.*

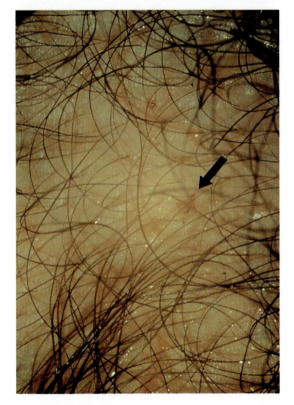

Figure 25-4   Pubic lice   *Pubic louse on a hair in a patient.*

PEDICULOSIS CORPORIS

Pediculosis corporis is caused by the body louse that lives on bedding and clothing but intermittently infests humans to feed.

Synonym   Body lice.

EPIDEMIOLOGY

Age   All ages.

Gender   M = F.

Incidence   Common.

Etiology   Caused by *Pediculus humanus corporis* (2- to 6-mm, six-legged louse).

Transmission   Spread by shared infested clothing or bedding.

HISTORY

Pediculosis corporis is transmitted when contaminated clothing or bedding touches another person. The louse feeds transiently on the skin, but deposits nits and eggs on the fibers of clothing, where they can remain viable for weeks. Furthermore, the louse can carry rickettsial organisms (typhus, trench fever) and transmit them to the human host while feeding. The infection is extremely pruritic.

PHYSICAL EXAMINATION

Skin Findings

Type   Macule, papule, or urticarial wheal at site of louse bite. Numerous body excoriations. Pinpoint white nits may be visible, especially in the seams of clothing (Fig. 25-5).

General Findings

Usually none present.

DIFFERENTIAL DIAGNOSIS

The diagnosis of pediculosis corporis is made by identification of louse or nits on person or more likely, clothing. The differential diagnosis includes eczema and scabies.

LABORATORY EXAMINATIONS

Microscopic Examination   *P. humanus corporis* can be visualized from infested clothes.

Wood's Light   Nits will fluoresce pearly-white.

COURSE AND PROGNOSIS

Undiagnosed pediculosis corporis can lead to worsening infection with worsening pruritus and increased risk of transmission to unaffected population.

MANAGEMENT

Because louse is rarely on the person's body, treatment is directed more toward patient education. Clothes and bedding should be washed in hot water and then dried on high heat.

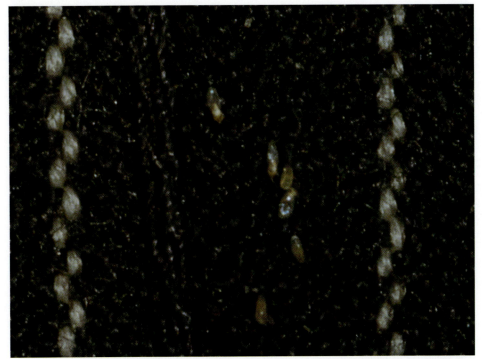

Figure 25-5 Body lice *Scattered nits seen on the seams of clothing.* (Reproduced with permission from TB Fitzpatrick et al., Color Atlas and Synopsis of Clinical Dermatology, 4th edition. New York: McGraw-Hill, 2001).

SCABIES

Scabies is an infestation by the mite *Sarcoptes scabiei,* characterized by severe pruritus and transmitted by close proximity to the infested person.

Synonym   Seven-year-itch.

EPIDEMIOLOGY

Age   Children < 5, adolescents, young adults (sexually transmitted), bedridden elderly patients.

Gender   M = F.

Incidence   Common.

Etiology   *Sarcoptes scabiei,* which can only survive and replicate on human skin. The mite is 400 μm in size and lays eggs and feces under the skin as it burrows.

Transmission   Mite can be transmitted to anyone in close proximity. Commonly seen in children playing together, families, or health care workers. Persons sharing a bed are also at risk. The mites and eggs can remain alive for 1 to 2 d on clothes or bedding.

Risk Factors   Crowded living conditions, immunosuppression.

PATHOPHYSIOLOGY

For pruritus to occur, there must be sensitization to the *Sarcoptes scabiei* mite. The widespread rash is usually caused by less than 10 mites jumping from site to site on the body. In infants or debilitated patients with more severe infestation, mites can exceed hundreds in number.

HISTORY

One month after first exposure, the infested person begins with intractable itching at the site with mite infestation. Itching is widespread and severe, often interfering with sleep. Often family members or caretakers will also report severe itching.

PHYSICAL EXAMINATION

Skin Findings

Type   Intraepidermal burrows or vesicles (Fig. 25-6), may have overlying excoriations, scale, or crust.

Color   Gray or flesh-colored, sometimes with a visible black dot at one end (the mite) with surrounding erythema.

Distribution   Web spaces of the fingers, wrists, elbows, umbilical area, genital area, feet. Usually spares the face and neck. In young infants, the infestations can be widespread and involve the head and neck.

Variants

Nodular Scabies   5- to 10-mm, red or brown, nodular lesions can be seen at the site of mite infestations, especially on the scrotum, back, or feet of children (Fig. 25-8).

Crusted or Norwegian Scabies   Seen in young infants or immunosuppressed patients. Widespread mite infestation causing a hyperkeratotic and/or crusted generalized rash.

DIFFERENTIAL DIAGNOSIS

The diagnosis of scabies is made by history, especially if other family members report recent, intractable pruritus, and by demonstration of the mites, eggs, or feces in the skin. The differential diagnosis includes impetigo, papular urticaria (insect bite), psoriasis, atopic dermatitis, or pediculosis.

LABORATORY EXAMINATIONS

Dermatopathology   Scabetic burrow located in the stratum corneum. Scabetic mite, eggs, or feces. Spongiosis may be seen near the mite. Dermis shows a diffuse eosinophilic infiltrate.

Scabies Prep   A scraping of the linear burrows can reveal mites, eggs, and feces (Fig. 25-7). Skin fragments can be placed on a glass slide with mineral oil and a cover slide and examined under low magnification for signs of mites (400-μm round mites with protruding legs), eggs (100-μm oval particles), or feces (10-μm small oval particles).

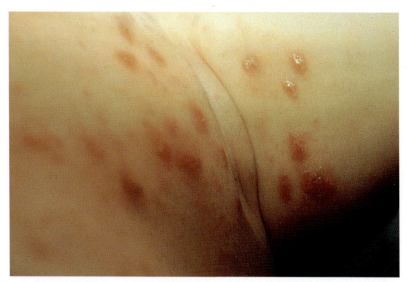

Figure 25-6   Scabies   *Papular and vesicular lesions in the axilla of a child infested with scabies.*

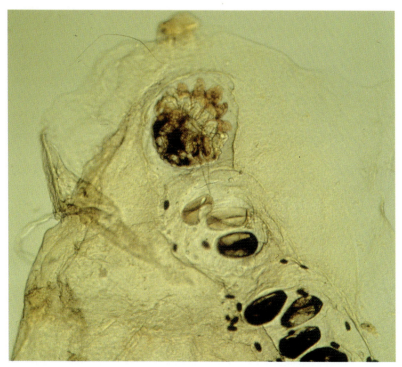

Figure 25-7   Sarcoptes scabiei   *Mite, 400 μm in size, alongside ova (large black ovals) and feces (scattered smaller black dots).*

COURSE AND PROGNOSIS

Scabies pruritius persists for weeks even after adequate treatment, and nodular lesions can take months to years to resolve.

MANAGEMENT

1. Permethrin 5% cream (Elimite) is applied from neck to toes, left on for 8 h, and then washed off.
2. All family members and close contacts should be treated simultaneously.
3. Treatment can be repeated in 1 week to ensure successful eradication.
4. More than two applications are typically not necessary. Residual pruritic symptoms and nodules are typical postscabetic and do not indicate persistent infection.
5. For infants and young children with whole-body involvement, permethrin, 10% crotamiton, or 6 to 10% sulfur ointment should be applied to all body surface areas.
6. For pruritus, emollients and topical steroids can be used for symptomatic relief.
7. Bedding and clothing should be machine washed in hot water and machine dried on high heat.
8. Infested articles can also be stored in an air-tight garbage bag for > 72 h so the mites will die.

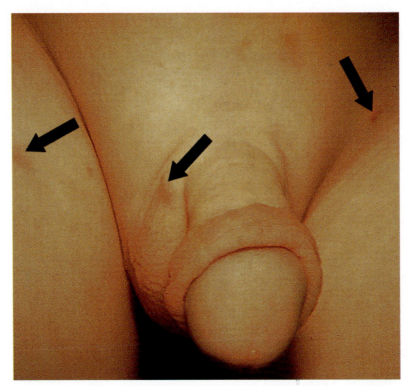

Figure 25-8   Scabies   *Nodular lesions (see arrows) on the genitalia of a child infested with scabies.*

PAPULAR URTICARIA

Papular urticaria is an immunologic-mediated reaction, to flea bites, characterized by an intensely pruritic eruption occurring at the bite sites hours to days after the bites. Of note, patients are often unaware of having been bitten.

EPIDEMIOLOGY

Age Any age, but more common in children.

Season Summer in temperate climates.

Etiology Cat fleas (*Ctenocephalides felis*), dog fleas (*C. canis*), human fleas (*Pulex* species, *Xenopsylla* species), fowl fleas (*Ceratophyllus* species).

PATHOPHYSIOLOGY

Papular urticaria follows an insect bite and is mediated by injected foreign antigens.

HISTORY

Incubation Period CRFB appears hours to days after the bite.

Duration of Lesions Days, weeks.

Skin Symptoms Individuals are not aware of being bitten by fleas. Most patients associate fleas with poor housekeeping practices, or poor personal hygiene. Dog or cat fleas commonly live in carpeting, and emerge and bite the lower legs. Additionally, some family members do not react to bites or are not as highly exposed as the children (do not hold or sleep with pets as much). Reactions to flea bites in infants on first exposure may be mild but upon subsequent exposure, young children (age 1 to 5) have a more severe response. Then the reactions subside as the child grows older.

PHYSICAL EXAMINATION

Skin Findings

Types

Erythematous macules. Occur at bite sites and are usually transient.
Papular urticaria. Persistent urticarial papules (Fig. 25-9), often surmounted by a vesicle, usually less than 1.0 cm (lesions persist more than 48 h). Excoriations and excoriated urticarial papules, vesicles. Excoriated or secondarily infected lesions may heal with hyper- or hypopigmentation, and/or raised or depressed scars, especially in more darkly pigmented individuals.
Vesiculobullous lesions. Tense vesicles or bullae with clear fluid on a slightly inflamed base at site of bite.

Color Red. Bullae have clear amber fluid.

Shape Round, domed.

Arrangement Usually in groups of three ("breakfast, lunch, and dinner").

Distribution The most common sites are the legs from ankles to knees. Thighs, forearms and arms, lower part of trunk, and waist, but sparing anogenital area and axillae.

DIFFERENTIAL DIAGNOSIS

The diagnosis of papular urticaria is a clinical one that is at times confirmed by skin biopsy. The differential diagnosis includes allergic contact dermatitis, especially to plants such as poison ivy or poison oak. Papular urticaria also follows the bites of mites, bedbugs, or mosquitoes.

LABORATORY EXAMINATIONS

Dermatopathology Skin biopsy shows edema and scattered spongiotic vesicles. The dermis has a deep inflammatory infiltrate with scattered eosinophils.

COURSE AND PROGNOSIS

Papular urticaria is self-limited. Bacterial superinfection is common and should be monitored and treated appropriately. Rarely, fleas are the vectors for more serious infections: bubonic plague, tularemia, murine typhus, boutonneuse fever, Q fever, lymphocytic choriomeningitis, tick-borne encephalitis.

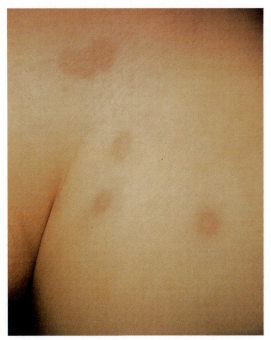

Figure 25-9   Papular   *Persistent erythematous papules on the buttock of a child bitten by fleas.*

Topical steroids offer symptomatic relief. For numerous lesions, oral antihistamines and/or steroids may be needed.

Cats and dogs should be checked and treated for fleas.

Household may need to be "flea-bombed" if wall-to-wall carpeting or furniture is infested.

FIRE ANT STING

Fire ant stings are caused by ants of the *Solenopsis* species and are characterized by burning, painful stings that flare immediately and then vesiculate with purulent fluid of the puncture site.

EPIDEMIOLOGY

Age Any age.

Gender M = F.

Incidence Common, especially in endemic areas.

Geography Imported from South America, fire ants now inhabit most of the southern U.S.

Etiology Fire ants (*Solenopsis saevissima, S. richteri,* and *S. invieta*) produce a venom more potent than the venom of any other hymenopteran (bees, wasps, or ants).

HISTORY

Fire ants will swarm on a person and bite ferociously, leaving hemorrhage puncta at the site of puncture. Then they pivot around their grasping jaws and sting with their tail. With each sting, they inject venom from glands located on their abdomen, leading to immediate flaring around the bite site followed by vesiculation. Systemic fever, GI distress, urticaria, and respiratory symptoms are common.

PHYSICAL EXAMINATION

Skin Findings

Type Macule to papule to wheal to purulent vesicle (Fig. 25-10A).

Color Red to fading pink with a central clear-white vesicle (Fig. 25-10B).

Size 1 to 3 mm with 1- to 3-cm surrounding flare.

Distribution Legs, torso, arms.

DIFFERENTIAL DIAGNOSIS

The diagnosis of fire ants is usually straightforward since the ants are commonly seen at the time of the injury. The differential diagnosis includes other insect bites, a viral exanthem, and varicella.

COURSE AND PROGNOSIS

Once bitten, the patient can feel quite ill, and the skin is very itchy and painful at the sites of bites. Systemic reactions can be quite severe and even life-threatening, especially in small children with numerous bites.

MANAGEMENT

1. Local application of cool compresses, calamine lotion, or topical steroids can alleviate the burning, stinging pain.
2. A papain solution of ¼ meat tenderizer and 4 parts water, applied topically, can also relieve the itch and burn.
3. Systemic antihistamines, steroids, or epinephrine may be needed in severe cases with signs of respiratory distress.
4. Patients with a known allergy to fire ant bites should carry an epinephrine pen or 15 mg sublingual tablet of isoproterenol for immediate use.

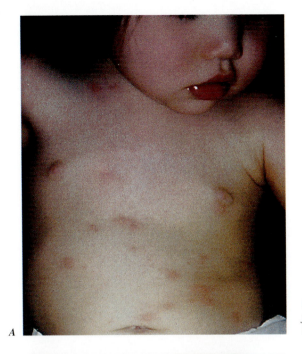

A

Figure 25-10 Fire ant stings *(A) Diffuse erythematous papules on a child bitten by numerous fire ants.*

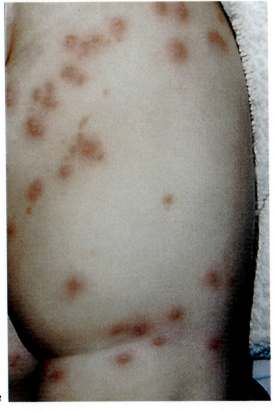

B

Figure 25-10 Fire ant stings *(B) Erythematous macules with central pustule formation 24 h after bites in the same child.*

INDEX

A

Abscesses
  of apocrine sweat glands, 140-142, 141*f*, 143*f*
  furuncles, 460-461, 461*f*
Acanthosis nigricans (AN), 428-429, 429*f*
Accessory nipple, 28, 29*f*
Acne
  infantile, 136, 137*f*
  keloidalis, 462*t*
  neonatorum, 12, 13*f*
  vulgaris, 132–135, 133*f*
    epidemiology, 132
    management, 134–135
    pathophysiology, 132
    physical examination, 132, 133*f*
Acquired melanocytic nevocellular nevi (moles), 144
  compound nevus, 149, 150*f*
  dermal nevus, 147, 148*f*
  junctional nevus, 145, 146*f*
Acrochordon, 250, 251*f*
Acrodermatitis enteropathica (AE), diaper area, 72–73, 73*f*
Acute febrile neutrophilic dermatosis, 348–349, 349*f*
Acute guttate parapsoriasis, 302–305, 303*f*, 305*f*
Acute sun damage (sunburn), 372–374, 375*f*
  epidemiology, 372–373
  management, 373–374
Adiposis dolorosa, 255*t*
Adolescent-type atopic dermatitis, 54, 55*f*
Albers–Schonberg disease, 241*t*
Albinism, 268–269, 270*f*, 271*t*
Albright syndrome, 176*t*
Allergic contact dermatitis, 62–63, 63*f*
Allergic cutaneous vasculitis. *See* Hypersensitivity vasculitis
Alopecia areata, 434–437, 435*f*, 437*f*
  epidemiology, 434
  management, 434, 436
AN (acanthosis nigricans), 428–429, 429*f*
Anaphylactoid purpura, 356–357, 357*f*
Angioedema, 324–327
  epidemiology, 324
  management, 326
Angiokeratoma, 196, 197*f*
  circumscriptum, 196
  of Fordyce, 196

of Mibelli, 196
multiple, 196
solitary, 196, 197*f*
Angiolipomas, 254
Angioma
  cherry, 194, 195*f*
  spider, 192, 193*f*
Angiomatosis, cutaneous meningospinal, 187*t*, 191*t*
Aplasia cutis congenita, 22–23, 23*f*
Apocrine glandular disorders. *See* Sebaceous and apocrine glandular disorders
Apocrinitis, 140–142, 141*f*, 143*f*
Appendageal proliferations, benign, 222–239
  epidermal inclusion cyst (EIC), 238, 239*f*
  nevus comedonicus, 226, 227*f*
  nevus sebaceus, 222–224, 223*f*–224*f*
    management, 224
    physical examination, 222, 223*f*
  pilomatrixoma, 232, 233*f*
  steatocystoma multiplex, 234, 235*f*
  syringoma, 230, 231*f*
  trichilemmal cyst, 236, 237*f*
  trichoepithelioma, 228, 229*f*
Aquatic infestations, 598–609
  cercarial dermatitis, 600, 601*f*
  coral dermatitis, 608, 609*f*
  cutaneous larva migrans, 598–599, 599*f*
  jellyfish dermatitis, 606, 607*f*
  seabather's itch, 602, 603*f*
  sea urchin dermatitis, 604, 605*f*
Arterial spider, 192
Ataxia telangiectasia, 177*t*, 398–401, 399*f*, 401*f*
Athlete's foot, 514, 515*f*
Atopic dermatitis, 46–55
  adolescent type, 54, 55*f*
  childhood type, 52, 53*f*
  epidemiology, 46
  infantile, 50, 50*f*
  management, 47–49
Atrophoderma vermiculata, 106
Atypical nevus, 154, 155*f*

B

Bacterial infections, cutaneous, 454–501
  blistering distal dactylitis, 454–457, 455*f*, 457*f*
  carbuncles, 460–461
  cat-scratch disease, 488–489, 489*f*

L

LAMB syndrome, 168*t*
Lamellar ichthyosis, 102–104, 103*f,* 105*f*
 management, 104
 physical examination, 102, 103*f,* 105*f*
Langerhans cell histiocytosis (LCH),
 438–441, 439*f,* 441*f*
Larva migrans, 598–599, 599*f*
Leiomyoma, 252–253, 253*f*
Lentigines-associated syndromes, 166, 167*f,*
 168*t*–169*t,* 172–173, 173*f*
Lentigo simplex, 166, 167*f,* 168*t*–169*t*
LEOPARD syndrome (multiple lentigines syndrome), 167*f,* 168*t,* 172–173, 173*f*
Leprosy, 490–492, 491*f*
Leukoderma acquisitum centrifugum, 158,
 159*f*
Lice
 body, 616, 617*f,* 635*f*
 crab, 614–615, 615*f*
 head, 610–613, 611*f,* 613*f*
 pubic, 614–615, 615*f*
Lichenoid eruptions, 306–317
 lichen nitidus, 313–314, 315*f*
  management, 313–314
  pathopysiology, 313
  physical examination, 313, 315*f*
 lichen planus, 309–312
  differential diagnosis, 309, 312*t*
  physical examination, 309, 311*f*
 lichen sclerosis (LS), 306–308, 307*f*
 lichen sclerosis et atrophicus, 306–308, 307*f*
 lichen simplex chronicus (LSC), 56, 57*f*
 lichen striatus, 316, 317*f*
Linear and whorled nevoid hypermelanosis,
 278, 279*f*
Linear IgA bullous disease of childhood,
 128–131, 130*f*–131*f*
 management, 129
 physical examination, 128, 130*f*–131*f*
Linear nevus sebaceus, 216–217, 217*f*
 syndrome, 220–221, 221*f*
Lipoma, 254, 255*f,* 255*t*
 associated syndromes, 255*t*
Livedo reticularis (livedo racemosa, livedo annularis), 200–201, 200*f*–201*f*
Louis–Bar syndrome, 177*t,* 398–401, 399*f,*
 401*f*
LS (lichen sclerosis), 306–308, 307*f*
LSC (lichen simplex chronicus), 56, 57*f*
Lupus. *See* Neonatal lupus erythematosus;
 Systemic lupus erythematosus
Lyell's syndrome, 332–333, 333*f*
Lyme borreliosis, 497–501
 epidemiology, 497, 499*f*
 management, 500–501

physical examination, 497, 501*f*
Lymphangioma
 cavernous, 210, 211*f*
 circumscriptum, 208, 209*f*
Lymphatic disorders. *See* Blood and lymph
 vessels, disorders of
Lymphedema, 214, 215*f*
Lymphomatoid papulosis (LyP), 450–451,
 451*f*
Lymphoreticulosis, benign, 488–489, 489*f*

M

M. Marinum infection, 495, 496*f*
Maculopapular drug eruption, 320–323, 321*f,*
 323*f*
Madelung's disease, 255*t*
Mafucci's syndrome, 191*t*
Malherbe, calcifying epithelioma of, 232, 233*f*
Marine dermatitis, 602, 603*f*
Mastocytosis syndromes, 446–449, 447*f,* 449*f*
McCune-Albright syndrome, 176*t*
Measles, 582–585, 583*f,* 585*f*
Melanocytic disorders, 144–181
 acquired melanocytic nevocellular nevi
  (moles), 144
  compound nevus, 149, 150*f*
  dermal nevus, 147, 148*f*
  junctional nevus, 145, 146*f*
 blue nevus, 156–157, 156*f*
 congenital nevomelanocytic nevus (CNN),
  151–153, 152*f*
 dermal melanocytic disorders
  Mongolian spot, 178, 179*f*
  nevi of Ota and Ito, 180, 181*f*
 dysplastic melanocytic nevus, 154, 155*f*
 epidermal melanocytic disorders
  café-au-lait macules (CALM), 174, 175*f,*
   176*t*–177*t*
  ephelides, 164, 165*f*
  lentigines-associated syndromes, 166,
   167*f,* 168*t*–169*t*
  lentigo simplex, 166, 167*f,* 168*t*–169*t*
  multiple lentigines syndrome (LEOPARD
   syndrome), 172–173, 173*f*
  Peutz-Jeghers syndrome, 170–171, 171*f*
 halo nevus, 158, 159*f*
 nevus spilus, 160, 161*f*
 Spitz nevus, 162, 163*f*
Melanoma, juvenile, benign, 162, 163*f*
Meningococcemia, 482–483, 483*f*
Meningospinal angiomatosis, cutaneous, 187*t,*
 191*t*
Mibelli, porokeratosis of, 108, 109*f*
Michelin-tire baby, 255*t*
Milia, 10, 11*f*
Miliaria, newborn, 8–9, 9*f*

Mims syndrome, 220–221, 221*f*
Moles (acquired melanocytic nevocellular nevi), 144
  compound nevus, 149, 150*f*
  dermal nevus, 147, 148*f*
  junctional nevus, 145, 146*f*
Molluscum contagiosum, 574–575, 575*f*
Mongolian spot, 178, 179*f*
Monilial diaper dermatitis, 70–71, 71*f*
Moniliasis, 40, 41*f*, 522–523, 523*f*, 524–527, 525*f*, 527*f*
Mononucleosis, 594–595, 595*f*
Morbilliform drug eruption, 320–323, 321*f*, 323*f*
Morphea, 420–422, 421*f*
  physical examination, 420, 421*f*
Moynahan syndrome, 168*t*, 172–173, 173*f*
Mucha-Habermann disease, 302–305, 303*f*, 305*f*
Mucocutaneous lymph node syndrome, 368, 369*f*–370*f*
Multiple benign cystic epithelioma, 228, 229*f*
Multiple endocrine neoplasia, 177*t*
Multiple familial lipomatosis, 255*t*
Multiple hamartoma syndrome, 177*t*
Multiple lentigines syndrome (LEOPARD syndrome), 167*f*, 168*t*, 172–173, 173*f*
Multiple nevoid basal cell carcinoma syndrome, 394–397, 395*f*, 397*f*
Mycobacterial infections, 490–496
  cutaneous tuberculosis, 493–494, 494*f*
  leprosy, 490–492, 491*f*
  M. Marinum, 495, 496*f*
Mycosis fungoides, 452–453, 453*f*
Mycotic stomatitis, 522–523, 523*f*

N

NAME syndrome, 168*t*
Necrobiosis lipoidica diabeticorum (NLD), 430–431, 431*f*
Necrotizing vasculitis. *See* Hypersensitivity vasculitis
Neonatal hair loss, 6, 7*f*
Neonatal herpes simplex virus infection, 30–33, 31*f*
  course and prognosis, 32
  epidemiology, 30
  laboratory examinations, 32
  physical examination, 30–32, 31*f*
Neonatal lupus erythematosus (NLE), 18–21, 19*f*
  course and prognosis, 19
  epidemiology, 18
  management, 20–21
Neonatal syphilis, 38–39, 39*f*

Neurocutaneous disorders, 280–297
  hypomelanosis of Ito, 296, 297*f*
  incontinentia pigmenti (IP), 292–295
    course and prognosis, 294
    epidemiology, 292
    physical examination, 292, 293*f*, 295*f*
  neurofibromatosis. *See* Neurofibromatosis
  overview, 280
  tuberous sclerosis, 286–291
    differential diagnosis, 290
    management, 290
    physical examination, 286, 287*f*–289*f*, 291*f*
Neurofibromatosis (NF), 280–285
  differential diagnosis, 282
  physical examination, 280, 281*f*, 282, 283*f*, 285*f*
  type 1 (NF-1, von Recklinghausen disease), 176*t*, 280, 282
  type 2 (NF–2, central or acoustic), 176*t*, 280, 282, 284
  type 5 (NF–5), 176*t*
  type 6 (NF–6), 176*t*
Nevoid basal cell carcinoma syndrome, 394–397, 395*f*, 397*f*
Nevoid lentigo, 168*t*
Nevoxanthoendothelioma, 442–445, 443*f*, 445*f*
Nevus(i)
  achromicus, 272, 273*f*
  acquired melanocytic nevocellular (mole), 144–150
  anemicus, 274, 275*f*
  araneus, 192, 193*f*
  atypical, 154, 155*f*
  basal cell nevus syndrome, 394–397, 395*f*, 397*f*
  Becker's, 242, 243*f*
  blue, 156–157, 156*f*
  Clark's, 154, 155*f*
  comedo, 226, 227*f*
  comedonicus, 226, 227*f*
  compound, 149, 150*f*
  congenital nevomelanocytic, 151–153, 152*f*
  connective tissue, 240–241, 241*f*, 241*t*
  depigmentosus, 272, 273*f*
  dermal, 147, 148*f*
  dysplastic melanocytic, 154, 155*f*
  elasticus, 240–241, 241*f*, 241*t*
  epidermal, 216–217, 217*f*
    syndromes, 220–221, 221*f*
  epitheloid cell–spindle cell, 162, 163*f*
  flammeus, 184, 185*f*–187*f*
  fuscocaeruleus acromiodeltoideus, 180–181, 181*f*

NOTES

NOTES

NOTES

NOTES

NOTES

NOTES

NOTES

NOTES

NOTES

NOTES